Manual of Psychiatric Nursing Skills

Sudha C. Patel, DNS, MN, MA, BSN, RN

Associate Professor
Department of Nursing
College of Nursing and Allied Health Professions
The University of Louisiana at Lafayette
Lafayette, Lousiana

Kim A. Jakopac, MSN, BSN, ASN, RN, PPCNP

BSN Nursing Instructor
Department of Nursing
College of Nursing and Allied Health Professions
The University of Louisiana at Lafayette
Lafayette, Louisiana

JONES & BARTLETT
LEARNING

World Headquarters
Jones & Bartlett Learning
40 Tall Pine Drive
Sudbury, MA 01776
978-443-5000
info@jblearning.com
www.jblearning.com

Jones & Bartlett Learning
Canada
6339 Ormindale Way
Mississauga, Ontario L5V 1J2
Canada

Jones & Bartlett Learning
International
Barb House, Barb Mews
London W6 7PA
United Kingdom

Jones & Bartlett Learning books and products are available through most bookstores and online booksellers. To contact Jones & Bartlett Learning directly, call 800-832-0034, fax 978-443-8000, or visit our website, www.jblearning.com.

Substantial discounts on bulk quantities of Jones & Bartlett Learning publications are available to corporations, professional associations, and other qualified organizations. For details and specific discount information, contact the special sales department at Jones & Bartlett Learning via the above contact information or send an email to specialsales@jblearning.com.

The authors, editor, and publisher have made every effort to provide accurate information. However, they are not responsible for errors, omissions, or for any outcomes related to the use of the contents of this book and take no responsibility for the use of the products and procedures described. Treatments and side effects described in this book may not be applicable to all people; likewise, some people may require a dose or experience a side effect that is not described herein. Drugs and medical devices are discussed that may have limited availability controlled by the Food and Drug Administration (FDA) for use only in a research study or clinical trial. Research, clinical practice, and government regulations often change the accepted standard in this field. When consideration is being given to use of any drug in the clinical setting, the health care provider or reader is responsible for determining FDA status of the drug, reading the package insert, and reviewing prescribing information for the most up-to-date recommendations on dose, precautions, and contraindications, and determining the appropriate usage for the product. This is especially important in the case of drugs that are new or seldom used.

Production Credits
Publisher: Kevin Sullivan
Editorial Assistant: Rachel Shuster
Production Assistant: Sara Fowles
Marketing Manager: Meagan Norlund
V.P., Manufacturing and Inventory Control: Therese Connell
Composition: DataStream Content Solutions, LLC
Cover Design: Scott Moden
Cover Image: © B. Speckart/ShutterStock, Inc.
Printing and Binding: Malloy, Inc.
Cover Printing: Malloy, Inc.

Library of Congress Cataloging-in-Publication Data
Patel, Sudha C.
   Manual of psychiatric nursing skills / Sudha C. Patel, Kimberly A. Jakopac.
      p. ; cm.
   Includes bibliographical references and index.
   ISBN-13: 978-1-4496-1356-3 (pbk.)
   ISBN-10: 1-4496-1356-X (pbk.)
   1. Psychiatric nursing.   I. Jakopac, Kim A.   II. Title.
   [DNLM: 1. Mental Disorders—nursing. 2. Psychiatric Nursing—methods. WY 160]
   RC440.P37 2012
   616.89'0231—dc22
                                                                        2010037482

6048

Printed in the United States of America
15 14 13 12 11   10 9 8 7 6 5 4 3 2 1

Contents

14 Administration and Monitoring of Psychotropic
Medications: Antidepressants   347
Kim A. Jakopac

15 Administration and Monitoring of Psychotropic Medications:
Anticonvulsants/Anxiolytics   387
Sudha C. Patel

UNIT V   Appendices   481

Preface

This book has been designed for nursing students and nurses in general for basic psychiatric and mental health nursing practice. The content in this text is organized to provide nurses and nursing students with basic knowledge and specific skills in the area of psychiatric-mental health nursing for care of clients with specific psychiatric disorders. Substance abuse disorders are not addressed in this book. We hope our readers—both nurses and nursing students—find this book readable and meaningful for day-to-day practice.

Acknowledgments

The authors wish to thank the students and psychiatric-mental health nurses who inspired us to write this book. The authors also extend sincere appreciation to Dr. Tari Dilks and Dr. Nellie Prudhomme, psychiatric-mental health nursing colleagues who took time to review content, and share their expert knowledge and insight, which has made this book possible.

We are grateful to our colleagues with whom we worked every day for providing us support and encouragement in writing this book. Thank you for your encouragement and unconditional support.

We wish to express our sincere appreciation for the editorial, production, marketing direction, and general support of Rachel Shuster, Kevin Sullivan, Emily Ekle, Sara Fowles, Patricia Rosendale, and their colleagues.

About the Authors

Sudha C. Patel, DNS, MN, MA, BSN, RN

Sudha C. Patel is an associate professor, involved in teaching psychiatric-mental health nursing in the master's program for psychiatric nurse practitioners and generic nursing students in the BSN program at the University of Louisiana at Lafayette. She has also instructed accelerated option students for 5 years in psychiatric-mental health nursing clinical teaching and has taught psychiatric nursing since 1979, including in both diploma and undergraduate nursing programs in the United States. Her experience, in addition to being a faculty member, has been in working with a wide range of clients with psychiatric disorders from children to the elderly as well as working with substance abuse and dual diagnosis clients. She also has a community health nursing specialty. She has done presentations of research studies with a colleague at several local, regional, and national conferences in the United States as well as at the international conferences at Australia, Russia, China, and Canada. Her publications to date include collaborative projects, textbooks chapters, and a textbook, *Psychiatric Mental Health Case Studies and Care Plans* (Jones & Bartlett Learning, 2009).

Kim A. Jakopac, MSN, BSN, ASN, RN, PPCNP

Kim A. Jakopac is teaching psychiatric-mental health nursing in a BSN program at the University of Louisiana at Lafayette. Her specialty is psychiatric-mental health nursing and medical-psychiatric nursing. Over the past 20 years she has worked with a variety of clients ranging from children to the elderly and has experience working with substance abuse clients, dual diagnosis clients, and case management. She has conducted psychiatric-mental health and substance abuse evaluations in an emergency room setting and has worked as a hospital supervisor. The last 6 years of her nursing career have been in education. Publications to date include the book

Psychiatric Mental Health Case Studies and Care Plans (Jones & Bartlett Learning, 2009), research reviews, and a literature review for Dr. Sudha Patel and Dr. Ardith Sudduth on the healthy behaviors of freshman nursing students. She has been involved in research with Dr. Ardith Sudduth, Dr. Evelyn Wills, and Dr. Ina Koerner, and has had a podium presentation in Alexandria, LA.

Reviewers

Sattaria S. Dilks, DNP, FPMHNP-BC
Associate Professor
College of Nursing—Graduate Program
McNeese State University
Lake Charles, LA

Nellie Prudhomme, BSN, MPH, DNS, RN-BC, CPI
Clinical Faculty
Louisiana State University, Eunice
CPI Instructor
Eunice, LA

Ina Koerner, PhD, RN
Eunice, LA

Introduction

The *Manual of Psychiatric Nursing Skills* is designed as a basic or supplementary textbook for undergraduate students and for nurses in general to keep up with their essential psychiatric nursing skills, including those who provide care for medical–surgical patients who may have actual or potential psychiatric-mental illness. The authors have not yet come across a separate psychiatric nursing skill book in a manual format that is handy at the clinical site as a reference for nursing students or nurses. The aim of this book is to help nursing students to integrate their theoretical knowledge with psychiatric-mental health nursing skills during their clinical practice. Psychiatric nursing skills are essential and are the heart of psychiatric-mental health nursing practice. The approach to this book is in manual format to discuss psychiatric nursing skills. It will include descriptions of the situation, skills implementation, safety, legal–ethical implications, and nursing process. This book will be a supplementary text for undergraduate college level courses in psychiatric nursing and can be used as a resource book for practicing nurses. The features of this book include chapters with objectives and key terms, examples, sample review questions, and a glossary.

The student will have opportunities to practice and learn fundamental psychiatric nursing skills, including the use of a safe environment and therapeutic communication techniques to assess, diagnose, develop a plan of care, and provide nursing interventions for a variety of actual or potential biopsychosocial responses of the patient using the nursing process. This textbook provides a practical approach for learning essential skills and applying the critical content of psychiatric-mental health nursing practice.

This textbook is based on the premise that the practice of psychiatric-mental health nursing depends upon the level of competency in psychiatric-mental health nursing skills to provide quality care. This text book is designed in a concise way to provide essential information/knowledge about psychiatric-mental health nursing practice, use of the nursing process, and psychiatric nursing skills to assist students to incorporate learned concepts and skills into their practice.

ORGANIZATION

The textbook is organized into five units with 18 chapters and 8 appendices. Unit 1, Chapter 1, addresses psychiatric-mental health nursing practice and nursing process, and the next three units with 17 chapters address the essential psychiatric-mental health nursing skills. Unit V contains the appendices.

Unit I addresses the starting stages for the psychiatric-mental nursing practice. In Chapter 1, readers are introduced to psychiatric-mental health nursing as a specialty area for practice, and explore the population focus, philosophical belief, and theoretical frame work that make the practice unique. The roles of the psychiatric-mental health (PMH) nurse and standards of care and performance as per the American Nurses Association (ANA), as well as current trends, use of information technology, and simulation for practice are addressed. This unit also examines the legal–ethical dilemmas for practice.

Unit II presents psychiatric-mental health nursing skill-building techniques. The major focus of skill building in this unit is in the areas of the therapeutic use of self, therapeutic communication, therapeutic relationships, safe environment or milieu, interview techniques, mental status examination, and leading psychoeducation groups. Chapter 2 includes how the PMH nurse uses themselves as a therapeutic agent when providing care for the client. In Chapter 3, the authors examine how to modify the environment depending upon the situation for the safety of clients, staff, and others. In Chapter 4 techniques for conducting a psychiatric interview with the client are provided. Chapter 5 includes how to develop and maintain therapeutic relationships. In Chapter 6 the content for psychoeducation and a teaching plan as well as how to lead psychoeducation groups are provided.

Unit III focuses psychiatric-mental health nursing skill building in the area of nursing assessment and interventions for the client with a specific psychiatric disorder. This unit has nine chapters. The selected psychiatric disorders include (by chapter number): (7) severe anxiety, (8) major depression, (9) suicidal ideation/gesture/attempt, (10) bipolar disorder—acute manic phase, (11) schizophrenia, (12) restriction to isolation or seclusion, and (13–15) administration and monitoring of psychotropic medications—antipsychotics, antidepressants, and anticonvulsants/anxiolytics.

Unit IV provides specific skills/techniques for crisis intervention, psychiatric emergencies, domestic violence, and disaster situations. Students are assisted to apply the nursing process to identify factors contributing to each of these areas and design relevant psychiatric nursing interventions.

Chapters are organized with the following: learning objectives, key terms, and clinical examples in some chapters. Additional information (e.g., stages of development) is included in the appendices as well as a glossary and sample blank care plan form.

UNIT I

Psychiatric-Mental Health Nursing Practice and Nursing Process

CHAPTER 1

Basic Concepts for Psychiatric-Mental Health Nursing Practice

Sudha C. Patel

OBJECTIVES

The nursing student will be able to:
1. Define psychiatric-mental health nursing practice
2. Identify the basic concept for psychiatric-mental health nursing practice
3. Discuss the roles played by the psychiatric-mental health nurse
4. Describe the theoretical framework for psychiatric-mental health nursing practice
5. Identify legal–ethical issues in psychiatric-mental health nursing practice
6. Discuss the scope and standards of psychiatric-mental health nursing practice
7. Define the nursing process
8. Identify the steps in the nursing process
9. Differentiate between psychiatric nursing diagnosis and DSM-IV-TR diagnoses
10. Identify the most common priority of care in psychiatric-mental health nursing practice

KEY TERMS

Counselor
Milieu manager
Nursing process
Psychiatric-mental health nursing practice

Role player
Socializing agent
Standards of performance
Standards of practice

It is essential to know the basic concepts for psychiatric-mental health (PMH) nursing practice. The basic concepts include (1) definition of psychiatric-mental health nurse and nursing practice; (2) philosophical beliefs for practice; (3) psychiatric-mental health nurses' roles; (4) theoretical framework for practice; (5) legal–ethical issues; (6) standards of care and standards of performance. Understanding these fundamental concepts helps psychiatric-mental health nurses to improve their performance and provide safe, quality care for the patients within their scope of practice.

PSYCHIATRIC-MENTAL HEALTH NURSE

Psychiatric-mental health nurses are the registered nurses who have education preparation in nursing and have a license to practice in their respective state. A PMH nurse's education preparation includes a specialized knowledge in nursing, neurobiologic, pharmacologic, sociological, and psychological sciences as well skills and abilities for the care of persons with psychiatric disorders, mental health problems, and mental health issues. PMH nurses also demonstrate knowledge and competencies in information technology to improve quality of care. Psychiatric-mental health nurses are valuable resources for providing psychiatric-mental health services in many settings. PMH nursing has subspecialties in the areas of child, adolescent, adult, geriatric, consult/liaison, substance abuse, eating disorders, and forensics. The PMH nurse can acquire certification in any subspecialty through the American Nurses' Credentialing Center (ANCC) and various subspecialty professional organizations.

Education

A generalist PMH nurse holds a baccalaureate of science in nursing (BSN) degree, associate of science in nursing (ASN or AD) degree or diploma in nursing (RN). The other category of the PMH nurse is for one who is a registered nurse with additional preparation in psychiatric-mental health nursing, called a psychiatric-mental health registered nurse (RN-PMH), this nurse works at a basic level. The nurses who practice at an advanced level in psychiatric-mental health nursing are a specialized group at the graduate level in education, with masters or doctoral degrees; they are called advanced psychiatric-mental health nurses (APRN-PMHs), have met the requirement for ANCC certification, and have an advanced practice license from the state in which they decided to practice (APNA, 2007, p. 16).

Qualifications

A psychiatric-mental health nurse at the basic level of practice must possess a knowledge of nursing; biologic and psychological theories of mental health and mental illness; various psychotherapy modalities; substance abuse and dual diagnosis; care of vulnerable populations; therapeutic milieu; cultural practices; spiritual implications of mental health and illness; psychopharmacology; and legal, ethical, and technical issues in psychiatric-mental health nursing practice.

Knowledge and Required Skills

The psychiatric-mental health nurse must have proficiencies in the following areas:

1. Performing a comprehensive assessment of the biopsychosocial-spiritual aspects of the client
2. Utilizing therapeutic communication in dealing with actual or potential problems, responses, or behaviors
3. Establishing a therapeutic relationship with the client
4. Using oneself as a therapeutic agent
5. Providing psycho-education and health teaching for promotion and maintenance of mental health and prevention of mental illness
6. Administering and monitoring therapeutic and adverse effects of psychopharmacologic agents
7. Diagnosing and planning patient care with expected outcomes in measurable terms
8. Providing nursing interventions and evaluating nursing care for the client with: depression, suicidal ideation/gesture/attempt, manic disorder-acute phase, severe anxiety, assaultive behavior, chemical dependency, hallucinations, schizophrenia, manipulative behavior, crisis interventions, restriction to isolation or seclusion, psychotropic medications
9. Interdisciplinary collaboration
10. Identifying and coordinating appropriate resources for patients and families
11. Understanding of Diagnoses and the *Statistical Manual of Psychiatric Disorders* for psychiatric diagnostic classification

PSYCHIATRIC-MENTAL HEALTH NURSING PRACTICE

Psychiatric-mental health nurse (PMH) nursing practice occurs at various levels depending upon the PMH nurse's educational preparation. Their role, job description, work position, and practice settings further describe their practice (APNA, 2007, p. 1).

PMH nurses work in a wide array of inpatient and outpatient settings such as full or partial hospitalization; community-based or home care programs; and local, state, and federal mental health agencies. Other settings include school/college of nursing, private practice, military, primary care office, prison/jail, home health agency, and behavioral care company/HMO.

Essential components of practice for the PMH nurse include health and wellness promotion through nursing assessment of mental health issues; prevention of mental illness problems; and providing nursing interventions and treatment for psychiatric disorders with related health problems (APNA, 2007, p. 4).

Definition of Psychiatric-Mental Health Nursing Practice

Psychiatric-mental health nursing is committed to promoting mental health through the assessment, diagnosis, and treatment of human responses to mental health problems or psychiatric disorders. PMH nursing practice employs a wide range of nursing, psychosocial, and neurobiologic theories, as well as research or evidence-based practice and employs purposeful use of self as its art to promote and maintain clients' mental health functioning and provide care and treatment for persons suffering from psychiatric disorders (APNA, 2007). The practice of PMH nursing is delivered through an interpersonal process using therapeutic communication to build a therapeutic relationship with the client.

The definition of psychiatric nursing practice incorporates the general nursing definition provided by the American Nurses Association (ANA) that nursing is the protection, promotion, and optimization of health and abilities; prevention of illness and injury; alleviation of suffering through the diagnosis and treatment of human response; and advocacy in the care of individuals, families, communities, and populations (ANA, 2003, p. 6; ANA, 2004, p. 7).

PHILOSOPHICAL BELIEFS OF PSYCHIATRIC NURSING PRACTICE

The practice of psychiatric nursing is based in part on the fundamental philosophical belief system held by the nursing profession, which includes the following principles:

1. The individual has intrinsic worth and dignity, and each person is worthy of respect.
2. The goal of individual is one of growth, health, autonomy, and self-actualization.
3. Every individual has the potential for change.
4. All people have basic common human needs; these needs include, shelter, food, safety, love, belonging, self-esteem and self-actualization.

5. All behavior of the individual is meaningful. It arises from personal needs and goals, and can be understood only from a personal internal frame of reference and within the context in which the behavior occurs.
6. Behavior consists of perceptions, thoughts, feelings, and actions. From one's perceptions thoughts arise, emotions are felt, and actions are conceived; disruption may occur in any of these areas.
7. Individuals vary in their coping capabilities, which depend on genetic and environmental influences; nature and level of stress; and availability of support systems and resources.
8. All individuals have potential for both health and illness. Illness can be a growth-producing experience for the individual.
9. All people have a right to equal opportunity for adequate health care regardless of gender, race, religion, ethnicity, sexual orientation, or cultural background.
10. Mental health is a critical component of comprehensive healthcare services.
11. An individual has a right to participate in decision making regarding their physical and mental health.
12. An individual has the right to self-determination, including the decision to pursue health or illness.
13. The goal of nursing care is to promote wellness, maximize integrated functioning, and enhance self-actualization. Nursing care is based on healthcare needs and expected treatment outcomes mutually determined by the individual, families, groups, and communities.
14. An interpersonal relationship can be used to produce change and growth within the individual. It is the vehicle for the application of the nursing process and the attainment of the goal of nursing care.

ROLE OF PSYCHIATRIC-MENTAL HEALTH NURSE

Defining the roles of the PMH nurse depends on state laws, education qualification, and work setting as well as the nurse's personal factors or attributes (Stuart & Laraia, 2001, p. 9). The PMH nurse assumes several roles in relation to the patient's growth and adaptation, regardless of what setting they are practicing in. Peplau (1991) identifies several roles of the psychiatric-mental health nurse. PMH nurses function within their prescribed role or scope of practice as outlined by the ANA and their State Board of Nursing. Whatever role the PMH nurse plays, they must be knowledgeable and sensitive about the patient's cultural identity and must take into account the client's cultural diversity needs.

Role of PMH Nurse

1. Socializing agent

This role is played by the nurse while working with the patent on a one-to-one basis. The focus is to identify what difficulties the client has in communicating thoughts and feelings to others. The client gets the benefits of this role by adapting an appropriate expression of behavior and affect.

2. Teacher

In this role the psychiatric-mental health nurse provides health teaching or health education based on the client's needs, as well as a treatment plan. The focus for the health teaching needs to be on health promotion, illness management, and illness prevention. The teaching content may include a wide variety of topics from teaching basic living skills and safety to management of their health and illness. Management of illness, medications, healthy life style, nutrition, exercise, and stress management are also important teaching topics.

3. Change agent or model

Generally, individuals learn by adapting or imitating the person they like. Thus, modeling helps patients to see and adapt alternative ways of dealing with the situation. Modeling also provides patients with clarity in their understanding of the events and ability to communicate without any hesitation. The PMH nurse plays a vital role in being a model for the client; however, the PMH nurse must understand that they should not impose their own values upon the client.

4. Counselor

This is another vital role the PMH nurse has to play. Counseling is done usually during one-on-one sessions. The focus of the counseling is to help the client achieve mutually agreed upon specific goals and outcomes. The nurse as counselor provides opportunities for the patient to express thoughts, feelings, and behaviors related to the issues they are attempting to cope with. The client also will benefit by observing the nurse for their verbal and nonverbal communication patterns and trying to adopt these patterns and practices in order to learn effective ways to communicate with others. The PMH nurse can assess the patient's improved coping skills, increased self-confidence, and better understanding of how to deal with the conflicts and situations and seek appropriate resources.

5. Role player

The PMH nurse plays a vital role for the client by creating simulation exercises of past, present, or future situations or incidents. Here the client will be able to practice new behavior in a nonthreatening environment. The patient can express thoughts and feelings, and act out during role play a specific or real situation. The benefit of this exercise is that the client is able to build up self-confidence, learn to communicate better and in a more assertive way with others, and cope better in the given situation in the future. However, role play may not be suitable for some clients. The client with

	psychotic symptoms who thinks concretely may have difficulty with or exhibit limitations in understanding this role-play technique since they may not be able to transfer techniques learned from role playing to real life situations due to disturbed cognitive functioning and perceptions.
6. Leader or milieu manager	The PMH nurse has an opportunity to demonstrate leadership as a therapeutic milieu manager since the nurse has regular contact with the clients during inpatient, outpatient, or clinical settings. As a milieu manager, the nurse can monitor the safe physical environment and interactions between patients and health team members during one-to-one interactions or groups meetings. A major role for the PMH nurse is to maintain a safe environment for the safety of everyone and allow patients to learn new behaviors, improve coping skills, and enhance socialization for those who isolate. The benefits a client gets from this milieu is that the they are able to recognize behavior, understand the impact of their behavior on others, and feel safe in expressing thoughts, feelings, and behavior in a safe manner.
7. Advocate	In this role the PMH nurse acts as an advocate for the patients. The PMH nurse has opportunities to apply a variety of communication techniques to assist clients. The nurse acts as a liaison between clients and other people in the society. The nurse can play an active role to destigmatize attitudes towards mentally ill people. The nurse also allows patients to express thoughts and feelings and protects clients from making unsafe decisions.

Among the roles described in the table, the PMH nurse also must be familiar with the current trends and research in their field; in this 21st century there is a plethora of knowledge development through research in the area of psychiatric disorders, mental health, and in the neurobiologic and pharmacologic fields. There is also more evidence of the existence of comorbid medical problems and increased use of substances among patients with psychiatric disorders. The PMH nurse must keep their knowledge up to date with the current trends, research, and issues related to prevention of psychiatric disorders, promotion of mental health, and how to provide rehabilitative care using available resources. They also must provide care based on the evidence in practice by utilizing research study findings.

THEORETICAL FRAMEWORK FOR PMH NURSING PRACTICE

Psychiatric-mental health nurses need to have knowledge of the following psychodynamic and nursing theories and understand their implications for PMH nursing practice.

Psychoanalytical Theory

This is the oldest theory developed by Sigmund Freud. Freud discussed the structure of personality in terms of id, ego, and superego. The PMH nurse needs to have the ability to recognize the client's behavior associated with their personality structure as identified by Freud. This will help the PMH nurse to understand and assess the development level of the client. They also need to recognize the patient's ego defense mechanisms to assess and plan care to bring about positive change in the client's behavior.

Interpersonal Theory

Sullivan (1953) discussed the interpersonal relationship and its impact on personality and behavior. The PMH nurse applies this theory to build the therapeutic relationship with the patient and to assist the client to reduce anxiety, develop a sense of security, and thus, learn to be independent and improve interpersonal relationships with significant others.

Personality Development Theory

Erickson (1963) discussed the development of personality by discussing eight stages of life development and the crisis in each stage that a person will go through. Knowledge of this theory provides the PMH nurse a stepwise approach to assess the client's developmental level and plan interventions to assist the patient to learn tasks to move from one stage of development to the next successfully by learning to resolve the crisis.

Cognitive Development Theory

Piaget (1969) developed a concept of cognitive development from birth to adolescent stage. Application of this theory to PMH nursing is very much evident in current practice by the use of cognitive therapy for patients who have cognitive distortions and by teaching patients how to change automatic distorted thoughts.

Theory of Moral Development

Kohlberg (1968) identified three stages of moral development. Knowledge of this theory helps the PMH nurse to assess the stage of moral development in the patient and assist through nursing interventions to move the patient to the next level of maturity.

Nursing Model

Peplau (1991) discussed the development of the nurse–client relationship by applying the principles of Sullivan's interpersonal theory. She was a pioneer in developing a framework of psychodynamic nursing, a psychiatric-mental health nursing model. According to Peplau, interpersonal relationships are a learning stage for both patient and nurse, and both of these individuals benefit from the relationship. Peplau discussed psychodynamic nursing by indicating that nurse must understand their own behavior in order to help the client. Peplau identified six roles of the PMH nurse: resource person, counselor, teacher, leader, technical expert, and surrogate person. The stages of the nurse–client relationships are the hallmark of Peplau's work. She identified four development stages of the nurse–client relationship: Stage 1 is orientation, and in this stage the client and nurse meet to assess and identify the problem the patient has identified. In the second stage the patient is able to get clarity in to their problem and respond accordingly to the nurse. During the third stage the client feels secure enough to learn about available resources offered to them and accept the help given to them. The last stage is resolution. In this stage the patient becomes more confident in their ability to be independent and to resolve the problematic situation while learning positive coping skills.

LEGAL–ETHICAL ISSUES

Ethical Issues

The most prominent ethical issues that the PMH nurse will come across in practice are the right to refuse medication and the right to least restrictive treatment. These patient rights are derived from the American Hospital Association Patient's Bill of Rights (1992). However, in the psychiatric setting, the right to refuse medication may be taken away by the treatment team if the client meets the three criteria needed to force medication. There must be evidence of client behavior to be a danger to self or others, and evidence that with medication there is a chance to help client. Other ethical issues related to treatment modalities including electroconvulsive therapy (ECT) and providing safety measures such as restricting a patient's movements by placing them in seclusion and/or restraints.

Legal Issues

The psychiatric-mental health nurse also may come across legal issues while providing care to patients, regardless of the setting in which they work. Some of the legal issues include the right to privacy, maintaining confidentiality of the patient's information, providing informed consent for treatment, instituting restraint and seclusion, commitment issues, malpractice, and negligence. Problems occur due to failure to provide for or adhere to care based on PMH nursing scope and standards, and the Nursing Practice Act.

STANDARDS OF CARE AND STANDARDS OF PERFORMANCE

Standards of Care

The psychiatric-mental health nurse is concerned with the actual and potential psychiatric and mental health problems of their patients. They must perform care based on the scope of PMH nursing practice defined by the nurse's State Board of Nursing and the standards of care and performance outlined by the American Nurses Association (ANA) (APNA, 2007, pp. 104–113).

The scope of practice by the State Board of Nursing and standards of care for psychiatric and mental health nursing by the ANA and APNA are identified for public safety. It is a commitment by the board of nursing as a licensing agency, American Nurses Association, and American Psychiatric Nursing Association (APNA) that the nurse will perform the PMH nursing care within their scope and standards of practice.

The standards of PMH nursing practice address the nursing process. The nursing process provides a scientific approach and directions for clinical decisions and nursing actions. The stages of the nursing process include assessing, diagnosing, developing outcomes, planning, implementing, and evaluating the client's health status.

The psychiatric nurse must know their practice standards at their level of practice as they will be held accountable for practice according to the standards of care prescribed by the profession and the Nurse Practice Act.

Standards of Professional Performance

The PMH nurse is expected to maintain proficiency and competency for practice as prescribed within the scope and standards of performance of psychiatric and mental health nursing by the APNA (2007, p. 118). The PMH nurses must keep themselves updated with the current knowledge and practice in their practice area by attending professional conferences or meetings or by seeking continuing education hours. The standards of professional performance provided by APNA include quality care, performance appraisal, education, collegiality, ethics, collaboration, research, and resource utilization.

THE NURSING PROCESS

The nursing process is a scientific problem-solving approach designed to meet the needs of clients. The nursing process is composed of five steps: assessment, nursing diagnosis, planning/outcome development, implementation, and evaluation. The purpose of these steps is to resolve the identified nursing diagnosis by meeting the client's outcome.

The implementation of the nursing process in the PMH nursing practice is like all areas of nursing practice. The ANA mandated in 2000 in the *Scope and Standards of Psychiatric Mental Health Nursing Practice* that psychiatric-mental health nurses are to follow the prescribed standards of practice. These standards of practice incorporate the five components of the nursing process. PMH nurses are held accountable for upholding these standards legally and ethically.

STEPS IN THE PMH NURSING PROCESS

Nursing Assessment (Standard I)

This is the fundamental step of the nursing process that assists the PMH nurse to make sound decisions, diagnose problems, develop outcomes, provide interventions, and evaluate the client's progress. This step also provides the PMH nurse an opportunity to systematically collect subjective and objective data. Subjective data is collected through obtaining a psychiatric history from multiple sources: client, family and friends, medical records, healthcare providers, etc. Objective data is collected by performing physical and mental status examinations in order to identify any actual or potential mental or physical health problems. The clinical skills needed in this step include making purposeful observations, validating observations, therapeutic use of self, therapeutic communication, obtaining a biopsychosocial history, and conducting mental, physical, and environmental assessments. Refer to Unit II, Chapter 4 for details.

Nursing Diagnosis (Standard II)

Nursing diagnosis is the second step of the nursing process. It is a clinical judgment about individual, family, or community responses to actual or potential health problems. Nursing diagnosis provides the basis for the selection of nursing interventions to achieve outcomes for which the nurse is accountable (Carpenito, 2002). The PMH nurse performs the following functions:

1. Organizes, analyzes and summarizes the collected data

2. Identifies the client's actual or potential mental health problems as well as interpersonal, physical, or environmental factors that have influence on the client's mental health

The nursing diagnosis needs to be accurate and written in a concise statement form that indicates the client's condition and situation, primary or secondary causes of the condition, and nursing action needed to prevent, reduce, or eliminate the condition.

The nursing diagnosis in PMH nursing also needs to conform to the acceptable classification system from the North American Nursing Diagnosis Association (NANDA) or other nursing classifications, and the *Diagnostic and Statistical Manual of Mental Disorders—IV-TR* (APNA, 2007, p. 106). The *Diagnostic and Statistical Manual of Mental Disorders* (DSM-IV-TR, 2000) is a reference book that is widely used by healthcare professionals such as psychiatrists, psychologists, nurse practitioners, physicians, social workers, medical and nursing students, pastoral counselors, and other professionals. The title of the book is shortened to DSM, and an abbreviation indicates the edition, such as DSM-IV-TR; this means it is a fourth edition, text revision. The DSM-IV-TR addresses the classification of mental disorders, criteria for differential diagnosis, and numerical codes for medical recordkeeping. The DSM-IV-TR provides a guideline for clinical practice, tools for research, and aids to communication between "clinicians and researchers"; it also serves as "an educational tool for teaching psychopathology." The five diagnostic axes specified by DSM-IV-TR (2007) include:

- Axis I: Clinical Disorders
- Axis II: Personality Disorders and Mental Retardation
- Axis III: General Medical Conditions
- Axis IV: Psychosocial and Environmental Problems
  - Family Problems
  - Social Environment Problems
  - Educational Problems
  - Occupational Problems
  - Housing Problems
  - Economic Problems
  - Problems with Access to Health Care
  - Problems with the Legal System
  - Other Problems (war, disasters, etc.)
- Axis V: Global Assessment of Functioning (GAF)—rating the patient's general level of functioning is intended to help the doctor draw up a treatment plan and evaluate treatment progress.

The PMH nurse needs to pay attention to DSM-IV diagnostic categories. These categories will help the PMH nurse to formulate the nursing diagnosis. Key points to remember in formulating nursing diagnosis include:

1. Nursing diagnosis and risk factors are discussed and verified with the client, family members, and health team members.
2. The diagnosis identifies actual or potential psychiatric disorders and mental health issues of the client (APNA, 2007, p. 106).
3. The statement of the nursing diagnosis needs to be accurate and in a concise form of documentation that indicates the description of the client's condition and situation, causes of the condition, primary or secondary, and nursing action needed to prevent, reduce, or eliminate the condition.

The PMH nurse can develop a concept map for the identified nursing diagnosis or list the nursing diagnosis and designate the priority by numbering each item. The priority is to identify the most urgent and critical problem (see appendix A, a sample of a nursing diagnosis concept map).

Outcome Identification (Standard III)

Planning is the third step of the nursing process. The PMH nurse in this stage identifies expected client-centered outcomes. The outcomes give the PMH nurse directions for care.

The PMH nurse develops goals or the expected outcomes using standard classifications language for formulating the outcomes. The outcomes must be documented using measurable terms; that is, outcomes need to be specific, client centered, realistic and must include a time frame.

A key point to remember in identifying expected outcomes is that outcomes must derive from identified nursing diagnoses, be based on evidence, and be therapeutically attainable, realistic, and cost effective. In formulating the outcomes, the PMH nurse needs to include client, family, and other health team members whenever possible.

Plan of Care (Standard IV)

To formulate the plan of care for the client, the PMH nurse interacts with the client, family, and health team members. The planning consists of (1) identifying priorities, such as in the PMH setting the need for client safety as being of utmost importance over other needs; (2) setting goals; and (3) determining nursing actions and developing a plan of care format. The PMH nurse uses an evidence-based approach to develop therapeutic nursing interventions to meet the identified expected outcomes and goals. Key points to remember for the PMH nurse include:

1. The plan of care must set priorities in relation to identified expected outcomes.
2. Identified nursing interventions need to reflect current trends in nursing practice.
3. The nursing interventions must reflect the client's health beliefs and functional capabilities as well motivation level.
4. Nursing interventions need to include client teaching based on identified problems and teaching needs. Examples for teaching topics include stress management, coping skills, discharge planning for relapse prevention, medication management, building self-esteem, assertiveness-building skills, healthy life style, and knowledge of available community health resources.

Whatever format the PMH nurse uses for the plan of care, the format must include a nursing diagnosis, expected outcomes, nursing intervention, and evaluation. Some agencies use a standardized care plan and mark off appropriate boxes related to the client situation and date for the expected outcome and date for the outcome to be met. The purpose of developing a plan of care is to assist or guide clients to move toward a positive level of coping and functioning.

Implementation of Nursing Interventions (Standard V)

The PMH nurse in this stage actually implements the identified therapeutic nursing interventions. The PMH nurse incorporates the health promotion and illness prevention steps in the nursing interventions. The nursing interventions need to be in accordance with the PMH nurse's level and scope of practice. Specific nursing interventions stated in Standard V for the basic level of practice for the PMH nurse include:

1. Counseling
2. Milieu therapy
3. Promotion of self-care activities
4. Psycho–biologic interventions
5. Health teaching
6. Case management
7. Health promotion and health maintenance

The nursing interventions for an advanced level of practice include psychotherapy, prescriptive authority and treatment, and consultation.

PMH nurses must address all of the interventions outlined in Standard V of the APNA scope and standard for practice guideline (2007) for the client. There is a standardized classification of nursing interventions in *The Nursing Intervention Classification Book* (NIC). This book can be used by the PMH nurse as a guide for developing client-centered interventions. Key points to remember for the PMH nurse include (APNA, 2007, p. 110):

1. Continue to maintain therapeutic relationships with the client and family.
2. Implement if possible evidence-based nursing interventions for effectiveness of care.
3. Interventions need to be implemented depending upon the level of practice, education, and scope of practice.
4. Implement interventions promptly, in a safe manner with consideration of legal and ethical consequences in mind.
5. Interventions need to be revised as needed based on the client's change of health or stated needs.
6. Nursing interventions need to be documented in relation to identified expected outcomes.

Evaluation (Standard VI)

The PMH nurse in this last part of the nursing process evaluates the client for their achievement of the expected outcomes. There are two parts in the evaluation process, formative and summative. In the formative evaluation stage, the PMH nurse evaluates each step of the nursing process continuously and revises the nursing process as needed for outcome achievement; the nurse continuously monitors the impact of the nursing interventions and the prescribed treatment regime on the client's health. In the summative evaluation stage, the PMH nurse appraises the expected outcome and resolution of the client's actual or potential health problems. The summative evaluation is accomplished when the client is to be discharged.

The PMH nurse must document the care provided in each step of the nursing process in the client's chart. Crucial items for documentation include falls, seclusion, restraints, suicidal or homicidal ideation or attempt, or violent behavior (Fontaine & Fletcher, 2003, p. 42).

The following are the sample questions that the PMH nurse can ask themselves to evaluate nursing care:

1. Was the data collection process adequate to assess the client's actual or potential problems?
2. Was there accuracy in identifying the actual or potential nursing diagnosis?
3. What personal concerns were involved in setting goals and outcomes in attainable terms?

4. Did nursing interventions help the client according to expectations?
5. What changes were observed in the client's cognitive, emotional, and behavioral status in terms of the positive or negative outcome of the intervention or implemented treatment regime?
6. Was there a need for revising the nursing diagnosis, goals, outcomes, plan of care, interventions, or treatment plan?
7. Was the documentation of nursing care adequate?
8. Was self-evaluation conducted about feelings and thoughts toward the care of the client and its impact on self?

REFERENCES

American Nurses Association (2003). Nursing's social policy statement, (2nd ed.). Washington, DC: Nursesbook.org

American Nurses Association (2004). Nursing: Scope and standard of practice. Silver Spring, MD: 2nd ed. Washington, DC: Nursesbook.org

American Psychiatric Nursing Association (2007). *Psychiatric mental health nursing, scope and standards of practice.* Silver Spring, MD: Author.

American Psychiatric Association (2007). *Diagnostic and statistical manual of mental disorders* (4th ed., text revision). Arlington, VA: Author.

Carpenito, L. J. (2002). Nursing diagnosis: Application to clinical practice. Philadelphia, PA: Lippincott, Williams & Wilkins.

Fontaine K. & Fletcher, J., (2003). *Mental health nursing* (5th ed.). Upper Saddle River, NJ: Prentice Hall.

Stuart, G., & Laraia, M. (2001). *Principles and practice of psychiatric nursing* (7th ed.). St. Louis, MO: Mosby, Inc.

Townsend, M. (2006). *Psychiatric mental health nursing* (5th ed.). Philadelphia, PA: F. A. Davis Co.

SUGGESTED READINGS

American Nurses Association (2006). *The American Nurses Association scope and standards of psychiatric mental health nursing practice.* Washington, DC: Author.

Boyd, M. (2008). *Psychiatric nursing* (4th ed.). Philadelphia, PA. Lippincott, Williams, & Wilkins.

Fetter, M. S. (2009). Improving information technology competencies: Implication for psychiatric mental health nursing. *Issues in Mental Health Nursing, 30,* 3.

Fountain, K. (2009). *Mental health nursing* (6th ed.). Upper Saddle River, NJ: Pearson Education, Inc.

Lego, S. (1984). *The American handbook of psychiatric nursing.* Philadelphia, PA: J. B. Lippincott Co.

Sadock, B. J., & Sadock. V.A. (2008). *Kaplan & Sadock's concise textbook of clinical psychiatry* (3rd ed.). Philadelphia, PA: Lippincott, Williams, & Wilkins.

Videbeck, S. (2008). *Psychiatric mental health nursing* (4th ed.). Philadelphia, PA: Lippincott, Williams, & Wilkins.

UNIT II

Therapeutic Communication and Building Safe Environment Skills

CHAPTER 2

Therapeutic Use of Self

Kim A. Jakopac

OBJECTIVES _____

The nursing student will be able to:

1. Define the concept of the therapeutic use of self
2. Give examples of therapeutic listening skills or attending skills
3. Explain the therapeutic use of self in the context of Hildegard Peplau's nursing theoretical framework
4. Describe how the nurse uses the self as a healing agent

KEY TERMS _____

Attending skills
Empathy
Empathetic linkage
Healing agent
Interpersonal

Psychodynamic nursing
Self-system
Therapeutic listening skills
Therapeutic use of self

Therapeutic Use of Self is defined as the conscious use of a nurse's own unique personality and empathy as therapeutic tools to assist the client to develop a positive relationship and provide structure to nursing interventions. It also involves the nurse being aware of their own values, attitudes, and beliefs regarding life and death, and acceptance of the uniqueness of and differences in the client. The nurse evaluates how their values, attitudes, and beliefs affect clients. According to Keltner, Schwecke, and Bostom (2007), therapeutic listening is included in the concept of the therapeutic use of self (p. 91).

EXAMPLES OF THERAPEUTIC LISTENING SKILLS

The nurse should take into consideration cultural differences and the client's mental state related to eye contact and interpersonal space, to include the following techniques:

- Making eye contact without staring
- Facing the client
- Leaning forward towards the client at arm's length
- Open body posture
- Avoiding invading the client's personal space
- Focusing on what the client is saying
- Paying attention to body posture and behavior
- Avoiding letting thoughts stray
- Using nonjudgmental, accepting tone of voice
- Remaining objective and open
- Employing empathetic facial expression
- Being genuine and sincere
- Using verbal and nonverbal encouragement to continue (e.g., "please continue," "go on," nodding head, appropriate use of silence)
- Clarifying information
- Being sensitive to important cues
- Summarizing important information and events
- Giving feedback as needed

PSYCHIATRIC-MENTAL HEALTH NURSING THEORY—PEPLAU

Hildegard Peplau developed an interpersonal relations nursing theoretical framework. According to Peplau, each person is "a unique biological-psychological-spiritual-sociological" being with their own unique reaction to others and life events (George, 1995, p. 50). Nursing is an interpersonal process between nurses and clients involving mutual respect for each other as unique individuals. This interpersonal process is influenced by how the nurses view themselves because their self-concept influences how they view the world, communicate, and make decisions about others. Therefore, self-awareness is an integral part of nursing and the therapeutic use of self (Williams, 2008, p. 17).

Nursing is therapeutic because it is a healing art with nurses acting as healing (therapeutic) agents to help reduce clients' anxiety by providing positive, accepting, nonjudgmental relationships in which the healing process can occur. Peplau also emphasized the power of empathy and the importance of environment, and introduced the nurse–client relationship (Boyd, 2008, p. 68–69).

Case Example #1

Susan, a 24-year-old divorced mother of two young children has been referred for a psychiatric evaluation by her primary care provider (PCP) for symptoms of major depression including suicidal thoughts. Following the psychiatric evaluation, she is admitted to a psychiatric-mental health unit on a voluntary basis. The nurse's first encounter with Susan occurs in the admission interview room. Susan avoids eye contact by looking at the floor and displays a closed body posture. The nurse sits across from Susan and tries to establish eye contact while facing her, leaning forward, and introducing herself. The nurse assesses Susan's slumped shoulders, arms folded in front of her body, and crossed legs. She uses silence therapeutically to give Susan a chance to speak. Susan nods her head when the nurse states that she understands Susan was referred by her PCP.

The nurse begins by greeting Susan, introducing herself, and offering her a chair.

> Nurse: (using a gentle, empathetic tone of voice) "Tell me more about the symptoms you reported to your family doctor."
>
> Susan: (hesitates a moment before replying) "Well, lately I've been so tired and just don't want to get out of bed in the morning." (Briefly makes eye contact.)
>
> The nurse nods her head and has a concerned facial expression. Using therapeutic silence, the nurse gives Susan a chance to think about anything else she wants to say. When it becomes clear that Susan is not going to say anything else, the nurse continues, "Have you been having any thoughts of harming yourself?"
>
> Susan: (becomes tearful and in a whisper) "yes."
>
> Nurse: (focusing on Susan's verbal and nonverbal responses, hands her a tissue) "How were you thinking of harming yourself?"
>
> Susan: "My husband has a bottle of sleeping pills. I was thinking of taking those."
>
> Nurse: "Have you ever attempted suicide before?"
>
> Susan shakes her head.
>
> Nurse: "Are you having thoughts of suicide now?"
>
> Susan: "No, not now, but I was when I saw my family doctor."

The nurse tells Susan that she is glad she sought help today and obtains a verbal no-self-harm contract with her.

Case Example #2

Ted, a 32-year-old male with a history of chronic paranoid schizophrenia, has been admitted to a state mental health psychiatric unit for a 3-month period. This is his third week on the unit. He is awake and dressed at 6 a.m. and starts pacing in the hallway. The night shift mental heath technician (MHT) ignores him. He starts pacing more quickly and begins talking to himself in an angry tone of voice. Ted stands in front of the locked door to the unit and stares out of the small Plexiglas opening.

The night shift nurse, Ellen, who has been working the past four nights, sees Ted standing by the door and calls his name as she slowly walks toward Ted. "What's wrong, Ted?" she asks in a concerned tone of voice while makes eye contact. Ted says, "Where's Michelle? I want to see Michelle." His affect is anxious. Ellen explains that Michelle will come at 7 a.m. because she is scheduled to work the day shift. She reminds Ted that it is only a little after 6 a.m. and offers to sit and talk with him before Michelle comes to work. Ted waits a few minutes and then follows her to a corner of the dayroom and sits down. He fidgets with his fingers, makes brief eye contact, and his affect is still anxious.

> Ellen: "What are you thinking about, Ted?"
>
> Ted: "I think something's happened to Michelle."
>
> Ellen: "What do you think has happened?"
>
> Ted: "I think someone has hurt her and that's why she's not here."
>
> Ellen: Leans forward, but remains at an arm's length away from Ted and says empathetically, "I know you like talking to Michelle and trust her, but do you remember I said she comes to work at 7 a.m.?"
>
> Ted: "I guess so."
>
> Ellen: "What time is it now?" and points to the wall clock in the dayroom.
>
> Ted: Turns to look at the clock, squints and says, "6:30."
>
> Ellen: "Yes."

She continues to stay with Ted and ask him about what he is thinking and feeling. She reinforces reality and offers him a cup of decaffeinated coffee.

REFERENCES

Boyd, M. A. (2008). *Psychiatric nursing: Contemporary practice* (4th ed.). Philadelphia, PA: Wolters/Kluwer, Lippincott, Williams, & Wilkins.

George, J. B. (1995). *Nursing theories* (4th ed.). Norwalk, CT: Appleton & Lange.

Keltner, N. L., Schwecke, L. H., & Bostrom, C. E. (2007). *Psychiatric nursing* (5th ed.). St. Louis, MO: Mosby, Elsevier.

Williams, C. L. (2008). *Therapeutic interaction in nursing* (2nd ed.). Sudbury, MA: Jones and Bartlett.

SUGGESTED READINGS

Dexter, G., & Wash, M. (1997). *Psychiatric nursing skills: A patient-centered approach* (2nd ed.). Cheltenham, UK: Stanley Thorns Publishers Ltd.

Fontaine, K. L. (2009). *Mental health nursing* (6th ed.). Upper Saddle River, NJ: Pearson Education Inc.

Kwiatek, E., McKenzie, K., & Loads, D. (2005). Self-awareness and reflection: Exploring the "therapeutic use of self." *Learning Disability Practice, 8*(3), 27–31.

Mohr, W. K. (2009). *Psychiatric-mental health nursing: Evidence based concepts, skills, and practices* (7th ed.). Philadelphia, PA: Wolters Kluwer/Lippincott, Williams, & Wilkins.

O'Brien, P. G., Kennedy, W. Z., & Ballard, K. A. (2008). *Psychiatric mental health nursing: An introduction to theory and practice.* Sudbury, MA: Jones and Bartlett.

Sheldon, L. K. (2009). *Communication for nurses* (2nd ed.). Sudbury, MA: Jones and Bartlett.

Smoyak, S. A. (2008). Psychiatric nursing as gift giving. *Journal of Psychosocial Nursing, 46*(12), 8–9.

Stuart, G. W., & Laraia, M. T. (2005). *Principles and practice of psychiatric nursing* (8th ed.). St. Louis, MO: Mosby, Elsevier.

Townsend, M. C. (2009). *Essentials of psychiatric mental health nursing: Concepts of care in evidence based practice* (6th ed.). Philadelphia, PA: F. A. Davis Company.

Varcarolis, E. M., Carson, V. B., & Shoemaker, N. C. (2006). *Foundations of psychiatric mental health nursing: A clinical approach* (6th ed.). St. Louis, MO: Saunders, Elsevier.

CHAPTER 3

Modification of the Environment

Kim A. Jakopac

OBJECTIVES _____

The nursing student will be able to:
1. Explain the difference between therapeutic and nontherapeutic environments
2. List important aspects of the therapeutic environment
3. Discuss ways to modify the environment to provide safety, reduce anxiety, enhance communication, and stimulate interaction
4. Explain ways to manage or alter the milieu related to client's needs per diagnoses and symptoms

KEY TERMS _____

Anxiety
Contraband
Cultural awareness
Cultural competence

Environment
Milieu
Nontherapeutic
Therapeutic

---

*E**nvironment** is defined as a group of external conditions that influence a person (see **Figure 3-1**). These external conditions can be physical, biologic, cultural, and social (APA, 2007, 334). *Therapeutic environment* is an environment that exerts a curative, healing, or beneficial effect on the client. A nontherapeutic environment does not promote healing or is not beneficial and can even be harmful. Also, according to nursing theorist Martha Rodgers, the nurse is viewed as part of the client's external environmental energy field and works *with* the client in a mutual relationship rather than *for* the client. The nurse uses their own positive energy to help move the client toward achieving their maximum potential as a human being (Frisch & Frisch, 2002, p. 39).

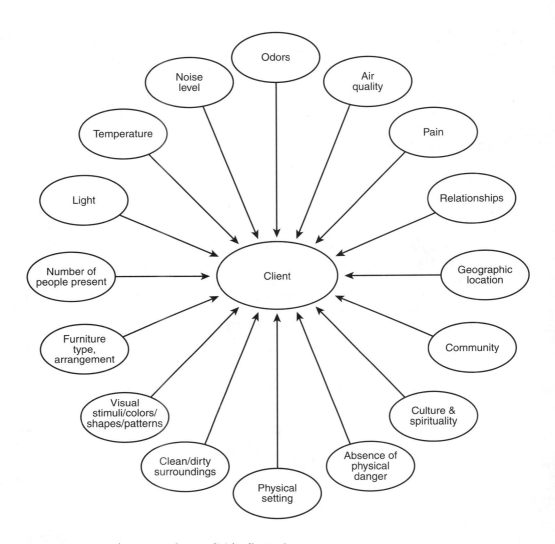

FIGURE 3-1   Elements of an Individual's Environment

A person's culture includes learned and shared beliefs, values, norms, and roles a person uses to function, understand, and interpret life (Keltner, Schwecke, & Bostrom, 2007, p. 164). Western culture focuses on the importance of the individual in the development of personal identity, whereas Eastern culture focuses on the importance of family for the development of one's identity, and indigenous cultures focus on the importance of the larger concept of the tribe for the development of personal identity (Varcarolis, Carson, & Shoemaker, 2006, p. 101–102). Cultural groups may be formed according to ethnicity, religion, occupation, socioeconomic status, geographical location, sexual orientation, and even abilities versus disabilities (Varcarolis, Carson, & Shoemaker, 2006, p. 100). Latinos receive less in terms of mental health services than other cultural groups even though the incidence of mental illness is relatively the same. Some of the disparities in services are related to beliefs about mental illness, decreased reporting of symptoms, language barriers, and suspicion of healthcare providers. Cultural differences may pose a barrier to seeking, accepting, or having access to mental health services (Shattell, Hamilton, Starr, Jenkins, & Hinderliter, 2008, p. 352). Also, Latino clients may present with and seek care for physical symptoms rather than psychiatric symptoms. African Americans depend upon social support from their church and family. They may use folk remedies rather than seek professional help. Asians fear being stigmatized, which may delay their seeking help until symptoms are severe. Native Americans and African Americans may consult a folk healer, root doctor, or shaman who combines spiritual and folk healing practices (APA, 2000, p. 897; O'Brien, Kennedy, & Ballard, 2008, p. 312). It is imperative that nurses strive to be culturally aware and develop cultural competence to enhance their abilities to modify the therapeutic environment to assist in developing improved therapeutic relationships with clients that will ultimately result in high quality nursing care.

In a psychiatric-mental health clinical setting, the environment is referred to as the *milieu* or the *therapeutic milieu*. It is an important part of treatment and is modified or manipulated by the nurse for the therapeutic benefit of the client. It is utilized as a safe community to promote healing and interaction between clients and staff, provide education, reinforce adaptive coping methods, and offer a place to learn and practice new adaptive behaviors.

There are general and more specific modifications of the environment or ways to manage the therapeutic milieu according to client and staff safety needs as well specific needs of the client per diagnoses or symptoms. Medical–psychiatric units have additional equipment depending on the needs of their clients.

GENERAL MODIFICATIONS

- Physical structure
- Safety
- Unit rules/expected norms
- Program structure
- Consistency

Physical Structure

The physical structure of the unit will be determined by the type and setting of the facility (e.g., free-standing vs as part of a general hospital) as well as the regulations of the Occupational Safety and Health Administration (OSHA), local fire department, and state building codes. The majority of psychiatric-mental health units are locked units, but there are open units depending on clients' needs and the program structure. Furniture, lighting, floor materials, décor, and color schemes are chosen for safety needs—including fall prevention—and aesthetic value as much as possible. Use of materials such as Plexiglas, electric door locking devices, cameras, and entry/exit intercom systems are common. Break-away railings and enclosure devices surrounding toilet plumbing help prevent suicide attempts. Televisions and telephones are located in central or common areas on the unit rather than in individual clients' rooms to promote interaction. Furniture in larger areas such as the dayroom and dining room is arranged to promote interaction rather than social isolation. There are also quieter areas where clients can temporarily go when anxious or becoming agitated to decrease environmental stimuli (i.e., noise, crowding) and help regain control. These areas would be within view of the nursing staff and provide an alternate area to their individual rooms. Smoking areas are located either in rooms with specialized air flow on the unit or in enclosed outside areas adjacent to the unit. Some facilities have a gymnasium and/or pool where clients can exercise. Seclusion/restraint or behavioral control rooms (BAC) are located near the nurses' station. The physical structure of locked units is adapted to decrease the chance of clients leaving on their own. Unit policies include performing environmental safety rounds at least every 24 hours. Typically the doors to medication rooms are modified so that only the top half may be opened during medication administration. Clients go to the medication room rather than a nurse taking a medication cart or tray down the hallway. The nurses' station is centrally located, and there are intercom systems in each client room to make the nursing staff more accessible.

Safety

The safety of the environment includes procedures for the control of and removal of personal objects, anything sharp, glass containers, weapons, and substances including alcohol and illegal drugs that may pose a danger to clients, members of the healthcare team, and visitors. These objects and substances are referred to as "contraband." Not all clients are suicidal or aggressive towards others, but some clients are under the influence of alcohol/substances, psychotic, confused, or have dementia. These clients could accidentally harm themselves or someone else if they had access to contraband. Sharp containers and gloves are placed only in strategic areas on the unit such as the medication room, physical exam room, and nurses' station. Paper rather than plastic garbage bags are used. For occasions requiring plastic and biohazard bags, these bags are taken to a locked storage area on the unit until they can be removed from the unit for permanent disposal. Due to the principal of least restrictive treatment and maintaining as much normalcy as possible, clients are allowed to wear their own clothing, with the exception of belts and shoestrings. A calm atmosphere is promoted and disruptive behavior is dealt with quickly. Visitors are required to remain in larger areas where they are easily visible, such as the dayroom, in order for staff members to be available if needed and to discourage passing contraband to clients or inappropriate sexual behavior between visitors and clients. Staff members are also available to provide emotional support when clients express strong emotions during visitation or request staff to be present when discussing emotionally charged topics with their visitors. If further privacy is needed (e.g., meeting with a lawyer), a room near the nurses' station (e.g., interview room, psychotherapy group room) would be appropriate, but not clients' rooms. It is not advisable to use clients' rooms because this is their personal space and because of safety concerns for visitors, staff, and clients. Procedures to keep track of where clients are at all times (i.e., client safety rounds) are another form of safety. There are plans for how to protect and, when needed, remove clients to a safe area in the event of a fire or other type of disaster.

Unit Rules/Expected Norms

Unit rules or expected norms provide psychosocial structure, clarify expected behavior, promote socially acceptable behavior and a sense of therapeutic community, support clients' rights, maintain clients' dignity, and help decrease clients' anxiety. Unit rules help make it possible for clients to live together in close quarters and get along with each other. Clients with problems related to social appropriateness or interaction benefit from unit expectations.

Program Structure

Program structure is an important part of the therapeutic environment as well as in the treatment of psychiatric-mental health disorders. Many different types of groups such as community meetings, psychotherapy, psycho-education, occupational therapy, activity therapy, art/music therapy, pet therapy, and gardening are usually offered. Community meetings in the morning and evening (sometimes referred to as "wrap-up" groups) are common. In group therapy not only is the topic of these groups important, but the number of clients that attend, which specific clients attend, the number of groups during the day, when these groups are conducted, and the length of time each group meets are also very important. Clients of different cognitive (high or low) functioning levels may meet in separate groups. Small breaks of time between groups, scheduling of meals, medication times, time for personal hygiene needs, smoking, visiting times, telephone times, and free time are part of the program structure and therapeutic milieu. Interdisciplinary treatment team meetings are regularly scheduled as part of the program. Clients are made aware of the daily and weekly program schedule by having it posted in larger common areas on the unit (e.g., dayroom). A copy of the daily program schedule is also provided for clients in a folder that is given to them on admission.

Consistency

Consistency is a key element of the therapeutic environment. It applies to many aspects of the unit environment including the program schedule, unit rules including application of the rules; responding to certain behaviors, maintaining therapeutic boundaries, visitation, confidentiality, staffing, and any form of communication. Consistency is part of the overall structure of the unit. Many clients diagnosed with psychiatric-mental health problems lack consistency in their lives and home environments and, therefore, greatly benefit from it in the treatment setting. **Tables 3-1** and **3-2** provide information on leading nursing groups as part of the therapeutic milieu as well as setting up and managing the therapeutic milieu.

TABLE 3-1 Nurse-led Groups in the Therapeutic Milieu		
Therapeutic groups	**Interventions**	**Rationales**
1. Community meetings	1a. Introduce self and others and state the purpose of the community meeting.	1a. Clients have the right to know who is providing care for them. This is how the nurse provides structure for the meetings.

(continues)

Therapeutic groups	Interventions	Rationales

TABLE 3-1 Nurse-led Groups in the Therapeutic Milieu (continued)

Therapeutic groups	Interventions	Rationales
	b. Review meeting rules if needed for new members.	b. The rate of admission/discharge varies. New clients will not know what is happening or what to do unless the rules are reviewed. Other clients may need the rules reviewed, especially if they are having problems with disorientation, psychosis, or behavioral control problems.
	c. Encourage clients to be assertive and express their views.	c. Clients need to be actively involved in their treatment, and some clients have difficulty being assertive. These meetings provide a safe environment for them to practice expressing their views and being assertive.
	d. In morning meetings ask clients to set goals for the day.	d. It is very important for clients to be actively involved in their treatment. Goal setting helps clients choose a direction and have some control over their treatment and progress.
	e. Discuss solutions for problems related to day-to-day functions on the unit (e.g., linen supply, meals/snacks, telephone access, television privileges, smoking privileges).	e. It is inevitable that problems will arise when several people live in close proximity to each other. Facilities deal with suppliers and cost containment issues that may alter the availability of supplies. Discussing problems with clients not only involves them in their care, but also helps provide them with practice using the steps of general problem solving that is a skill needed for daily living; many clients have difficulty with basic problem solving.

(continues)

TABLE 3-1   Nurse-led Groups in the Therapeutic Milieu *(continued)*

Therapeutic groups	Interventions	Rationales
	f. Refer to appropriate staff members, therapists, or psychiatrist for other problems.	f. Not all problems are appropriate to be discussed in community meetings. However, the nurse leader should not ignore a client's questions or report of problems. Referrals to the appropriate members of the treatment team assure that the client's question or problem will be addressed and maintains the structure of the community meeting.
	g. For evening meetings or "wrap-up" groups, review how clients felt about their day and whether or not goals were attained; discuss what helped or hindered goal attainment.	g. This format provides feedback from the nurse leader and the therapeutic community of other clients as to what worked best for a client and other possible ways to meet goals if they were not met. Positive or negative visits from family or friends are discussed. A client may feel neglected if they did not receive a visitor and is given emotional support from the group. This group also provides emotional/psychological closure for the day.
Psychoeducation groups	2a. Provide education on a variety of topics (refer to chapter on leading psychoeducation groups).	2a. Nurses are required by ANA and Psychiatric-Mental Health Nurse Scope and Standards to provide education to clients. Clients need education to be involved in treatment decisions to the best of their ability and have as much control of their symptoms as possible. Information is made available to the family as much as possible without breaching client confidentiality.

(continues)

TABLE 3-1   Nurse-led Groups in the Therapeutic Milieu (continued)

Therapeutic groups	Interventions	Rationales
Creative writing groups	3a. Allow clients to choose appropriate theme and write one or two pages about the chosen theme.	3a. This type of group provides opportunities for clients to express their thoughts and feelings in a different way. Clients may not be aware of their own ability to express themselves in this way. Writing exercises a different portion of the brain than speaking.
	b. An alternative to writing would be drawing pictures/symbols.	b. This would be useful for clients with literacy problems or for whom English is not their primary language. It also may benefit clients who have had a CVA.

Table 3-2   Specific Management of the Therapeutic Milieu

Major Depression

Technique	Rationale
1. When possible assign the same primary nurses and other mental health staff to the same set of clients.	1. This helps provide consistency in the milieu, which in turn helps promote the development of trust between clients, nurses, and other mental health staff.
2. Encourage clients to remain out on the unit rather than isolating in their own rooms.	2. Isolating from others is a symptom of major depression. Clients may insist on staying or lying down in their own room versus going to the day room or dining room. They may also complain of fatigue, which is another symptom of major depression. Although clients initially only wish to spend time with the nurse, it is more therapeutic to encourage remaining out in the unit.

(continues)

Table 3-2   Specific Management of the Therapeutic Milieu *(continued)*

Major Depression

Technique	Rationale
3. Arrange chairs in small groups of three or four and invite clients to sit and talk, play cards/board games, or watch television/movie with nurse.	3. Smaller groups in a more informal atmosphere may be less intimidating to clients who frequently have problems with low self-esteem and low energy levels.
4. Monitor television programs, movies, and music, and avoid anything with sad, depressing themes.	4. This type of stimuli will reinforce and increase a depressed mood.
5. Orient the client to the dining room area and explain that clients eat together rather than alone in their own rooms.	5. Clients diagnosed with major depression not only isolate themselves from others, but also may experience decreased appetite. Eating with others decreases social isolation, encourages imitation of the behavior of others, and can stimulate appetite. On some units all clients eat on the unit, but on other units clients earn privileges to go to the hospital cafeteria.
6. In severe cases with clients who refuse to leave their rooms even to eat, the door to the client's room may be locked (in some facilities this is a treatment team decision versus a decision by the nurse).	6. Allowing clients to isolate in their rooms while ruminating about their problems is not therapeutic and can worsen their depressed mood.

Suicidal Thoughts/Gestures/Attempts

Technique	Rationale
1. Move clients to a room as close to the nurses' station as possible if current rooms are farther away.	1. Although general environment modifications and management are in place, these clients may need even more supervision to prevent any further self-harm.
2. Place clients on 1:1 observation or constant observation (CO) if unable to verbally contract to refrain from harming themselves. This will require a staff member to remain with an individual client at an arm's length at all times. Arrangements may need to be made for additional staffing to provide care for the remaining clients on the unit.	2. Clients who are unable to at least verbally contract to refrain from harming themselves are at high risk for attempting suicide. Even though psychiatric-mental health units take special general safety precautions regarding the physical environment and contraband, unfortunately sometimes clients do find ways to harm themselves.

(continues)

| Table 3-2   **Specific Management of the Therapeutic Milieu** *(continued)* | |

Suicidal Thoughts/Gestures/Attempts

Technique	Rationale
3. Assign only staff (i.e., MHTs, CNAs, LPNs, or RNs) that have been educated and have experience providing care for clients on 1:1 observation or COs.	3. Inexperienced staff lacking education related to working with psychiatric–mental health clients unfortunately have contributed to unsafe environments, and clients have attempted suicide because these staff members were not able to provide appropriate supervision and care for these clients. This becomes a delegation problem and legal–ethical liability issue for the nurse as well as the facility.
4. In severe cases bed linens may be ordered to be removed and the client provided with a heavy blanket and pillow without a pillowcase. The client may also be placed in a hospital gown without strings (snap closure only).	4. Clients may try to hang themselves by tying bed linens together and then placing them over the top of a door or around a piece of furniture or toilet plumbing.
5. Perform mouth checks when administering medication to these clients.	5. Clients may cheek (hold) medication tablets, capsules or small amounts of liquids/elixirs in their buccal pouch or under their tongue and spit the medication out later. Tablets or capsules can be hidden in their clothing or in their rooms to be stored up and taken as an overdose at a later time.
6. If the nurse suspects clients of storing up medications to overdose with or of hiding other types of contraband in their clothing or in their rooms, the nurse may initiate a clothing and/or room search (in some facilities this is a standing policy; in other facilities the psychiatrist may wish to be notified before proceeding).	6. Nurses must balance clients' rights, including privacy, with safety needs. Two staff members should be present at all times. When searching clothing, the client is covered with a hospital gown without strings (snap closure only) or bed sheet for privacy while the staff searches their clothing including the pockets, hems, and lining of all pieces of clothing. There are separate policies, specific criteria, and orders for body cavity searches (refer to individual facility policies and procedures). Body cavity searches are *not* routinely done. When performing a room search the client must be present as well as

(continues)

Table 3-2   Specific Management of the Therapeutic Milieu *(continued)*

Suicidal Thoughts/Gestures/Attempts

Technique	Rationale
	two staff members and a security guard if the facility has their own security personnel. Documentation of any search must be completed according to facility policies.

Bipolar Disorder

Technique	Rationale
1. Refer to previous techniques listed for major depression for the depressed phase of bipolar disorder.	1. Bipolar disorder is typically characterized by two phases: a depressed phase and a manic phase.
2. For clients experiencing a manic phase, reduce the environmental stimuli by turning off the TV or radio; moving clients to a quieter area where they can pace; or taking them to an exercise area.	2. In a manic phase, clients are extremely sensitive to the environment and display symptoms such as psychomotor agitation, hyperactivity, impulsiveness, irritability, and distractibility. Decreasing the stimuli and providing an area and activities that use gross motor movements can help dissipate the excess energy they feel during this phase.
3. Maintain consistency by reinforcing unit policies, limit setting, and scheduling of nursing and other mental health staff.	3. Clients experiencing a manic phase can easily create conflict among other clients and staff. Typical behavior includes testing limits, blaming others, arguing over perceived discrepancies in unit policies, staff behavior, or communication. Consistent staffing helps ensure that clients receive the same responses when testing limits as well as establishing and maintaining trust.
4. Monitor television programs, movies, and music and avoid anything with violent or sexual themes.	4. Television programs, movies, and music with violent or sexual themes can cause increased agitation in clients experiencing a manic phase of bipolar disorder.

(continues)

Table 3-2 Specific Management of the Therapeutic Milieu *(continued)*

Severe Anxiety States

Technique	Rationale
1. Provide a quiet room with less stimulation.	1. There will be less stimuli for clients to react to, and it will be easier to engage them in relaxation exercises and discussion of their thoughts and feelings in a quieter area. Also, clients who are overwhelmed with excess stimuli and their own feelings may actually begin to feel suicidal. They may do something impulsively to stop the overwhelming feelings and thoughts.
2. Move the client away from the dayroom, dining room or other activity areas.	2. See item 1.
3. Stay with the client and reassure that they are safe.	3. The nurse's presence has a calming effect on the client. This also provides an opportunity to further assess the client.
4. Monitor the client for a reduction in anxiety.	4. The steps of the nursing process include evaluation of interventions implemented. The nurse needs to evaluate if the milieu modifications are effective or not. Further changes will be implemented if the client's anxiety level remains unchanged.
5. Provide an area and activities that use gross motor movements, such as riding a stationary bicycle, walking, or use of the facility's gymnasium to play basketball or volleyball.	5. Physical activity can help dissipate excess energy clients experience during high anxiety or panic states.
6. Monitor the client for a reduction in anxiety.	6. See item 4.
7. Offer medication if medication is ordered.	7. Some clients may need medication if removing them to a quieter area and staying with them is not effective (see nursing interventions such as deep breathing in Unit IV).
8. Continue to monitor the client for a reduction in anxiety.	8. If the client is not experiencing a reduction in their level of anxiety, the nurse will notify the psychiatrist.

(continues)

Table 3-2   Specific Management of the Therapeutic Milieu *(continued)*

Aggressive or Assaultive Behavior

Technique	Rationale
1. Provide a quiet room with less stimulation than occurs in the day room or dining room.	1. The legal–ethical principle of "least restrictive treatment" guides management of the therapeutic milieu. There will be fewer stimuli for clients to react to, and it will be easier to engage them in relaxation exercises and discussion of their thoughts and feelings in a quieter area. This area may also be used for time-out sessions to help clients regain control of their own behavior. Aggressive clients may feel so overwhelmed or angry that they become physically assaultive.
2. Remove other clients from the area of the assaultive client.	2. This provides safety for the other clients on the unit and is a step towards containing the assaultive client in one area of the unit.
3. Move chairs and other small pieces of furniture out of the immediate area when possible.	3. This helps provide more space for other staff members coming to provide a show of force.
4. Place assaultive client in seclusion room or BCR that has previously been prepared according to regulations when other less restrictive interventions have not been successful, including offering medication. Use of physical restraints may also be necessary.	4. The purpose of the seclusion room or BCR is to provide safety and decrease stimuli for aggressive/assaultive clients themselves and the other clients on the unit who are in danger of assault by these clients. Physical restraints offer a higher level of safety if clients strike or kick the walls, door, bed, or staff members while in the seclusion room.
5. Clients in the seclusion room or BCR are automatically placed on 1:1 observation or constant observation (CO). Because this will require a staff member to remain with an individual client at all times, arrangements may need to be made for additional staffing to provide care for the remaining clients on the unit.	5. Clients in the seclusion room or BCR are at high risk to harm others or themselves and must be supervised very closely. Clients who are physically restrained are vulnerable to injury by other clients, potential aspiration, or neurovascular complications from the restraints themselves. They need assistance with drinking, eating, toileting, position changes, and constant supervision to be sure they do not somehow remove the restraints themselves. Documentation will

(continues)

Table 3-2 Specific Management of the Therapeutic Milieu *(continued)*

Aggressive or Assaultive Behavior

Technique	Rationale
	need to be done according to Joint Commission regulations and the facility's policies.
6. Assign only staff (i.e., MHTs, CNAs, LPNs, RNs) who have been educated and have experience providing care for clients.	6. Inexperienced staff lacking education related to working with psychiatric-mental health clients unfortunately have contributed to unsafe environments, and clients have been injured while in the seclusion room or BAC as a result.

Schizophrenia and Psychosis

Technique	Rationale
1. Additional care is taken to avoid the use of bright colors, including red and abstract patterns in wallpaper, paintings, furniture coverings, drapes, and flooring.	1. Clients diagnosed with schizophrenia and/or experiencing psychosis are very sensitive to bright colors, including red and abstract patterns. They have difficulty distinguishing between reality and nonreality, and use of these items can cause increased anxiety and possible agitation. For example, a pattern may be misinterpreted as faces, and this may be frightening to clients who are suspicious and paranoid.
2. Provide a calm, nonthreatening environment.	2. Clients diagnosed with schizophrenia and/or experiencing psychosis experience fear and an increase in symptoms such as hallucinations and delusions when exposed to environmental chaos and excessive stimuli.
3. Maintain consistency of the program schedule and staffing of nurses and other mental health staff members.	3. Variations in the program schedule can cause increased anxiety and paranoia for clients diagnosed with schizophrenia and/or experiencing psychosis. Consistent staffing of nurses and other mental health staff members helps establish trust, which is especially important when working with paranoid clients. Subtle changes in clients' mental

(continues)

Table 3-2   Specific Management of the Therapeutic Milieu *(continued)*

Schizophrenia and Psychosis

Technique	Rationale
	status will be more easily recognized when nurses are able to work with clients on a consistent basis.
4. Encourage clients to remain out on the unit versus isolating in their own rooms.	4. Isolating from others is a symptom of schizophrenia. Clients do not experience the same emotional rewards from social interaction that others do. Increased isolating behaviors may indicate that clients are experiencing increased psychotic symptoms.
5. Arrange chairs in small groups of two or three and invite clients to sit and talk, play cards/board games, or watch television/ movie with nurse.	5. Smaller groups in a more informal atmosphere may be less intimidating to clients who frequently have problems with social skills and low self-esteem. Smaller groups are also less stimulating.
6. Monitor television programs, movies, and music, and avoid anything with violent or sexual themes.	6. Television programs, movies, and music with violent or sexual themes can cause increased agitation in clients diagnosed with schizophrenia and/or experiencing psychosis.

Chemical Dependency

Technique	Rationale
1. Additional care is taken regarding the potential presence of contraband on the unit.	1. Unfortunately, visitors have brought illegal drugs and alcohol to clients during visiting hours. This demonstrates a need for more education regarding chemical dependency with family members and friends of clients receiving treatment.
2. Monitor television programs, movies, music, reading material to avoid anything with violent, sexual, or substance abuse themes.	2. Television programs, movies, music, and reading materials with violent, sexual, or substance abuse themes can cause increased agitation, escalation of inappropriate behavior or cravings to use/drink.

(continues)

Table 3-2 Specific Management of the Therapeutic Milieu *(continued)*	
Chemical Dependency	
Technique	**Rationale**
3. Maintain consistency in reinforcement of unit rules, limit setting, and personal accountability for behavior.	3. Many clients with chemical dependency problems have learned to manipulate and circumvent rules to meet their needs. Many avoid personal accountability for their behavior. Consistency regarding unit rules, responses to behavior, limit setting, and staffing is needed to provide a therapeutic environment for these clients.
4. Assign primary nurses and other mental health staff to the same clients.	4. Assigning the same (primary) nurses and other mental health staff assures consistency.
5. If the nurse suspects clients of having or receiving contraband, they may initiate a clothing and/or room search per facility protocol without violating clients' rights (in some facilities this is a standing policy; in other facilities the psychiatrist may wish to be notified before proceeding).	5. Nurses must balance clients' rights, including privacy, with safety needs. Two staff members should be present all times. When searching clothing, the client is covered with a hospital gown without strings (snap closure only) or bed sheet for privacy while the staff searches their clothing including the pockets, hems, and lining of all pieces of clothing. There are separate policies, specific criteria, and orders for body cavity searches (refer to individual facility policies and procedures). Body cavity searches are *not* routinely done. When performing a room search the client must be present as well as two staff members, and a security guard if the facility has their own security personnel. Documentation of any search must be completed according to facility policies.

REFERENCES

American Psychiatric Association (2000). *Diagnostic and statistical manual of mental disorders* (4th ed.), *text revision*. Washington, DC: Author.

American Psychological Association (2007). *APA dictionary of psychology*. Washington, DC: Author.

Frisch, N. C., & Frisch, L. E. (2002). *Psychiatric mental health nursing* (2nd ed.). Albany, NY: Delmar/Thomas Learning, Inc.

Keltner, N. L., Schwecke, L. H., & Bostrom, C. E. (2007). *Psychiatric nursing* (5th ed.). St. Louis, MO: Mosby, Elsevier.

O'Brien, P. G., Kennedy, W. Z., & Ballard, K. A. (2008). *Psychiatric mental health nursing: An introduction to theory and practice*. Sudbury, MA: Jones and Bartlett.

Shattell, M. M., Hamilton, D., Starr, S. S., Jenkins, C. J., & Hinderliter, N. A. (2008). Mental health service needs of a Latino population: A community-based participatory research project. *Issues in Mental Health Nursing, 29*, 351–370.

Varcarolis, E. M., Carson, V. B., & Shoemaker, N. C. (2006). *Foundations of psychiatric mental health nursing: A clinical approach* (5th ed.). St. Louis, MO: Saunders, Elsevier.

SUGGESTED READINGS

Dunn, K., Elsom, S., & Cross, W. (Feb., 2007). Self-efficacy and locus of control affect management of aggression by mental health nurses. *Issues in Mental Health Nursing, 28*(2), 201–217.

CHAPTER 4

Interview Techniques and the Biopsychosocial Nursing Assessment

Kim A. Jakopac

OBJECTIVES

The nursing student will be able to:
1. Explain how to conduct a client interview
2. Discuss the application of nursing process and critical thinking using information obtained during the client interview
3. Compare therapeutic communication and nontherapeutic communication techniques
4. Describe how to perform a mental status examination and its importance in the application of nursing process and critical thinking
5. Describe important elements of a biopsychosocial nursing assessment
6. Discuss the application of the nursing process as well as critical thinking when analyzing the information obtained from the biopsychosocial nursing assessment

KEY TERMS

Abstinence	Clang association	DSM-IV-TR	Insight
Abstract thinking	Cognition	Dystonia	Intelligence
Affect	Complementary	Echolalia	Intensive outpatient
Akthesia	Compulsion	Echopraxia	program
Alternative	Concentration	Ego defense	Judgment
Ameliorating	Concrete	mechanisms	Latency
Apathetic	Confabulation	Flight of ideas	Linear
Appearance	Congruent	Grandiose	Memory
Assessment	Critical thinking	Hallucinations	Mental status
Attention	Day treatment	Hyperactive	Monotone
Biopsychosocial	Delusions	Hypervigilant	Mood
Bizarre	Depersonalization	Hypoactive	Negativism
Blackouts	Derailment	Ideas of reference	Neologism
Catatonic	Derealization	Illusions	Nursing process
Circumstantial	Dissociation	Incongruent	Obsession

Orientation	Pressured speech	Tardive dyskinesia	Thought removal
Paranoid	Psychomotor	Thought blocking	Tics
Partial	Psychotherapy	Thought	Unintelligible/
hospitalization	Rambling speech	broadcasting	incoherent
Perseveration	Rumination	Thought content	Word salad
Phobia	Somatic	Thought insertion	
Poverty of speech	Tangential	Thought processes	

The *client interview* is a specific communication process with the goals of meeting the client where they are in their life situation, gaining their cooperation, establishing a rapport, and obtaining factual information from the client's perspective related to the reasons for entering the healthcare system. This information provides the initial database that will be used in the nursing process to make clinical decisions. The interview occurs during the assessment phase of the nursing process (see **Figure 4-1**) and meets requirements of Standard I of the American Nurses' Association (ANA) Scope and Standards of Psychiatric-Mental Health Nursing Practice (Fontaine, 2009, p. 25). See Chapter 1 for more detailed information.

The client interview may also be referred to as the *assessment* or *behavioral intake assessment* depending on the healthcare system the nurse functions in. Prior to the interview, the nurse must examine their own assumptions about the client, their situation, lifestyle, and any information that is available prior to meeting the client. The interview consists of three phases: initial, middle, and termination. During the initial phase, the nurse introduces themselves by first name including title/credentials, makes sure the client is as comfortable as possible while taking into consideration safety needs, assures the client of confidentiality, and begins to build rapport with the

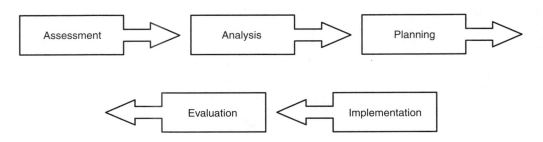

FIGURE 4-1   Nursing Process

client. The nurse also clarifies their reason for meeting with the client and provides general information regarding the healthcare setting. Asking the client if the nurse may write down information for accuracy during the interview conveys respect for the client and shows that the nurse values the importance of what the client has to say. Explaining that writing down information is in the client's best interest related to achieving an accurate diagnosis and planning treatment can help reduce any suspicions the client may have. During the middle phase of the interview, the nurse obtains assessment data and provides information about the client's rights, unit policies, and the program schedule. In the termination phase assessment data is summarized, any remaining questions are answered, and the initial nursing plan of care is formed with as much collaboration with the client as possible (O'Brien, Kennedy, & Ballard, 2008, pp. 49–50). As soon as it is appropriate, the client is shown their room and given a tour of the unit.

The setting in which the client interview takes place should be private, but allow for safety precautions (see Chapter 3) for everyone such as being within the view of others, having another staff member present or waiting just outside of the door, telephone access, more than one exit, and a panic/emergency button should the situation suddenly escalate. Some clients may be in such a severe crisis situation that additional assistance may be required quickly. Furniture and chairs are arranged to promote eye contact and communication. The nurse conducting the interview should attempt to place themselves at eye level to provide a sense of equality in relation to the power component of the relationship. The nurse sits or stands at a 90° angle or beside the client rather than directly opposite to promote the client's psychological comfort and decrease the intensity of the situation or feeling of being interrogated (Varcarolis, Carson, & Shoemaker, 2006, pp. 172–173; Mohr, 2009, pp. 161–162). In situations where the client is paranoid, the nurse will have to allow for additional personal space to avoid physically cornering the client, which could lead to agitation.

The nurse must pay strict attention to nonverbal as well as verbal communication and use all their observation skills during the interview because much of the information the client reports will be subjective. Permission to validate the information obtained during the interview will have to be obtained in writing from the client. Clinical skills needed to complete the interview include the following:

- Observation
- Validation
- Therapeutic use of self
- Use of therapeutic communication
- Ability to obtain a biopsychosocial history

- Ability to perform a mental status examination (neuropsychiatric assessment)
- Ability to perform a physical assessment

(Fontaine, 2009, p. 25; Mohr, 2009, p. 145)

OBSERVATION

The nurse will observe the client's affect and behavior during the interview. The following questions will help guide the nurse's observations:

1. What exactly is the client doing at this time (sitting, standing, pacing, restlessness/fidgeting, using hand gestures, shaking, crying, laughing, displaying bizarre behavior, responding as if someone/something else is in the room, displaying slow motor movements)?
2. Is the behavior dangerous to the client or others present?
3. How would you describe the client's affect?
4. Does the client make eye contact?
5. Is the client alert, oriented/disoriented, psychotic or aware of your presence? Does the client tolerate your presence?
6. Is the client capable of interacting with you at this time?
7. Is the client willing to be interviewed at this time?
8. Does the client speak or remain silent? Do they ruminate about a specific situation or topic?
9. Can you follow what the client says? Are there reoccurring themes in the client's speech?
10. Is the client dressed appropriately for the situation and season of the year?
11. Has the client been medicated and is, therefore, currently experiencing drowsiness that would affect the quality of the interview?
12. If family members/significant others are present, are they supportive of the client and allow the client to answer questions?
13. Do family members/significant others sit appropriately close together or far apart?

VALIDATION

1. Does the client clarify information when asked?
2. Is the client able to state their mood?
3. Is the client willing to give written permission to contact family members or friends to obtain and give information?

4. Are prior psychiatric and medical records available? Is the client willing to give written permission to obtain these records?
5. Does the client have any sensory aids needed with them from home?
6. How does your information compare with information obtained by other members of the current treatment team?

THERAPEUTIC COMMUNICATION

Therapeutic communication may be defined as the purposeful use of certain techniques or procedures with the goals of enhancing the therapeutic nurse–client relationship; promoting healing and change; and assisting the client to disclose information as well as express feelings or thoughts (Keltner, Schwecke, & Bostrom, 2007, p. 90; Townsend, 2009, p. 132). Therapeutic communication is an active process that includes empathy and active listening while maintaining objectivity and professional boundaries. Professional boundaries and the therapeutic nurse–client relationship will be discussed in Chapter 5. The client is the focus of therapeutic communication, whereas in social communication the focus is on all participants for everyone's personal benefit. It is important for the nurse to keep their communication nonjudgmental and congruent to promote trust and avoid misinterpretation. Therapeutic communication techniques are used in virtually all interactions with clients. Nursing students may use an Interpersonal Process Recording (IPR) to help remember conversations with clients, identify specific therapeutic communication techniques, identify themes, and avoid nontherapeutic communication techniques. See Appendix E for an IPR form.

The psychiatric-mental health (PMH) nurse must pay attention to both overt or obvious and covert or hidden messages when interacting with and interviewing clients. How language is used; the semantics or meaning; voice tone, pitch, or inflection; slang or jargon; cultural influences; and the client's primary language all influence verbal communication (Arnold & Boggs, 2007, p. 187). Although it is important to obtain an interpreter when interviewing any client whose primary language is not English, it is imperative when dealing with a victim or survivor of any type of abuse, violence, or rape. Unfortunately, anyone accompanying the client could be involved in the abuse, violence, or rape, thus detracting from the accuracy of the information obtained if they are used as an interpreter. According to Arnold and Boggs (2007), most communication between individuals is nonverbal. This includes body language, gestures, touch, affect, eye contact, and amount of personal space between the client and interviewer or between the client and family members or friends (pp. 188–189). It is important to pay attention to what the client is *not* saying or is avoiding as well as what they are telling you. The nurse can revisit these issues or information at a later time after better rapport and trust have been established. For examples and rationales for therapeutic techniques and identification of nontherapteutic techniques, see **Table 4-1** and **Table 4-2**.

Table 4-1	Therapeutic Communication Techniques	
Techniques	**Examples**	**Rationales**
Accepting or active listening	Maintaining eye contact, facing the client, nodding head, "I can imagine how it might feel to be so sad."	This technique lets the client know that the nurse heard what was said and accepts what is said as the client's perception.
Broad opening	"What was happening at home before you came to the hospital?"; "What progress have you made so far?"	Provides an opportunity for the client to state in their own words what is happening. This technique emphasizes how important the client is to the interaction. It may also provide the nurse with a direction to pursue further for more information.
Clarifying	"I'm having trouble understanding how your son has been a 'problem' lately. Give me an example of what you mean by 'problem.'"	The nurse may make the mistake of assuming they know exactly what the client means and may inaccurately minimize or exaggerate the impact of a client's choice of words or statement. Asking the client to restate, give an example or more detail will help the nurse gain a clear understanding of what the client says to gain an accurate clinical picture in order to plan for appropriate nursing care.
Empathy	"I can hear how angry you are."; "I can hear how painful the news of your mother's death was for you."	This technique recognizes and focuses on the client's feelings as well as conveying the nurse's concern for the client.

(continues)

Table 4-1	Therapeutic Communication Techniques *(continued)*	
Techniques	**Examples**	**Rationales**
Encouraging comparisons	"How is this hospitalization different from the last time?"; "How is your depressed mood different from the day you were admitted?"	This technique helps the client compare situations that may reoccur in their life.
Encouraging consideration of options or decisions	"How would going to outpatient therapy three times a week help you versus one time a week?"; "How would moving in with your daughter benefit you versus returning to live in your own home after discharge?"; "Of all the options you have been given, which one do you think would work the best for you?"	This technique assists the client to look at the pros and cons of treatment options and life situations and promotes decision making without the nurse telling the client what they should do.
Encouraging descriptions of perceptions	"What do you think is your main stressor at work?"; "What do you think is happening to you right now?"; "What do you think the voices are telling you right now?"	The technique helps the nurse determine how the client views a stressor, situation or relationship. It can also be used to obtain more information about the client's thought processes and content.

During the initial interview/assessment it is important to know what type of delusions, hallucinations or illusions the client is experiencing. This is followed with presenting/reinforcing reality. |
| Encouraging evaluation | "How important is it to you at this time to make a change in your lifestyle?"; "How important is this relationship to you?" | This technique clarifies the client's view of the meaning or importance of change or a life situation. |
| Encouraging the formulation of a plan | "What else can you do the next time you get angry or feel anxious?"; "What else do you need to do to find a more permanent place to live?" | This technique guides the client step-by-step through planning future actions. |

(continues)

Table 4-1   Therapeutic Communication Techniques *(continued)*

Techniques	Examples	Rationales
Exploring	"Tell me more about your suicide attempt."; "Please tell me more about your relationship with your boss."	This technique helps get the client involved in managing their own feelings or situation and can help increase a feeling of control for the client. It also encourages the client to take some responsibility for themselves.
Feedback	"I thought you were assertive when you told your husband how you felt about wanting to go back to college."; "You sounded angry when a peer in the morning community group accused you of stealing."; "You did a great job with the progressive relaxation exercise today."; "I think you need to practice more listening skills when interacting with your spouse. What do you think?"	It is important for a client to know when they are doing well and when they need more practice at certain skills or information. It is easier to correct a technique or misinterpretation while learning a new behavior/skill/information than after the behavior/skill/information has been learned. Also, the therapeutic milieu and therapeutic nurse–client relationship provide a safe, nonjudgmental environment for the client to practice new behaviors/skills and gain confidence.
Focusing	"Let's get back to what you were saying about your son's relationship with his father."; "I'd like to hear more about how you felt when you failed your college entrance exam."	This technique helps obtain more information especially when a client provides only superficial information. If, however, the client resists giving more information, the nurse does not continue to ask because it would be considered "probing." Probing is not therapeutic. The client may be more open to this technique after a trusting relationship has been established. There are also times when a client provides a good deal of information or moves from one topic to another. This technique can help the nurse concentrate on a more specific portion of information, word, or theme.

(continues)

Table 4-1   Therapeutic Communication Techniques *(continued)*

Techniques	Examples	Rationales
General leads	"I'm listening, go on."; "And then what happened?"; "Yes."	The use of emotionally neutral expressions is used to encourage the client to continue talking.
Giving recognition	"I see you've combed your hair today."; "I see you changed into clean clothes."; "That's a pretty dress you have on."; "You've been using journaling lately."	This technique shows the nurse is aware of the client's efforts and provides recognition of progress without sounding judgmental.
Identifying themes	Client: "I feel so far away from everyone as if I've way out in the ocean." Nurse: "You sound like you are feeling lonely." -or- Client: "I feel as if I'm down in a deep well and I can't get out." Nurse: "You sound very depressed."	This technique conveys the nurse's perception of the client's behavior or words and important issues the client is dealing with either consciously or unconsciously.
Interpreting	"You seem to get in trouble when you go out with your brother."	This technique conveys the nurse's perception of the client's behavior or words.
Making observations	"You look uncomfortable."; "You are pacing more often and look tense."	This technique verbalizes the nurse's observations. It encourages the client to be more aware of their own behavior and how others perceive their behavior. It also provides an opportunity for the client to express feelings and thoughts to the nurse.
Offering self	"I'll stay (sit) with you for awhile."	This technique shows the client that the nurse is available, concerned, and considers spending time with them to be important.
Placing an event in sequence or time	"When did your son leave?"; "How is this connected with the loss of your job?"; "Did this happen before or after you relocated?"	This technique helps both the client and nurse gain a sense of time, sequence and connection of events. The timing of events can be very important to the development

(continues)

Table 4-1	Therapeutic Communication Techniques *(continued)*	
Techniques	**Examples**	**Rationales**
		or worsening of the client's symptoms. For example, specific events may have preceded the client's depressed mood, suicidal thoughts, hearing of voices, or use of illegal substances.
Presenting/ Reinforcing reality	"I understand that you believe (I know you think) you see someone, but the only people I see are you and myself."; "I understand you believe (I know you think) you are hearing voices, but the only voices I hear are yours and mine."; "I see a shadow reflection on the floor because of the angle of the light in your room."; "I hear the voices from the television program other people are watching in the dayroom."	This technique acknowledges the client's perception without arguing, which could cause the client to become agitated, or being judgmental, which would erode the client's trust. The nurse defines reality by stating facts and by their presence.
Reflection or restatement	Client: "What do you think I should do about my son's drinking?" Nurse: "What do *you* think you should do?" -or- Client: "I can't stop thinking about how much fun my friends are having tonight going out and partying." Nurse: "You're worried you are missing all the fun and they don't miss you?" Client: Laughs, "Yeah, something like that. " -or- Client: "I can't go to that job interview. What if I don't get hired?"	The client's words, statements, questions, thoughts are repeated back so that the client knows that they have been understood. The client now has an opportunity to continue or clarify what they have said. This also allows the client to think about the validity of what they have said. This technique is useful when a client asks the nurse for advice.

(continues)

Table 4-1 Therapeutic Communication Techniques (continued)

Techniques	Examples	Rationales
	Nurse: "You are afraid to go to the job interview because you don't think you will get the job and will be a failure."	
Seeking validation	"Did I understand you correctly when you said you were sexually abused by both your father with your mother's boyfriend?"	The nurse attempts to obtain and clearly understand what the client's reports to ensure accurate information.
Silence	Avoiding speaking just to fill the void, maintaining eye contact, focusing attention on client, conveying concern with an empathetic facial expression.	Purposefully avoiding talking or asking questions allows the client time to think about what they are going to say and reflect on what they already have said or what questions you have asked them.
Suggesting collaboration	"Let's try to come up with a daily home schedule for you together."; "Let's see if working together we can come up with a better way to handle your anxiety."	The nurse offers to help the client and by working together decrease the client's feelings of not knowing where to start or of feeling overwhelmed.
Summarizing	"So far we have talked about the death of your son, your divorce, and how you felt abandoned by the rest of your family. All this has caused an increase in your depressed mood. Is there anything else I should know about?"	This technique is used to review main topics of information and any conclusions that have been made.
Supportive confrontation	"I know it is difficult for you to think about contacting your sister, but you need to at least give it a try."; "You are slipping back into old ways of dealing with stress. Try using one of the new relaxation techniques you learned yesterday."; "I know you don't like to go to group, but you do need to at least try going to at least one group this morning."	This technique pushes the client to act while acknowledging it is difficult.

(continues)

Table 4-1	Therapeutic Communication Techniques *(continued)*	
Techniques	**Examples**	**Rationales**
Verbalizing the implied	Client: "I'm wasting time cooped up here. Nobody is listening to me." Nurse: "Are you feeling like no one understands you or your situation?" Client: Silence. Nurse: "It must be very difficult for you losing your job and house so suddenly."	This technique puts into words what a client has indirectly said or implied. It helps make the client's meaning more explicit or clear and shows the nurse is listening and is empathetic.
Voicing doubt	"I know you believe that she is staring at you, but I think she is looking at the clock on the wall behind you."; "I know you think you are hearing voices, but do you think you are hearing the radio that your roommate is listening to?"; "Is there another explanation for what you think you are hearing?"; "Is there another interpretation of that person's behavior?"	This technique expresses uncertainty of the client's perceptions without arguing, which could cause the client to become agitated or being judgmental which would erode the client's trust. It also can stimulate the client to question the validity of their perceptions.

Sources: Keltner, Schwecke, & Bostrom, 2007, pp. 93–95; Fontaine, 2009, pp. 133–136; Townsend, 2009, pp. 132–137.

Table 4-2	Nontherapeutic Communication Techniques	
Techniques	**Examples**	**Rationales**
Belittling expressed feelings or minimizing problems	Client: "My mother always held me back." Nurse: "You shouldn't feel that way about your mother." -or- Client: "I wish I were dead. There's no reason for me to live."	The nurse comes across as lacking empathy and being uncaring due to misjudging how uncomfortable the client is. Telling a client how they should or should not feel is nontherapeutic. It is also nontherapeutic to tell a client they should "just snap out of it" or "keep look-

(continues)

Table 4-2	Nontherapeutic Communication Techniques *(continued)*	
Techniques	**Examples**	**Rationales**
	Nurse: "I feel that way sometimes. We all feel down at times." -or- "That was 2 years ago. It shouldn't bother you now."	ing up." These statements minimize the client's problems and degree of discomfort. A better technique would be "You must be very sad or upset. Tell me what you are feeling." Or "What is it about the situation that still bothers you?"
Challenging	"What in the world would make you want to go back there?"	This technique will cause a defensive reaction from the client or cause the client to agree with the nurse rather than express true feelings. It may also cause the client to stop talking to the nurse.
Changing the topic	Client: "I'm afraid something terrible is going to happen to my husband." Nurse: "Are you having any side-effects from your medication?"	This technique blocks communication and further discussion of the client's feelings. It also minimizes the client's fears.
Denying the problem	Client: "I'm worthless." Nurse: "You're not worthless. Everyone is worth something."	This technique blocks communication and denies that the client is experiencing a problem. A better technique would be "It sounds as if you're feeling that no one cares for you." Or "Tell me what you mean by 'worthless.'"
Disagreeing or arguing	"There's no reason for you to feel this way."; "You're not hearing voices."; "No, there aren't any spirits here."	This technique can be belittling, judgmental, or block communication. In other instances it can cause a client who is delusional or experiencing hallucinations to become agitated and potentially escalate into a physically dangerous situation.

(continues)

Table 4-2   Nontherapeutic Communication Techniques *(continued)*

Techniques	Examples	Rationales
Giving advice or imposing personal values	"I think you should divorce your husband (wife)."; "I think you should " send your child to a private school to get him away from kids who use drugs."; "I sure wouldn't put up with that kind of abuse." -or- Client: "I had planned to go on vacation, but my sister is coming to stay with me." Nurse: "You must be looking forward to seeing her.	Giving advice implies that the nurse knows what is best in the client's situation and implies that the client is not capable of making independent decisions. This encourages dependence rather than independence and goes against psychiatric-mental health nursing principles (see Chapter 1). Imposing personal values not only encourages dependence, but is judgmental. Making assumptions about how the client feels blocks communication and causes the client to agree rather than state how they really feel and risk disagreeing with the nurse who is perceived to be in a position of authority. A better technique would be to ask the client what they think they should do or how they feel about the situation.
Making stereotyped comments or using clichés	"Hang in there, things are bound to get better."; "Keep the faith."; "Keep a stiff upper lip."; "What doesn't kill you makes you stronger." -or- Nurse: "How are you feeling today?" Client: Silence. Nurse: "What's the matter? Cat's got your tongue?"	These expressions are meaningless, discourage expression of feelings or thoughts, and can be belittling. It is better to ask the client how they feel or what they are thinking. Also, if the nurse truly does not know what to say it is better to be honest and tell the client that you want to help them, but are not sure what to say at this time.

(continues)

Table 4-2   Nontherapeutic Communication Techniques *(continued)*

Techniques	Examples	Rationales
Probing	Continuing to ask for more information on a topic or pushing the client for answers to a question that is obviously emotionally painful for the client.	This technique can disrupt the trusting nurse–client relationship and is nontherapeutic. A better approach would be to wait until a later time when the client is more comfortable, has been in treatment for a longer period of time or willingly brings the topic up on their own.
Providing false reassurance or false hope	"I'm sure everything will be fine."; "I wouldn't be worried about that if I were you."	This technique presumes that the nurse can predict the future. No one knows exactly how a situation will turn out. The client may blame the nurse when the situation does not turn out as expected. It is better to provide emotional and spiritual support and encourage the client to discuss what facts they have in the situation. The nurse also could ask who they usually turn to for help when they have similar situations.
Requesting or insisting on an explanation	"Why did you say (do) that?"; "Why do you think that?"	Using the word "why" places the nurse in the role of interrogator, which is not therapeutic. A better technique is to ask "What reason did you have for saying that?" or "What do you think caused you to do that?" Also "What do you think makes you feel that way?" or "Please tell me more about your thoughts."

Sources: Varcarolis, Carson, & Shoemaker, 2006, pp. 186–193; Keltner, Schwecke, & Bostrom, 2007, pp. 93–95; Fontaine, 2009, pp. 133–136; Townsend, 2009, pp. 132–137.

BIOPSYCHOSOCIAL NURSING ASSESSMENT

The biopsychosocial nursing assessment consists of the admission diagnosis, biopsychosocial history, mental status examination, and the physical assessment. According to Jensen, Decker, and Anderson (2006), clients with chronic mental illness have higher morbidity and mortality rates than the general population even when suicide attempts are excluded (p. 617). Therefore, it is vitally important that a holistic, accurate nursing assessment be completed on each client.

Biopsychosocial History

The content of the psychosocial history begins with demographic information, such as the client's name/room number, age, gender, marital status, primary language, education level completed, racial/ethnic identification, admission status (i.e., voluntary or involuntary), and the chief complaint or the client's reason for seeking help in their own words. If the client is not seeking help voluntarily, the client's view or understanding of the reason they are being hospitalized is documented. If the client refuses to answer, is mute, or too confused to answer, this is also documented.

A history of the present illness (HPI) describes in chronological order the client's symptoms including onset, duration, frequency, any changes over time, possible precipitating events (i.e., negative or positive stressful events), any self-treatment the client has attempted, and anything that helps alleviate (ameliorate) the symptoms or makes them worse (aggravate).

Past psychiatric treatment, chemical dependency including use of nicotine and caffeine, medical history including allergies, and developmental history are also recorded. Information regarding the client's prenatal, infancy, childhood, and adolescent periods of development, as well as temperament, may shed light on the client's current problems especially if it is known that the client's mother had problems during pregnancy or delivery; if there were any physical or mental abnormalities; developmental delays; impulse control problems; learning difficulties; and any type of abuse (Boyd, 2008, pp. 156–157; O'Brien, Kennedy, & Ballard, 2008, p. 43).

It is also important to obtain a family history. In the past the family was blamed for causing a client's mental illness, but currently there is more evidence for biologic etiologies. That does not mean that the client is not affected by the environmental influence of their family and vice versa, but the family is viewed in a more positive light. Families may be able to provide the client much needed social and financial support, and there is recognition of the need for family education regarding mental illness. Due to the emphasis on biologic etiologies, there may be family members who are affected by mental illness. A genetic component has been identified, especially with disorders such as major depression, bipolar disorder, schizophrenia, and attention deficit disorder (O'Brien, Kennedy, & Ballard, 2008, p. 43).

The social, occupational, legal, and educational history provide valuable information regarding how the client currently, and in the past, functions in relationships with family, friends, and coworkers; their ability to maintain employment and obtain adequate housing; and what type of education strategies would be beneficial. The ethnic/cultural, spiritual, sexuality related, coping, and social support portions of the biopsychosocial history also provide important information. There are more detailed assessments for ethnicity, culture, and spirituality also available to expand upon the general information usually included in a biopsychosocial history. The client's ethnic background, cultural and spiritual beliefs and practices can be of help or hindrance to the client in seeking and accepting treatment. For example, the client may believe a higher power or external source in the universe is a source of strength or that they are being punished by said higher power. The client's culture may discourage them from seeking mental health treatment and/or prohibit certain types of treatment. The client may have specific dietary restrictions/requirements or prayer times/rituals that are consistent with their culture and spiritual beliefs that should be supported as much a possible within the unit safety requirements as long as they do not contribute to current symptoms. The type of coping skills (adaptive versus maladaptive) and amount of social support have a direct influence on the client's symptoms and also affect their prognosis. A suicide/homicide/domestic violence risk assessment should also be performed as part of the biopsychosocial history (Boyd, 2008, pp. 156–157; O'Brien, Kennedy, & Ballard, 2008, pp. 40–46).

Mental Status Examination

The mental status examination assesses several areas and provides valuable information related to the client's illness. These areas include general appearance, behavior, mood, affect, orientation, concentration, memory, speech pattern, thought processes, thought content, intellectual functioning, insight, judgment, abstract reasoning, impulse control, and motivation for treatment (Keltner, Schwecke, & Bostrom, 2007, p. 114; Boyd, 2008, 156–157; O'Brien, Kennedy, & Ballard, 2008, p. 46–49; Fontaine, 2009, p. 27; Mohr, 2009, pp. 171–176). The mental status examination is also performed separately from the full biopsychosocial nursing assessment as part of the ongoing assessment while the client is still receiving inpatient or outpatient treatment.

Physical Assessment

The physical assessment is the same basic assessment involved in a body systems review included in nursing curriculum physical assessment courses and, therefore, will not be repeated in this text. However, there are medical disorders that can produce symptoms similar to some psychiatric illnesses or exacerbate the psychiatric symptoms. These medical disorders will be mentioned with specific psychiatric illnesses in Unit IV. It is important to note any physical abnormalities, especially in the cardiovascular (e.g., arrhythmias, hypertension, hypotension); respiratory; neurologic (e.g., alertness, orientation, cranial nerve assessment, seizures, head trauma, abnormal muscle movements or reflexes, paresthesias, recent personality changes, olfactory hallucinations, recent onset disorientation/confusion, signs of possible brain tumor); endocrine (e.g., diabetes mellitus, hypothyroidism, hyperthyroidism); and integumentary (e.g., open areas, rashes or lacerations of skin, wounds, scars, bruising/bleeding, infestations, signs of abuse) portions of the physical assessment, as well as any type of pain or symptoms of withdrawal from chemical substances (Mohr, 2009, p. 170). These abnormalities should be reported to the appropriate attending psychiatrist and medical physician to determine if further follow-up is necessary. Any medical problems for which the client is already under a physician's care should also be documented, and the psychiatrist or medical physician notified. These are areas of nursing liability and cannot be ignored simply because the client is seeing help for a psychiatric-mental illness.

Also included in this area are results of any laboratory, x-ray, computed tomography (CT), magnetic resonance imaging (MRI), magnetic resonance spectroscopy (MRS), positron emission tomography (PET), or other diagnostic test results. Nutrition and hydration status, sleep pattern, activity/exercise pattern, elimination pattern, and ability for self-care are assessed for this portion of the nursing assessment (Boyd, 2008, p. 158–159). See **Table 4-3** for an example of a biopsychosocial assessment form.

ADDITIONAL SCREENING TOOLS

In addition to the biopsychosocial nursing assessment, there are several screening tools to augment the assessment. Some of these screening tools may be used without having to obtain special permission, while for others permission must be obtained from the authors.

- CAGE for Alcohol Abuse
- Clinical Institute Withdrawal Assessment for Alcoholism (CIWA-Ar)
- Michigan Alcoholism Screening Test (MAST)

Table 4-3 Biopsychosocial Nursing Assessment

I. **Name/Room #:** *(For educational purposes and to protect the client's confidentiality use room number only)* _____

Admission date: _____

Age: _____ Male/Female: _____ Marital status: _____

Height: _____ Weight: _____ Vital signs: TPR/BP/O2 sat _____

Prosthesis: _____

Ambulatory aids: _____

Sensory aids: _____

Primary language: _____

Education level completed: _____

Racial/Ethnic identification: _____

Health insurance: _____

Physical/mental disabilities: _____

Physical deformity: _____

Living Will/POA/Mental Health Living Will: _____

Admission status: _____

Safety check of personal belongings by: _____

Chief complaint: _____

II. **History of present illness:**

Symptoms: _____

Onset: _____

Duration/Frequency/Changes over time: _____

Precipitating event/situation: _____

Self-treatment including complementary/alternative treatment: _____

(continues)

Table 4-3   Biopsychosocial Nursing Assessment *(continued)*

Ameliorating/Aggravating factors: _____

Medical disorders/problems currently being treated for: _____

Allergies and specific type of reaction *(include medications, food, dyes, etc.)*: _____

III. **DSM-IV-TR admission diagnosis:**

Axis I: _____

Axis II: _____

Axis III: _____

Axis IV: _____

Axis V: _____

Prognosis: _____

Current psychiatric and medical disorder medications *(include OTC, herbal supplements, vitamins, etc.)*:

Name: _____   Dose/Frequency: _____   Route: _____   Last dose: _____

_____

_____

IV. **Mental status examination *(Circle appropriate description)*:**

1. General appearance *(compare to stated age, dressed appropriate to situation/weather, clean & neat versus dirty or slovenly appearance; smeared, sloppy makeup if female)*:

Age	Dress	Posture
Age appropriate	Appropriate	Normal
	Clothing matches	
Older	Mismatched clothing	Tense
	Untidy	
Younger	Dirty	Slumped

Comments: _____

2. Observed behaviors:

Attitude	Psychomotor	Eye contact
Cooperative Submissive	Agitated	Good Fair
Uncooperative Tearful	Restless/fidgeting	Poor Evasive
	Hyperactive	Darting Staring
Calm Hypervigilant		None
Bored Bizarre	Hypoactive	
Apathetic Hostile	Intoxicated	
Argumentative		

Comments: _____

3. Mood (*subjective*):

Angry   Sad   Depressed   Anxious   Tired

Happy   Euphoric   Labile   Even   Appropriate to situation   Other

Comments: _____

4. Affect (*objective*):

Flat   Blunted   Sad   Anxious   Angry

Happy   Labile   Appropriate to situation   Other

Comments (*include whether or not the observed affect is congruent with the client's reported mood and how it is different*):

_____

_____

(continues)

Table 4-3 Biopsychosocial Nursing Assessment *(continued)*

5. Cognition:

a. Orientation:

Yes	No
Self	Self
Person	Person
Place	Place
Time	Time
Situation	Situation

b. Attention/Concentration:

Yes	No	Alert
Yes	No	Lethargic
Yes	No	Able to complete a thought without wandering to another topic or stopping
Yes	No	Able to follow a set of directions correctly (e.g., Please pick up this glass of water with your left hand, take a drink, put the glass in your right hand, and put it back down)
Yes	No	Able to repeat five digits forward and backward

c. Memory:

Yes	No	Short-term/recent (e.g., 24-hour recall of events/diet; date came into the hospital; repeats four unrelated words after greater than 5 minutes)
Yes	No	Remote (e.g., recall past personal history/events anniversaries, birthdays, first job, high school attended)
Yes	No	Confabulation
Yes	No	Able to perform simple calculations (addition/subtraction) forward, backward

d. Abstract thinking:

Yes	No	Able to state the meaning of common proverbs such as "Don't cry over spilt milk.", "People who live in glass houses shouldn't throw stones." or "A stitch in time saves nine."

Yes   No   Able to identify common characteristics of objects such as an apple and an orange (fruit, round); a bicycle and a plane (transportation); or a table and a chair (furniture)

e. Intellectual functioning/intelligence:

Yes   No   Able to perform simple calculations (e.g., $2 \times 48 = 96$)

Yes   No   Able to state why the moon looks larger than the stars at night (closer objects look larger than farther away objects)

Yes   No   Able to name the current president and the president before that

Comments: _____

6. Speech pattern:

Form	Rate	Quality
Logical	Normal Slow	Appropriate Mute
Illogical	Fast/rapid	Pressured Loud
Rambling	Latency/delayed	Soft Monotone
Unintelligible/incoherent	Poverty of speech	Mumbling Slurred
Tangential		Stuttering Vocal tics
Circumstantial		

Comments: _____

7. Thought processes:

Appropriate Logical Linear Illogical Grandiose Derailment Loose Association Racing Echolalia Concrete Flight of Ideas Slowed Neologism Bizarre Clang Association Tangential Circumstantial Thought Blocking Word Salad Perseveration Other

Comments: _____

(continues)

Table 4-3   Biopsychosocial Nursing Assessment (continued)

8. Thought content:

Appropriate   Somatic   Complaints   Phobias   Minimizing   Panic   Derealization

Depersonalization   Dissociation   Unworthiness   Blaming   Negativism   Denial   Guilt   Worthlessness

Suicidal   Homicidal   Hopelessness   Helplessness   Powerlessness   Suspicious   Illusions

Delusional: Paranoid   Ideas of Reference   Thought broadcasting   Thought insertion/removal

Grandiose   Sexual   Religious   Magical thinking

Hallucinations: Auditory   Visual   Tactile   Gustatory   Olfactory

Are hallucinations or delusions congruent or incongruent with mood?   Yes   No

Obsessions   Compulsions   Rumination   Preoccupation   Other

Comments: _____

_____

9. Insight:

Yes	No	Aware of illness
Yes	No	Accepting of illness
Yes	No	Denies illness
Yes	No	Accepting of illness, but denies need for treatment

Comments: _____

_____

10. Judgment:

Yes	No	Future plans consistent with education/occupational background and resources
Yes	No	Able to appropriately decide what to do if someone reported a fire or if found a stamped ad-dressed envelope on the street
Yes	No	Accepts personal responsibility for own actions without blaming others

Comments: _____

11. Impulse control:

    Yes   No   Admits to problems with eating, sexual activities, spending, gambling, anger management, obsessions/compulsions, other

Comments: _____

12. Psychomotor function:

    Slow   Restless   Fidgeting   Akathesia   Pacing   Rigidity   Catatonic   Tremors   Choreatic

    Athetoid   Tics   Tardive Dyskinesia   Dystonia   Echopraxia   Avoidance of touching

    Stereotypical movements   Slow body movements   Pauses in verbal responses

    Decreased speech volume   Decreased speech amount or content

Comments: _____

13. Motivation/reasons for seeking treatment: _____

Comments: _____

V. **Suicide/homicide/domestic violence risk assessment:**

    Yes   No   History of suicide gestures/attempts

    If yes, describe: _____

    Yes   No   Suicidal ideations/homicidal (thoughts)

    If yes, describe: _____

(continues)

Table 4-3   Biopsychosocial Nursing Assessment (continued)

Plan

Yes   No

If yes, describe: _____

Lethality of plan: _____

Access to means to carry out plan

Yes   No

If yes, describe: _____

At least able to verbally contract to refrain from hurting self or others and notify staff when thinking of suicide

Yes   No

With whom? _____

Prevention action recommended: _____

What do you do when you become angry? _____

Have you ever pushed or hit anyone?

Yes   No

If yes, who? _____

Have you ever been arrested for assault/battery?

Yes   No

Has anyone you live with now, or in the past, ever pushed, hit, kicked, or harmed you in any way?

Yes   No

If yes, who? _____

Do you feel safe in your own home?

Yes   No

Comments: _____

VI. **Developmental stage and task (Erickson) according to biologic age:**

Trust vs Mistrust   Autonomy vs Shame & Doubt   Initiative vs Guilt

Identity vs Role Confusion   Generativity vs Stagnation   Integrity vs Despair

VII. **Psychiatric history/treatment** *(include inpatient & outpatient, dates; ECT):*

Yes   No   Are you aware of any problems during the prenatal, infancy, childhood, and adolescent periods of your physical/mental/psychosocial development? *(e.g., abnormalities, developmental delays, temperament, impulse control problems, learning difficulties, academic problems, social anxiety, difficulty making friends, any type of abuse, sexual promiscuity, use of alcohol/drugs, fighting, bullying, setting fires, stealing, cruelty to animals, etc.):*

If yes, please describe: _____

Yes   No   Are you aware of any problems your birth mother may have had during pregnancy or delivery?

If yes, please explain: _____

VIII. **Medical-surgical history/treatment** *(include inpatient & outpatient, dates):*

IX. **Current/Past chemical use/dependency:**

Age when started drinking: _____ Age when started using illegal drug/prescription pills/other substances: _____

Current or past IV use: circle   yes   or   no

Preferred type of alcohol, amount & frequency: _____

Preferred type of drugs, amount & frequency _____

Last date/time drank or used, what specifically, and amount: _____

Experience blackouts: circle   yes   or   no.

Withdrawal symptoms experienced including DTs, seizures: _____

(continues)

Table 4-3   Biopsychosocial Nursing Assessment (continued)

Longest period of abstinence (*days, months, years*): _____

Dates: _____

Factors that precipitate/trigger use: _____

Do you or have you ever attended AA or NA meetings? _____

Do you or have you ever had a sponsor? _____

X.   **Review of systems/physical & sensory function (*place a check mark under correct indication*):**

	WNL	Receiving Treatment	Untreated
Cardiovascular			
Respiratory			
Neurologic			
Endocrine			
Musculoskeletal			
Nutrition/weight			
Hydration			
Genitourinary			
Skin			
Activity/exercise			
Sleep/rest			
Sexuality			
Pain			
Fatigue/energy			
HEENT			
Self-care ability			

Are DTRs WNL?   Yes   or   No.   If no, who was this reported to? _____

Are cranial nerves II-XII grossly intact?   Yes   or   No.   If no, who was this reported to?

Comments *(if pain is present ask client to rate pain on a scale of 0= no pain to 10= extremely severe pain; describe sleep pattern if abnormal including usual # of hours, # of times awakens at night, difficulty falling asleep, middle of the night awakening, early morning awakening, methods used to help fall asleep)*:

For female clients: Yes   No.   Is there any chance you could be pregnant?

Results of physical examination: WNL   or   abnormal

Comments:

Are there any abnormal laboratory/diagnostic tests results? If yes, who were the results reported to? If a female client within child-bearing age, is the urine pregnancy test negative? If positive what physician was notified?

Attach abnormal laboratory/diagnostic tests results information to this form.

XI.   **Family psychiatric/chemical dependency/medical history & treatment:**

Is there a specific psychiatric medication or treatment that was helpful or caused an adverse reaction for your family member?

XII.   **Social/occupation/legal/education history:**

Yes   No   Problems in relationships including family members, friend, coworkers?

If yes, with who?

Who do you obtain support from or confide in during times of stress/crisis?

Describe social roles and ability or inability to fulfill these currently:

Yes   No   Current employed?

Yes   No   Problems obtaining or maintaining employment?

Yes   No   Adequate housing?

Yes   No   Current or past legal problems?

Yes   No   Do you have a pending court date?

If so, when and for what reason?

(continues)

Table 4-3 Biopsychosocial Nursing Assessment *(continued)*

Education background: _____

_____

Comments: _____

_____

XIII. Ethnic/cultural/spiritual/coping/support/history:

Yes _____ No _____ Do you follow any special ethnic/cultural rules or practices regarding your health?

If yes, describe: _____

Yes _____ No _____ Do you have a specific religious affiliation or spiritual practices?

If yes, describe: _____

Describe stressors identified: _____

Describe perception of stressors *(e.g., realistic, minimized, exaggerated)*: _____

Describe usual conscious coping strategies: _____

List client's strengths *(e.g., education, high motivation for treatment, good/fair insight, cooperativeness, resources, support system, etc.)*: _____

List factors that may hinder the client's progress in treatment *(e.g., poor insight/judgment, low motivation, uncooperativeness, limited resources, poor support system, physical problems, etc.)*: _____

Yes _____ No _____ Are you satisfied with your quality of life?

Comments: _____

_____

Impression of reliability of client as a historian: Good   Fair   Poor

Comments (include any interfering factors): _____

_____

XIV. Ego defense mechanisms

Compensation   Schizoid Fantasy   Projection   Repression   Undoing   Denial

Identification   Rationalization   Splitting   Displacement   Intellectualization

Reaction   Formation   Sublimation   Dissociation   Introjection   Regression   Suppression

Comments: _____

XV. Community resources and discharge planning

List current community resources used: _____

_____

Follow-up recommended *(include appointment and contact information)*: _____

Psychiatrist: _____

Medical Physician: _____

Psychotherapy with Psychologist/Social Worker/APRN: _____

Partial Hospitalization/Day Treatment/Intensive Outpatient Program/Community Mental Health Clinic: _____

Client Teaching Needs: _____

Housing Needs: _____

Transportation Needs: _____

Support Groups: _____

Family Teaching/Psychotherapy/Support Groups Needs: _____

Other Needs: _____

Sources: Jarvis, 2004, pp. 108–109; Sadock & Sadock, 2005, Vol. 1, pp. 805–812; Boyd, 2008, pp. 157–158; Townsend, 2009, pp. 142–147.

- Holmes and Rahe Social Readjustment Scale
- The Hassles and Uplifts Scale
- Life Experiences Survey (LES)
- WHO Quality of Life Instrument
- Hamilton Depression Scale (HDS)
- Beck Depression Inventory (BDI)
- Zung Self Rating Depression Scale
- Geriatric Depression Scale
- Edinburgh Postnatal Depression Scale
- SAD PERSONS Scale
- Mood Disorder Questionnaire (MDQ)
- Young Mania Rating Scale (YMRS)
- MiniMental State Examination (MMSE) or Folstein—for dementia
- Brief Psychiatric Rating Scale
- Wong-Baker FACES Pain Rating Scale
- Index of Independence in Activities of Daily Living
- Instrumental Activities of Daily Living
- Functional Activities Questionnaire

A separate cultural assessment, including spirituality, may be used to identify and explore further cultural issues (Keltner, Schwecke, & Bostrom, 2007, p. 171). After conducting the client interview, the nurse will use critical thinking to analyze the information obtained and formulate a nursing care map and plans individualized to meet identified client needs. The nurse will evaluate the effectiveness of interventions and progress made towards planned outcomes and revise as needed. A short admission note should be documented in the client's medical record and copies of a living will, medical power of attorney (POA), and mental health living will should also be placed on the record as soon as the family provides these.

CHILDREN AND ADOLESCENTS

Children and adolescents are usually accompanied by at least one parent. A parent or guardian will be responsible for signing voluntary admission paperwork (agreeing to the admission) unless the adolescent is an emancipated minor. There are also some states where laws allow teenagers younger than age 18 to sign themselves into the hospital voluntarily for psychiatric treatment (e.g., age 14 in Pennsylvania), although a parent or guardian is still responsible for the payment of any treatment the adolescent receives. Also, permission must be obtained from a parent or guardian to begin psychiatric medications. The same criteria for involuntary admissions of adults applies to children and adolescents. Arrangements for school work may need to be made while maintaining confidentiality. Certified teachers or tutors may be available as part of the facility's treatment program to help prevent the child or adolescent from falling behind academically. Arrangements may also be made by the child or adolescent's parents to collect homework from their school.

When assessing children and adolescents, the nurse usually meets with the child/adolescent along with the parents or guardian and then separately (Boyd, 2008, p. 597). This provides opportunities for the nurse to get to know the child/adolescent better, for the child/adolescent to say or ask something they may not feel comfortable with in front of the parents or guardian, and for the parents or guardian to say or ask something they would not feel comfortable with in front of the child/adolescent. A separate assessment time also is valuable when there is suspected abuse. In a case of suspected abuse, the nurse would notify their immediate supervisor and the psychiatrist as well as referring to the individual facility and state reporting guidelines (see Chapter 15 for more details regarding domestic violence and abuse). It is normal for a child/adolescent to initially be wary of the nurse or staff member, but soon this reaction should pass and the client should begin to be more comfortable. The nurse may reassure the client that if they want to they can come back and check on the parents or guardian. Play therapy using dolls, puppets, or action figures is extremely helpful in assessing and interacting with younger children (Sadock & Sadock, 2005, pp. 3051–3052). Assessing how children treat their toys may provide a clue to aggressiveness that is not verbally expressed. It also is normal for adolescents to act indifferent, suspicious, or angry when asked to meet with the nurse separately. Adolescents may be afraid that their symptoms are abnormal or that they will be blamed for their problems (Boyd, 2008, p. 597). Encouraging the use of drawing or art supplies to express feelings is also helpful in assessment and later on in intervention. Asking about hobbies and favorite music or movies can help show the adolescent that the nurse is interested in them as a person. Being genuine and respectful with children/adolescents is the best approach to building rapport and trust. Children/adolescents are able to quickly identify when an adult is not genuinely interested in them. Establishing rapport with the parents or guardian also helps establish rapport with their children/adolescents. It is also important to observe how the child/adolescent and parents or guardian interact, for evidence of attachment, communication patterns, and openness in the relationship. Do the parents or guardian provide all of the assessment information or do they encourage the child/adolescent to speak freely about how they feel and what they think is happening?

During the assessment the nurse should use language that is age appropriate and focus on common terms. The younger the child, the more concrete (i.e., literal, simple) the language and thinking processes will be. For example, if a child is being assessed for symptoms of depression, a more common word such as a "sad" should be used when asking about how they feel. Encouraging free-hand drawing of feelings and thoughts is useful when language skills are limited. "By age 3 years, children should be able to draw some facial features and limbs, but their drawings have an "x-ray" quality, in which clothing is transparent and the body can be seen underneath" (Boyd, 2008, p. 609). Drawings also can be used to determine self-concept and relationships. Drawings are processed (discussed) with the child as to their meaning. The nurse should openly acknowledge any signs of fear, anger, discomfort, or any other emotions that they are observing, invite further discussion while clarifying any misinformation, and reassure that the nurse truly wants to help.

The biopsychosocial nursing assessment for children/adolescents will be similar to the one for adults, but will include information from the pediatrician or primary care provider (PCP), including immunization record, a physical developmental history such as the Denver II-Revision and Restandardization of the Denver Developmental Screening Test (DDST), and childhood illnesses. The DDST screening tool (Jarvis, 2004, p. 33–34) is used for infants and preschool-age children who may exhibit developmental lags that could be symptoms of neurologic problems. A physical developmental history is important when assessing children/adolescents, as well as noting any problems their birth mother experienced during pregnancy or during labor and delivery. Anything that would affect oxygen supply, nutrition, or the physical safety of the fetus (e.g., trauma, accidents) during the prenatal and perinatal periods could affect brain development and have an impact on psychiatric-mental health symptoms. Children may exhibit temporary developmental regression (e.g., thumb sucking, wetting the bed, clinging behaviors) when under enough stress. Additionally, information from the school including IQ scores, grades, relationships with peers and teachers, and behavior will need to be obtained. Permission will need to be obtained from the parents or guardian for information from all of these additional sources. Examples of other screening tools used when assessing children and adolescents are provided in the following list. Specific permission from the author/developer may need to be obtained to use these screening tools.

- Behavior Assessment System for Children (BASC) for ages 4 to 18 years
- Child Behavior Checklist (CBDL) for ages 4 to 16 years
- Children's Yale-Brown Obsessive Compulsive Scale for ages 6 to 17 years
- Diagnostic Interview Schedule for Children (DISC)
- Pediatric Anxiety Rating Scale (PARS) for ages 6 to 17 years
- Schedule for Affective Disorders and Schizophrenia for Children (K-SADS)

- Minnesota Multiphasic Personality Inventory-Adolescent (MMPI-A)
- Milton Adolescent Personality Inventory (MAPI)
- Milton Adolescent Clinical Inventory (MACI)

In addition to performing a child/adolescent assessment, the PMH nurse would include the following areas in their collection of information:

- School
- Friends/peer relationships and social interaction
- Home
- Attachment to parents/caregivers and parental/caregiver reactions
- Temperament
- Self-concept
- Interests/Hobbies
- Fears and worries
- Losses including deaths, divorces, loss of pets, relocations
- Changes in socioeconomic status
- Positive changes including birth of siblings
- Somatic symptoms
- Memories and fantasy
- Sexual activity
- Use of alcohol, tobacco, illegal drugs, prescription medications prescribed for others
- Spiritual concepts
- Physical, sexual, emotional abuse
- Stereotypical, repetitive motor movement
- Ritualistic behaviors
- Poor impulse control

THE ELDERLY

There are a few additional things to consider when assessing elderly clients. These clients frequently have more medical illnesses, report somatic symptoms rather than psychiatric-mental health symptoms, and may need additional time to respond due to longer time to recall/retrieve information and sensory deficits. Any conditions that can affect oxygenation, cardiac functioning, electrolyte balance, or endocrine and metabolic/renal processes will affect the mental status of elderly clients. Elderly clients may appear to have symptoms of dementia, a condition referred to as "pseudodementia," when they are actually suffering from depression. The nurse should choose a quiet, private, comfortable place away from noises, and with adequate lighting. Offer the use of a bathroom before beginning the interview. The client may use sensory aides such as eye glasses or hearing aids that will be needed at this time. If the client does not currently have these with them, it may be necessary to repeat portions of the assessment later when they are available. Although it is important for the nurse to empty their mouth of gum, mints, or candy before beginning an assessment with any client, it is especially important when working with elderly clients who may have difficulty hearing and need to lip read. Speaking slowly and clearly while looking directly at these clients is helpful. Also, it is very important to avoid "Elderspeak" (APA, 2007, p. 319) or patronizing elderly clients by oversimplifying your speech, talking down to them or sounding as if you perceive them as unintelligent. Losses of hearing or eyesight do not diminish intelligence. On the other hand, the nurse must take into consideration a client's education level and culture when choosing words, phrasing questions, and providing information to obtain as accurate a clinical picture as possible.

Again, being genuine, respectful, open, truly listening, and providing time for them to tell their story will help build rapport and trust with elderly clients. Asking about self-care and health promotion behavior (e.g., use of seat belts, not smoking, avoiding alcohol/alcohol in moderation; annual physical examinations, gynecological exams for females, PSA testing for males) will provide an idea of self-esteem and opportunities for teaching. Many elderly clients have poor nutrition and may be dehydrated, which can lead to symptoms that may initially look like decreased mental function and fatigue, but which improve when normal nutrition and hydration needs are met. Dehydration can lead to electrolyte imbalances and interfere with normal neurologic and cardiac functioning, leading to abnormal behavior in some clients. Also, many elderly clients are prescribed several medications that at any time can interact or become toxic due to normal aging processes, resulting in decreased ability to metabolize and eliminate medications. Delirium can occur as a result of medications or an infectious process.

If an elderly client is accompanied by a spouse, adult children, or a caregiver, the nurse will also meet separately with the client and those who have accompanied the client. The client may not report information in front of someone else because they do not want to cause someone they care about additional concern. Unfortunately there may also be a case of suspected abuse, and the client may be afraid to report this in the presence of the abuser or anyone else. In such cases the nurse would report information to the physician and immediate supervisor, and follow the facility/agency reporting policies. Also, the people accompanying the client may have information or questions they feel more comfortable bringing up while the client is not present. A spouse or adult child may feel guilty for not bringing the client for evaluation sooner due to denial of the problem or not knowing the signs and symptoms of mental illness. They will need emotional support from the nurse at this time and information on support groups.

REFERENCES

American Psychological Association (2007). *APA dictionary of psychology*. Washington, DC: Author.

Arnold, E. C., & Boggs, K. U. (2007). *Interpersonal relationships: Professional communication skills for nurses* (5th ed.). St. Louis, MO: Saunders, Elsevier.

Boyd, M. A. (2008). *Psychiatric nursing: Contemporary practice* (4th ed.). Philadelphia, PA: Wolters/Kluwer/Lippincott, Williams, & Wilkins.

Fontaine, K. L. (2009). *Mental health nursing* (6th ed.). Upper Saddle River, NJ: Pearson Education Inc.

Jarvis, C. (2004). *Physical examination & health assessment* (4th ed.). St. Louis, MO: Elsevier, Saunders.

Jensen, L. W., Decker, L., & Andersen, M. M. (2006). Depression and health-promoting lifestyles of persons with chronic mental illness. *Issues in Mental Health Nursing, 27*, 617–634.

Keltner, N. L., Schwecke, L. H., & Bostrom, C. E. (2007). *Psychiatric nursing* (5th ed.). St. Louis, MO: Mosby, Elsevier.

Mohr, W. K. (2009). *Psychiatric-mental health nursing: Evidence based concepts, skills, and practices* (7th ed.). Philadelphia, PA: Wolters Kluwer/Lippincott, Williams, & Wilkins.

O'Brien, P. G., Kennedy, W. Z., & Ballard, K. A. (2008). *Psychiatric mental health nursing: An introduction to theory and practice*. Sudbury, MA: Jones and Bartlett.

Sadock, B. J., & Sadock, V. A. (2005) *Kaplan & Sadock's comprehensive textbook of psychiatry* (8th ed.). Philadelphia, PA: Lippincott, Williams, & Wilkins.

Townsend, M. C. (2009). *Essentials of psychiatric mental health nursing: Concepts of care in evidence based practice* (6th ed.). Philadelphia, PA: F. A. Davis Company.

Varcarolis, E. M., Carson, V. B., & Shoemaker, N. C. (2006). *Foundations of psychiatric mental health nursing: A clinical approach* (6th ed.). St. Louis, MO: Saunders, Elsevier.

SUGGESTED READINGS

American Psychiatric Association (2000). *Diagnostic and statistical manual of mental disorders* (4th ed., text revision). Washington, DC: Author.

Kaplan, B. J., & Sadock, V. A. (2003). *Kaplan & Sadock's synopsis of psychiatry: Behavioral sciences/ clinical psychiatry* (9th ed.). Philadelphia, PA: Lippincott, Williams, & Wilkins.

Lego, S. (1984). *The American handbook of psychiatric nursing*. Philadelphia, PA: Lippincott.

Pagana, K. D., & Pagana, T. J. (2007). *Mosby's diagnostic and laboratory test reference* (8th ed.). St. Louis, MO: Mosby, Elsevier.

Sheldon, L. K. (2009). *Communication for nurses* (2nd ed.). Sudbury, MA: Jones and Bartlett.

Stuart, G. W. & Laraia, M. T. (2005). *Principles and practice of psychiatric nursing* (8th ed.). St. Louis, MO: Mosby, Elsevier.

Varcarolis, E. M. (2006). *Manual of psychiatric nursing care plans* (3rd ed.). St. Louis, MO: Saunders, Elsevier.

Williams, C. L. (2008). *Therapeutic interaction in nursing* (2nd ed.). Sudbury, MA: Jones and Bartlett.

CHAPTER 5

Developing and Maintaining Therapeutic Relationships

Kim A. Jakopac

OBJECTIVES

The nursing student will be able to:

1. Identify key elements of therapeutic relationships
2. List potential obstacles to forming therapeutic relationships
3. Discuss the importance of maintaining professional boundaries when forming and continuing in therapeutic relationships
4. Describe the stages of therapeutic nurse–client relationships
5. Identify the goals of therapeutic nurse–client relationships
6. Recognize resistance behaviors and potential ways of dealing with them

KEY TERMS

Boundaries	Orientation stage	Therapeutic alliance
Collaboration	Rapport	Therapeutic encounter
Countertransference	Resistance behaviors	Therapeutic relationship
Empathy	Resolution stage	Transference
External locus of control	Self-awareness	Trust
Feedback	Self-disclosure	Unconditional positive regard
Genuineness	Social relationship	Values clarification
Internal locus of control	Termination stage	Working stage

The *therapeutic nurse–client relationship* is defined as an interaction between the nurse and client in which both participants contribute to promote a climate of healing and personal growth, and prevent further illness for the client. The relationship exists for and focuses on the needs of the client. It is the foundation on which psychiatric-mental health nursing is based (Varcarolis, Carson, & Shoemaker, 2006, p. 155; Townsend, 2009, p. 115).

Analysis of randomized clinical trials data from the National Institute of Mental Health Treatment of Depression Collaboration Research Program has demonstrated the development of a positive therapeutic alliance to be one of the best predictors for therapy outcomes for depression (Varcarolis, Carson, & Shoemaker, 2006, p. 155). Establishing a therapeutic nurse–client relationship is important in all nursing situations, but interpersonal interaction is the core of psychiatric-mental health nursing. The success of nursing interventions, improved medication adherence, and problem solving is based upon quality therapeutic nurse–client relationships (Dziopa & Ahern, 2009, p. 14).

A therapeutic relationship is very different from a social relationship. A social relationship exists for the benefit of everyone involved. The goals of a social relationship include increasing friendship, providing enjoyment, meeting dependency needs, and asking and receiving personal advice. A social relationship is also described as subjective in nature (Varcarolis, Carson, & Shoemaker, 2006, p. 156; Keltner, Schwecke, & Bostrom, 2007, p. 97). In a therapeutic relationship, the nurse uses themself therapeutically (see Chapter 2; Kwiatek, McKenzie & Loads, 2005, p. 27–31), employs therapeutic communication, and calls on personal strengths for the purpose of enhancing the client's personal growth and to further understand human behavior. A therapeutic relationship also is consistently focused on the client's needs, is objective, and is a helping relationship guided by a code of ethics used to care for human needs (Varcarolis, Carson, & Shoemaker, 2006, p. 156; Gamez, 2009, p. 126). The therapeutic nurse–client relationship embodies the psychiatric-mental health nursing principle that clients have the right to participate in goal setting and treatment decisions to the extent they are capable. The client is viewed as a partner in their own healing process (Dziopa & Ahern, 2009, pp. 16–17; Fontaine, 2009, p. 22). The therapeutic nurse–client relationship is strengthened with each therapeutic encounter whether the encounter is for only a brief amount of time or a longer time period.

There are four components to the therapeutic nurse–client relationship: physical, psychosocial, spiritual, and power. The physical component is made up of all the medical technical skills and procedures performed by the nurse (e.g., taking a blood pressure or changing a dressing). The psychosocial component includes the nurse's response to the client as one human being to another and the qualities the nurse brings to the relationship. These qualities include acceptance, positive regard, empathy, a nonjudgmental attitude, genuineness, and congruity of communication (see also Chapter 2). The nurse uses the psychosocial component when encouraging the client to express their thoughts and feelings about their perceptions, experiences, and expectations. The spiritual component is described as the feeling of connection between the nurse and the client and as the nurse being a part of something more than just themselves as well as the caring relationship piece. When conducting a spiritual assessment the nurse needs to include what traditions shape the client's spiritual life. The power component relates to the nurse and the client's belief in external or internal causes or loci for chances of success or failure (Fontaine, 2009, pp. 23–24).

ELEMENTS OF THERAPEUTIC NURSE–CLIENT RELATIONSHIP

There are important key elements in establishing and maintaining a therapeutic nurse–client relationship. These key elements include:

- Self-awareness
- Values clarification
- Genuineness
- Unconditional positive regard
- Therapeutic use of self
- Empathy
- Rapport
- Collaboration
- Trust
- Warmth
- Consistency
- Therapeutic listening skills
- Therapeutic communication
- Boundaries

Self-Awareness

Self-awareness is an integral part of psychiatric-mental health nursing. The nurse must examine their own feelings, biases, attitudes, emotions, thoughts, and actions (Stuart & Laraia, 2005, p. 17). Included in self-awareness is the concept of emotional intelligence. Emotional intelligence is defined as "the ability to notice, understand, and regulate one's emotions." (Williams, 2008, p. 3). The nurse must be aware of how their emotions affect others and avoid impulsive expression of strong emotions when interacting with the client. Emotions in one person can have a strong influence or psychological impact on another person in either positive or negative ways (Williams, 2008, p. 4).

Values Clarification

In order to develop good self-awareness, the nurse must be clear about their own set of values. An individual's values are established early in life from their family, friends, culture, education, work, and life experiences (Stuart & Laraia, 2005, p. 18; Townsend, 2009, p. 116). Values clarification is a process through which the nurse can discover their own values by exploring, assessing, questioning, and choosing what their values are and how these values will influence their attitudes, emotions, and actions. A value system provides a framework by which decisions are made. Many times the nurse and client's value systems are not in agreement and may clash. By clarifying values and suspending value judgments, the nurse can more easily avoid projecting or imposing their value system onto a client. If the nurse is unaware of certain values they may appear to be uncaring and viewed negatively by the client, which will make it more difficult to establish a therapeutic nurse–client relationship.

Genuineness

Genuineness may be described as being open, honest, oneself, or authentic in interactions with the client. Many clients can tell or feel when the nurse is not being genuine, which can prevent a therapeutic nurse–client relationship from starting or continuing to develop. Genuineness is needed for building rapport and trust with a client. Some ways to demonstrate genuineness include acknowledging how difficult the client's problems are for them and their efforts to change. Showing interest in the client's day-to-day progress, hobbies, or family members helps convey the nurse's genuine interest in the client as a person (Fontaine, 2009, p. 124; Sheldon, 2009, p. 54–55; Townsend, 2009, p. 120).

Unconditional Positive Regard

The concept of unconditional positive regard includes giving respect, remaining nonjudgmental, and believing in the worth and dignity of another individual. Unconditional positive regard makes it possible for the nurse to accept the client exactly as they are, even though they may have conflicting values, opinions, or lifestyles. What is truly important is that the client is a worthwhile human being. Many psychiatric-mental health clients have problems with self-worth, self-esteem, self-concept, feel rejected due to stigma, and lack self-respect. That is why it is so important for the nurse to convey unconditional positive regard. This can be demonstrated by calling the client by their name; allowing enough time to spend with the client; answering questions and talking about concerns; providing as much privacy as possible within the unit safety requirements; being open and honest with sometimes difficult topics; trying to understand the motivation behind the client's behavior; and taking into consideration the client's wishes when planning nursing care (Townsend, 2009, pp. 119–120).

Therapeutic Use of Self

The therapeutic use of self is vitally important in all interactions with a client including the initiation and continuing development of the therapeutic nurse–client relationship (see Chapter 2 for more details).

Empathy

Empathy encompasses the ability to feel in ourselves or recognize the feelings experienced by someone else as if they are our own. Empathy includes the ability to objectively understand someone else's point of view or communicate an intention to understand another person. Empathy is different from sympathy which is subjective and is a combination of kindness and compassion (Boyd, 2008, p. 143; Fontaine, 2009, p. 124; Sheldon, 2009, p. 56–57; Townsend, 2009, p. 120). Compassion involves the desire to relieve another person's suffering, and empathy is used in conjunction with compassion when providing nursing care. Sympathy may have the effect of impairing the nurse's judgment (Sheldon, 2009, p. 57). The nurse incorporates empathy to increase their understanding of the client and when collaborating with the client to set goals (Fontaine, 2009, p. 124).

Rapport

Rapport is a relaxed, warm relationship of mutual acceptance, understanding, respect, and harmony between people. Establishing a rapport with a client is essential to building trust and a therapeutic nurse–client relationship. Establishing a rapport also helps decrease the social isolation and loneliness many psychiatric-mental health clients experience (Boyd, 2008, p. 143).

Collaboration

Collaboration is an interpersonal process, act or relationship where two or more people work together showing cooperation and sensitivity to each other's needs. In psychiatric-mental health nursing the nurse and client work together when exploring the client's problems and needs; set goals, plan outcomes and ways to meet those goals; and evaluate the effectiveness of interventions as well as progress made towards meeting mutually established goals (Stuart & Laraia, 2005, p. 860; APA, 2007, p. 193).

Trust

Trust is a key building block in the initiation and development of a therapeutic nurse–client relationship. Trust may be defined as confidence in the worth, value, or truth of someone or something else. It is an important component of all types of relationships (APA, 2007, p. 960). Establishing a rapport and being genuine, consistent, and empathetic help build trust. Trust is both strong and fragile. If there is a strong bond of trust between the nurse and client, the nurse can use trust to help persuade the client to engage in treatment and behavior for their benefit even when they initially are not receptive to it. Trust is also fragile because once broken it may be very difficult to reestablish. A client who experiences paranoia will have great difficulty trusting others, and it will take longer for the nurse to build rapport and trust with this client.

Warmth

Warmth does not mean that the nurse is on intimate terms with the client, but is a nonverbal manner in which the nurse expresses interest in or concern for the client (Fontaine, 2009, p. 124). Warmth is conveyed by assuming a positive attitude, smiling, leaning forward, and listening actively.

Consistency

The concept of consistency includes sameness, maintaining a routine, being honest, following through with promises, responding in a predictable manner, reinforcing rules uniformly, and assigning the same nurse and other mental healthcare staff to the same clients (Varcarolis, Carson, & Shoemaker, 2006, p. 168). Many clients have problems with consistency in their lives. Consistency is vitally important to maintaining rapport and trust. There are situations that challenge the nurse's ability to maintain consistency depending on the needs of other clients on a unit, but the nurse preserves consistency to the best of their ability. If the nurse cannot meet the client at a prearranged time or fulfill a promise made, every effort must be made to explain the reasons why. This is important to maintain consistency as well as trust between the client and nurse.

Therapeutic Listening Skills

Therapeutic listening skills are invaluable when establishing a therapeutic nurse–client relationship.

Therapeutic Communication

Therapeutic communication is fundamental for any interaction with a client and especially in forming a therapeutic nurse–client relationship.

Boundaries

In psychiatric-mental health nursing, boundaries are psychological limits that protect the client and the nurse. Boundaries set realistic limits on behavior, communication, and interaction (APA, 2007, p. 131) so that the client knows what behavior to expect from the nurse and what behavior is expected of them. Boundaries are also used to mark territory that can include physical boundaries as in personal space; legal–ethical boundaries as in maintaining confidentiality and refraining from keeping secrets from other treatment team members; professional boundaries such as refraining from accepting personal gifts from a client or becoming overly emotionally involved with a client, using touch very judiciously *only with* a client's permission or refraining from engaging in inappropriate social or romantic/sexual behavior with a client, or self-disclosure. Self-disclosure or providing personal information or intimate details about oneself or one's life is generally discouraged because the focus of any interaction should be on the client rather than the nurse. Self-disclosure is also usually discouraged for the protection of both the nurse and client. It is easy to give more information than originally intended. Some authors agree that in rare instances it may be used, but should *always* be for the benefit of the client rather than for meeting the nurse's needs (Townsend, 2009, p. 123). Listening to feedback from other nurses and members of the treatment team helps the nurse maintain healthy boundaries, as does setting clear boundaries in the beginning of the therapeutic nurse–client relationship by clearly stating the nurse's role, expectations for both the nurse and client, and what is *not* included as part of the relationship. Also, being culturally aware and self-aware will help set healthy boundaries (Sheldon, 2009, p. 64).

STAGES OF THE THERAPEUTIC NURSE–CLIENT RELATIONSHIP

Interpersonal relationships are used by the psychiatric-mental health (PMH) nurse as the primary interventions with clients in any setting. Peplau's nursing theoretical framework is based in the interpersonal theory of Sullivan. A therapeutic interpersonal relationship or therapeutic nurse–client relationship is the vehicle for implementing the nursing process According to Peplau, the therapeutic nurse–client relationship is composed of distinct stages, with each stage having specific tasks and goals to be accomplished. However, realistically there may be some overlapping of tasks, especially when time is limited (Townsend, 2009, p. 121). These stages also apply to the client interview and leadership of psychoeducation groups.

Orientation Stage

The orientation stage is where the initial encounter occurs between the client and the PMH nurse. This is the initial stage of Peplau's therapeutic nurse–client relationship. Another name for this stage is the "introductory" stage. In some psychiatric-mental health nursing textbooks this stage is preceded by a "pre-interaction" or "pre-orientation" stage when information about the client is obtained from the medical record, other members of the healthcare team, or significant others. However, most PMH nursing textbooks include this step as part of the orientation stage. The orientation stage begins when the nurse has gathered information about the client, introduces themselves to the client, establishes the purpose of the meeting, and respectfully acknowledges the client by their preferred name (Sheldon, 2009, p. 52):

> Nurse: "Hello, my name is Lisa. I am an RN and will be working with you today. By what name do you prefer to be called?"
> Client: "Hi. Janice would be fine."

According to Townsend (2009), the goals for the orientation phase are to explore the client's perceptions of themselves, establish trust, and formulate a contract for intervention (p. 121). Tasks for the orientation stage include:

- Obtaining information from the medical record, other members of the healthcare team or significant other

- Meeting the client
- Clarifying the purpose for meeting
- Informing the client of the nurse's role
- Establishing the client's preferred name to be addressed by
- Creating a setting that is comfortable and conducive to establishing a rapport and trust with the client
- Establishing rapport
- Gathering initial assessment data
- Identifying the client's strengths and limitations
- Mutually identifying problems to address
- Formulating nursing diagnoses
- Setting mutual realistic goals
- Planning reasonable outcomes and interventions to meet set goals
- Establishing a contract (may be verbal) that includes responsibilities and expectations of both the client and the nurse as well as a time frame for the duration of care
- Reviewing client's rights and reinforcing confidentiality
- Discussing and exploring feelings and concerns of both the client and the nurse regarding what has happened so far and for the near future in this healthcare setting

(Stuart & Laraia, 2005, p. 22; Keltner, Schwecke, & Bostrom, 2007, p. 99–101; Boyd, 2008, p. 149; Williams, 2008, p. 36; Fontaine, 2009, p. 22; Sheldon, 2009, p. 60–62; Townsend, 2009, p. 121)

Working Stage

The second stage of Peplau's therapeutic nurse–client relationship is referred to as the working stage. In this stage therapeutic "work" towards the goals set in the orientation stage begins and progresses. The goal for this stage is promoting healthy personal change for the client (Townsend, 2009, p. 121). Tasks for the working stage include:

- Maintaining rapport and trust
- Promoting the client's perception of reality and insight
- Promoting the client's independence
- Continuing to gather data
- Exploring relevant stressors
- Promoting the client's self-esteem and problem-solving skills

- Providing education
- Overcoming the client's resistance behaviors that may occur in response to anxiety when dealing with psychologically painful issues and clinging to previous defenses
- Promoting practice of alternative coping, adapting behaviors
- Facilitating change in behaviors
- Evaluating effectiveness of interventions and progress made toward goals

(Stuart & Laraia, 2005, pp. 22, 24; Keltner, Schwecke, & Bostrom, 2007, pp. 101–104; Boyd, 2008, p. 150; Williams, 2008, p. 36; Fontaine, 2009, pp. 22–23; Sheldon, 2009, p. 62; Townsend, 2009, pp. 121–122)

Termination Stage

The termination stage is the third or last of Peplau's therapeutic nurse–client relationship, depending upon the author. This stage may also be combined with the resolution stage in some psychiatric-mental health nursing textbooks. The time frame of the duration of care was established during the orientation stage. A high level of trust and learning has been attained by this stage of the therapeutic nurse–client relationship, and memories of time together are shared. Any progress the client has made, no matter how great or small, is summarized and reviewed. It is normal for the client to experience and express feelings of sadness and loss due to the ending of the time spent with the nurse and loss of this relationship (Stuart & Laraia, 2005, p. 23). It is also normal for the nurse to experience feelings of sadness and loss when someone they care about leaves (Varcarolis, Carson, & Shoemaker, 2006, p. 167). It is important to be empathetic and emphasize that the client will have support from their outpatient treatment team. The goals for this stage are evaluating to see if the goals set in the orientation stage were met and ensuring that there is a therapeutic closure or ending to the client and nurse's time together (Townsend, 2009, p. 121). Tasks for the termination stage include:

- Review of symptom relief and progress made
- Identifying attainment of goals
- Recognizing accomplishments such as improved social functioning, greater independence, and development of healthy, adaptive behaviors
- Acknowledging problems that may need to be resolved after discharge with future outpatient therapy and care
- Establishing the reality of separation and end of your time together
- Exploring feelings of loss, separation, rejection, anxiety, or anger

- Avoiding addressing new problems the client unexpectedly presents or resurrection of old problems as a way of extending your time together
- Thanking the client for the opportunity of working together
- Reinforcing that there will be support available from the client's outpatient treatment team

(Stuart & Laraia, 2005, pp. 23–24; Keltner, Schwecke, & Bostrom, 2007, pp. 104–105; Boyd, 2008, pp. 150–151; Williams, 2008, p. 36; Fontaine, 2009, p. 23; Sheldon, 2009, pp. 62–63; Townsend, 2009, pp. 121–123)

Resolution Stage

The resolution stage is the last phase of Peplau's therapeutic nurse–client relationship. This phase may also be combined with the termination stage or listed in place of the termination stage in some psychiatric-mental health nursing textbooks. The goals and tasks of the resolution stage are essentially the same as the termination stage. When four stages are listed, the termination stage focuses on summarizing progress made and review of time spent together (Boyd, 2008, pp. 150–151; Sheldon, 2009, p. 63).

During the therapeutic nurse–client relationship some unique problems may be encountered. The most common problems include the phenomena of transference, countertransference, resistance behavior, and difficulty ending the therapeutic nurse–client relationship.

TRANSFERENCE AND COUNTERTRANSFERENCE

Transference and countertransference commonly occur in the working stage of the therapeutic nurse–client relationship. In transference the client displaces or projects unconscious feelings, desires, or actions from a person in their life onto the nurse or other healthcare provider (Varcarolis, Carson, & Shoemaker, 2006, pp. 159–160; APA, 2007, p. 952; Keltner, Schwecke, & Bostrom, 2007, pp. 107–108; Fontaine, 2009, p. 23; Townsend, 2009, p. 122). In countertransference the opposite is true. The nurse or other healthcare provider displaces or projects unconscious feelings, desires, or actions from a person in their life onto the client (APA, 2007, p. 239; Keltner, Schwecke, & Bostrom, 2007, pp. 107–108; Fontaine, 2009, p. 23). Both phenomena are used by psychoanalytic therapists in psychoanalysis therapy. These therapists receive education and training in how to use transference and countertransference therapeutically to help the client address problematic issues. However, PMH nurses at the basic level have a different role, education, and training that does not include the therapeutic use of transference and countertransference; the exception being advanced practice nursing. The occurrence of transference and countertransference in the therapeutic nurse–client relationship can be problematic and nontherapeutic because it can block communication, interfere with identifying the client's needs, erode professional boundaries, interfere with the healing process, and may lead to power struggles and resistance behaviors (Varcarolis, Carson, & Shoemaker, 2006, pp. 159–160; Boyd, 2008, p. 150). The best way to deal with transference and countertransference is to be aware that they may occur, recognize them as soon as possible, identify them, talk about them with the client and other nurses or members of the treatment team, and accept feedback.

RESISTANCE BEHAVIORS

In the working stage problems such as power struggles and resistance behaviors may occur (APA, 2007, p. 792). During power struggles either the client or the nurse may attempt to exert more control over the relationship or compete for control over the relationship. This may occur because of the existence of transference or countertransference (Varcarolis, Carson, & Shoemaker, 2006, pp. 159–160). Common resistance or testing behaviors include:

- Shifting the focus of conversation to the nurse/staff member
- Asking personal questions
- Making sexual comments or advances
- Making statements just to see the nurse's reaction
- Acting out anger inappropriately
- Withdrawing socially
- Intellectualizing or denying identified problems and behavior
- Using manipulation—trying to get attention, sympathy, or control, or being dependent rather than independent
- Continuing to arrive late for appointment, group ("forgets" you were supposed to talk now)
- Trying to get the nurse/staff to do things for them that they are capable of, or making decisions for them that they can make on their own

When dealing with resistance or testing behaviors, the nurse should clearly state what they observe and attempt to engage the client in exploring reasons behind the behavior. Reinforcing acceptable or appropriate social behavior, what the nurse knows the client is capable of doing for themselves, stating what the nurse is uncomfortable with, reinforcing factual information, and possibly leaving the situation temporarily are ways the nurse can deal with resistance (Varcarolis, Carson, & Shoemaker, 2006, pp. 165–166).

DIFFICULTY ENDING THE THERAPEUTIC NURSE–CLIENT RELATIONSHIP

There may be times when it is difficult to end the therapeutic nurse–client relationship or achieve therapeutic closure. As previously stated, both the client and nurse may feel and express sadness and loss due to the ending of the time spent with the nurse and loss of this relationship (Stuart & Laraia, 2005, p. 23). The client's anxiety level may increase or they may become angry as well. These are natural human responses and should be acknowledged rather than ignored. The client may also state that previously resolved problems have resurfaced or report new problems or symptoms in an effort to extend the time together. As previously stated when dealing with the termination or resolution phase, the nurse should acknowledge the client's reactions and admit that not all problems may be completely resolved, but these can be further dealt with in outpatient treatment. The nurse should avoid addressing new problems and reinforce what the client has learned when dealing with resurfacing old problems as well as progress made. The nurse should also explain that it is common for clients to experience increased anxiety before discharge because they are leaving a safe, comfortable place and having to reenter situations that previously were overwhelming to them. Reinforcing that the client now has more adaptive ways to cope with problems or stress can help reassure the client as well as emphasizing that there will be support from the client's outpatient treatment team. Finally, thanking the client again for the opportunity to work together, but firmly stating that their time has ended and that the nurse is confident that the client can work with their outpatient treatment team is very important.

When the PMH nurse experiences problems "letting go," they should discuss these feelings with fellow nurses or other members of the healthcare/treatment team. It is important to acknowledge the assistance that the nurse was able to provide the client, reinforce the importance of the client's independence, and accept appropriate feedback. Again, countertransference may be a reason for the nurse's feelings and may need to be explored further (Stuart & Laraia, 2005, pp. 23–24; Keltner, Schwecke, & Bostrom, 2007, pp. 104–105; Boyd, 2008, pp. 150–151; Williams, 2008, p. 36; Fontaine, 2009, p. 23; Sheldon, 2009, pp. 62–63; Townsend, 2009, pp. 121–123)

REFERENCES

American Psychological Association (2007). *APA dictionary of psychology.* Washington, DC: Author.

Boyd, M. A. (2008). *Psychiatric nursing: Contemporary practice* (4th ed.). Philadelphia, PA: Wolters/Kluwer/Lippincott, Williams, & Wilkins.

Dziopa, F., & Ahern, K. (2009). Three different ways mental health nurses develop quality therapeutic relationships. *Issues in Mental Health Nursing, 30,* 14–22.

Fontaine, K. L. (2009). *Mental health nursing* (6th ed.). Upper Saddle River, NJ: Pearson Education Inc.

Gamez, G. G. (2009). The nurse-patient relationship as a caring relationship. *Nursing Science Quarterly, 22*(2), 126–127.

Keltner, N. L., Schwecke, L. H., & Bostrom, C. E. (2007). *Psychiatric nursing* (5th ed.). St. Louis, MO: Mosby, Elsevier.

Kwiatek, E., McKenzie, K., & Loads, D. (2005). Self-awareness and reflection: Exploring the "therapeutic use of self." *Learning Disability Practice, 8*(3), 27–31.

Sheldon, L. K. (2009). *Communication for nurses* (2nd ed.). Sudbury, MA: Jones and Bartlett.

Stuart, G. W., & Laraia, M. T. (2005). *Principles and practice of psychiatric nursing* (8th ed.). St. Louis, MO: Mosby, Elsevier.

Townsend, M. C. (2009). *Essentials of psychiatric mental health nursing: Concepts of care in evidence based practice* (6th ed.). Philadelphia, PA: F. A. Davis Company.

Varcarolis, E. M., Carson, V. B., & Shoemaker, N. C. (2006). *Foundations of psychiatric mental health nursing: A clinical approach* (6th ed.). St. Louis, MO: Saunders, Elsevier.

Williams, C. L. (2008). *Therapeutic interaction in nursing* (2nd ed.). Sudbury, MA: Jones and Bartlett.

CHAPTER 6

Leading Psychoeducation Groups

Kim A. Jakopac

OBJECTIVES

The nursing student will be able to:

1. Explain the PMH nurse's roles when working with psychoeducation groups
2. Discuss therapeutic, curative, or beneficial factors of psychoeducation groups
3. Identify topics appropriate for PMH nurse led psychoeducation groups
4. Describe the phases of group development
5. Identify the tasks of the PMH nurse group leader and group members in each phase
6. Describe communication and intervention techniques used by the PMH nurse group leader to facilitate group process
7. Identify roles clients may assume during group process and ways to deal with common problems affecting group members, including resistance or testing behaviors
8. Identify key elements to include when documenting a psychoeducation group

KEY TERMS

Boundaries	Group process
Curative factors	Group themes
Deviant behavior	Group therapy
Feedback	Psychoeducation
Group	Resistance behaviors
Group content	Social microcosm
Group dynamics	Subgrouping
Group norm	Therapeutic factors

Psychoeducation groups provide information on a range of topics that benefit the client and anyone else involved in the client's care or life. Goals include increasing understanding and empowerment. Psychoeducation groups are utilized in both inpatient and outpatient settings.

ROLES OF THE PMH NURSE

The psychiatric-mental health (PMH) nurse assumes many roles including those of teacher, leader, counselor, and change agent (see Chapter 1). The PMH nurse assumes these roles when leading psychoeducation groups. The group leader maintains confidentiality and adheres to ethical principles such as beneficence, autonomy, nonmaleficence, and informed consent. Leadership styles include autocratic, democratic, and laissez-faire. An autocratic leader takes control of the group, does not encourage much member participation, and rarely seeks input from group members. A democratic leader encourages group member participation, interaction, decision making, and problem solving. A laissez-faire leader exerts little or no control over group members. An autocratic leader may be helpful in emergency situations and may achieve high productivity, but they also may limit the personal growth of group members and cause either hostility or dependence from them. A laissez-faire style may not be helpful for clients who need more direction and structure, which is often the case with many inpatient psychiatric-mental health clients (Mohr, 2009, p. 244; Townsend, 2009, p. 165). A democratic leadership style seems to be the most helpful, but may be limited in effectiveness by the amount of time needed to hear every member's views and define and accomplish the group's goals. In situations where quick decisions or immediate actions are needed, this leadership style would not be as effective as the autocratic style. The PMH nurse group leader has to assess the group's needs, resources available, and the setting to determine which style would work best. The leader assumes a neutral, nonjudgmental attitude and affect. Qualities that contribute to being an effective leader include:

- Attentiveness
- Therapeutic use of self
- Therapeutic listening skills
- Flexibility
- Confidence
- Enthusiasm
- Creativity
- Having a clear set of therapeutic boundaries
- Ability to limit set with a consistent approach
- Appropriate use of humor
- Ability to tolerate frustration
- Ability to receive as well as give feedback
- Ability to instill hope in clients for their own recovery
- Being honest and having trust in clients' own ability and potential for recovery

The nurse also selects topics to be presented and must be knowledgeable and able to present information in ways clients can understand. Clients may come from varied ethnic and cultural backgrounds, education levels, and age groups, and have varied psychiatric-mental health diagnoses. Some clients may have problems with literacy or may be literate, but English is not their primary language. The PMH nurse must take all these variables into consideration, especially when working in general psychiatric-mental health settings and programs rather than in more specialized treatment programs that group clients by diagnosis or problem. The nurse may also lead groups that include significant others, family members, and friends of clients whose needs may differ from those of clients.

THERAPEUTIC FACTORS

Clients receive many therapeutic factors or benefits from meeting in psychoeducation groups in addition to one-to-one interaction with PMH nurses. Client education is included in the American Nurses Association (ANA)'s PMH nurse scope and standards of practice and is required by the nurse practice act of individual state boards of nursing. Client education is an important intervention in enhancing treatment, increasing treatment adherence or compliance, improving attitudes toward treatment (Tay, 2007, p. 29), and symptom relapse prevention (Keltner, Schwecke, & Bostrom, 2007, p. 144). Client education is provided both individually and in groups. Psychoeducation groups are also provided for significant others, additional family members, or friends. A psychoeducation group is not psychotherapy, but provides valuable health teaching to clients in a group setting where group process and therapeutic factors occur. Advanced practice registered nurses (APRNs) can provide psychotherapy. There are additional educational and clinical requirements as well as guidelines for APRNs who provide psychotherapy, including advanced degrees, additional education, and clinical experience (Townsend, 2009, p. 167).

Psychotherapist Irvin Yalom identified therapeutic factors he called "curative" that are achieved through interpersonal interaction between group members and occur to some degree in most groups (Yalom, 2005, pp. 1–18; Townsend, 2009, p. 164) (see **Table 6-1**). Yalom also thought that interpersonal learning takes place during groups, and that groups over time develop into a social microcosm (Yalom, 2005, pp. 19, 31–32). Characteristics and behaviors that clients may not be consciously aware of become obvious to group members who can help each other identify maladaptive behaviors and provide information. More adaptive behaviors

Table 6-1	Curative Factors of Groups
Universality	Realization that one is not alone or that others experience illness, problems, concerns, or feelings provides relief from anxiety.
Instillation of Hope	Hope and optimism are gained from observing that others in the group have received help with problems or some benefit from being in the group; increase of faith in treatment being offered.
Imparting of Information	Knowledge is obtained about areas of need through formal instruction and from the advice of group members.
Cohesiveness	Development of a sense of belonging, bonding, value, and acceptance occurs.
Development of Socializing Techniques	Maladaptive social skills and behaviors are identified through interaction with and feedback from group members. Adaptive skills and behaviors are learned and practiced.
Interpersonal Learning	Opportunities are provided for clients to learn how their behavior is perceived by and affects others in the group. Insight is gained.
Imitative Behavior	Clients can choose to model healthy, adaptive behaviors of the leader or other group members who have mastered psychosocial skills and act as role models.
Corrective Capitulation of the Primary Family Group	Clients may re-experience early development family conflicts that remain unresolved. Dysfunctional patterns of relating can be identified. Group members can help by providing feedback and exploring problems together. Healthier patterns of relating can be learned and practiced.
Catharsis	Expression of strong positive and negative feelings that may never have been expressed before is encouraged in appropriate ways in a safe, supportive, nonthreatening environment. Insight and changes in cognition may follow catharsis experiences.
Altruism	Through mutual sharing of experiences or what has worked for them, clients experience feelings of being helpful to others, self-growth, and positive self-image.
Existential Factors	Clients share concerns about quality of life, morality, loneliness, separation, death, acceptance of lack of control over some life situations, and taking responsibility for their own lives.

Sources: Yalom, 2005, pp. 1–2; Keltner, Schwecke, & Bostrom, 2007, p. 143; Mohr, 2009, pp. 253–254; Townsend, 2009, p. 164; Fontaine, 2011, pp. 178–180.

can be learned during group interaction and relationships. In psychoeducation groups the PMH nurse provides information on a variety of topics and promotes learning as well as encouraging clients to attempt new behaviors with the support of group members. While it is true that there are some disadvantages to group therapy, such as potential problems with confidentiality, there are many therapeutic benefits.

TYPES OF GROUPS

There are many different types of groups that may be formed by specific diagnosis or problem, topic, age, gender, degree of intellectual ability, degree of physical ability, or extent of personality disorganization. One group may also be composed of a mixture of diagnoses, ages, genders, or degrees of abilities (heterogeneous) depending on the type of program offered and resources available. Clients who are experiencing a high degree of psychosis, mania, or disorientation may be overly simulated by a group setting and have much difficulty focusing, and therefore would not be candidates initially for psychoeducation groups. These clients would benefit more from individual psychoeducation using simple concepts until they start experiencing relief from their symptoms.

Groups are also referred to as *open* or *closed*. Open groups accept new members when current members leave. Closed groups do not accept new members and continue to meet with the remaining members until the end of the total agreed-upon sessions. Ideally a recommended group size is seven to nine members, not including the leader, which allows everyone to have a chance to participate. It is helpful to have an uneven number of group members when situations or decisions requiring group members to vote occur since the leader usually abstains from voting. Frequently the group leader and members sit in a circle to encourage eye contact and provide a symbol of equal power among members. Even though it is usually best not to have any physical barriers such as a table between group members, there are times when a table may be used if members will need to write, play a board game, or perform other tasks where a table would be useful. Some treatment programs use behavioral modification systems including a token economy. In a token economy system, clients are given tokens or points for engaging in appropriate or positive behavior that leads to more long-lasting change. The tokens or points are later exchanged for extra privileges (Keltner, 2007, p. 566). Tokens or points may be given for attending and participating in group.

PSYCHOEDUCATION GROUP TOPICS

The following topics are commonly used for psychoeducation groups:

- Diagnosis—signs/symptoms, possible treatment
- Medications
- Stress management/relaxation techniques
- Coping skills
- Guided imagery
- Problem-solving/decision-making skills
- Healthy communication/assertiveness
- Improving sleep pattern
- Balanced nutrition
- Social skills
- Time management
- Exercise
- Relapse prevention and illness management
- Anger management
- Smoking cessation
- Aromatherapy
- Community resources/support groups
- Parenting skills
- Other health promotion/healthy life style topics

PHASES OF GROUP DEVELOPMENT

Just as the therapeutic nurse–client relationship occurs in phases, so do groups, including psychoeducation groups. Each phase includes tasks for both the PMH nurse group leader and group members. There are four phases in group development: initial/orientation, working, maintenance/mature, and termination (see **Table 6-2**). Each phase includes separate tasks for the leader and group members to work towards completing (Varcarolis, Carson, & Shoemaker, 2006, pp. 721–722; Mohr, 2009, pp. 245, 250–251). During short inpatient hospitalizations, groups may meet only once or a few times. Therefore, it may be difficult to see a group progress through all four phases. If only the first two phases occur, the PMH nurse group leader may follow up with clients on an individual basis to determine retention of information or provide opportunities to practice skills and provide feedback. The nurse will implement the principles of the termination stage of the therapeutic nurse–client relationship and psychoeducation group's phases on an individual basis.

Table 6-2   Phases and Tasks of Psychoeducation Groups

Phases	Tasks
1. Initial/Orientation Phase	1.a. Leader: —Prepares the physical environment/setting including seating arrangements, temperature, light, controlling noise —Introduces self, including credentials —Establishes atmosphere of respect, trust, and confidentiality —Fosters a milieu that encourages development of therapeutic alliances with all group members —Provides structure by explaining group purpose, time frame, and rules —Introduces topic material b. Group members —Give input related to group purpose —If an outpatient group, may have input into the time and number of weeks to meet —Get to know each other —Help each other be comfortable and relax —Initial conversation is superficial as members begin to get to know each other
2. Working Phase	2.a. Leader —Ensures the group starts and ends on time —Reminds group members of confidentiality, rules, and time frame —Encourages and facilitates group members' communication and working together —Keeps members focused on topic and goals —Gives advice if appropriate —Helps motivate all group members to participate by expressing hopefulness and confidence in the group, encouraging members to try new skills, and reminding of progress made —Encourages cooperation and handles conflict among members —Intervenes/redirects as needed —Assists members to process/talk about feelings, difficult issues, and thoughts —Assists members to apply learning to daily activities —Summarizes work done during each session

(continues)

Table 6-2 Phases and Tasks of Psychoeducation Groups *(continued)*	
Phases	**Tasks**
	b. Group members —Work cooperatively and support each other —Allow every member opportunity to participate —Handle conflict, power struggles, and control issues
3. Maintenance/Mature Phase	3.a. Leader —See "Working Phase"; may not need reminding of rules —Keeps members focused on topic and goals b. Group members —Encourage members to accept each other's differences —Develop functional norms —Develop a sense of identity —Actively participate to achieve goals —Adapt to changes and learn new skills to cope with loss of, addition, or illness of a member
4. Termination Phase	4.a. Leader —Acknowledges contributions of each member —Acknowledges individual member as well as entire group's experience —Provides feedback and evaluates whether the purpose of the group was accomplished —Explores group members' feelings of the experience and impending separation —Ensures all problems/conflicts are resolved or that there is follow-up —Summarizes the most important issues and reinforces learning that has taken place throughout the entire time the group has met (i.e., during entire inpatient hospitalization or several weeks of outpatient meetings) b. Group members —Deal with and accept closure —Acknowledge goals met —Accept progress made on goals still working on

Sources: Varcarolis, Carson, & Shoemaker, 2006, pp. 721–722; Mohr, 2009, 245, pp. 250–251.

GROUP LEADER'S FACILITATION TECHNIQUES

The PMH nurse as a group leader uses communication and intervention techniques to facilitate group process. Some of these techniques are similar to the therapeutic communication techniques presented in Chapter 4, and the group leader does use therapeutic communication techniques (see **Table 6-3**), and themselves therapeutically as described in Chapter 2.

Table 6-3	PMH Nurse Group Leader Communication and Intervention Techniques	
Techniques	**Descriptions**	**Examples**
1. Acceptance	1. Openly receiving communication or conveying an attitude that recognizes the client's worth *(but not necessarily agreeing with or approving of actions)*	1. Leader: "Yes, Don, I heard you say that you didn't think you would get much out of coming to this group." -or- "Yes, Don, it's okay for you to be angry with me for asking you to come to group."
2. Approval	2. Encouraging a feeling, action or attitude	2. Don: "I decided to ask my brother to move so I'm not tempted to keep drinking with him." Leader: "That sounds like a good decision."
3. Clarification	3. Restating the content of what a client said	3. Don: "I was upset when she said I was a hopeless case!" Leader "You were upset by what she said?" Don: "Yes, I guess I was upset . . . hurt and angry."
4. Confrontation	4. Challenging, but in a supportive environment to help a client learn more about themselves, help group members deal more openly with each other or help reduce disruptive behavior	4. "Don, this is the third time you've changed the subject. Is something going on?"

(continues)

Table 6-3	PMH Nurse Group Leader Communication and Intervention Techniques *(continued)*	
Techniques	**Descriptions**	**Examples**
5. Encouraging comparison	5. Asking members to compare and contrast their feelings, thoughts, and experiences with other group members	5. Leader: "Did anyone in the group handle their problem the same way Don did? Who handled it differently?"
6. Encouraging description and exploration	6. Moving deeper into a feeling/ thought/experience or moving from considering one aspect of a situation to another	6. Leader: "How did you feel when your wife left?" or "Tell us about how you handled your wife leaving you."
7. Encouraging expression of thoughts or feelings	7. Conveying it is okay or desirable to talk about thoughts or feelings	7. Don: "Lately it seems to take so long to get out of bed in the morning." Leader: "Does anyone else in the group feel like this?" -or- "Can anyone else in the group relate to Don's experience?"
8. Encouraging evaluation	8. Asking the group or an individual member to judge their experience	8. Leader: "How did we do with helping Don with his problem?" -or- "Did you feel better when Lisa gave you support during group today?" -or- "Do you feel you will be able to cope better with stress now that you have learned some relaxation techniques?"
9. Focusing	9. Concentrating on a single topic or issue	9. Leader: "What is the biggest problem you have staying on medication?"
10. Giving information	10. Stating group topic and providing facts and explanations	10. Leader: "Today I will be sharing information with you about major depression."

(continues)

Table 6-3 PMH Nurse Group Leader Communication and Intervention Techniques *(continued)*

Techniques	Descriptions	Examples
11. Giving recognition	11. Acknowledging, sharing awareness, congratulating	11. Leader: "We have a new group member today. This is Susan." -or- "Today is Don's one year anniversary of sobriety."
12. Interpretation	12. Explaining or finding the significance of information	12. Don: "All we are doing is talking. Just a waste of time." Leader: "Don, you sound annoyed." Don: "I feel like there is no hope for me, no way out, and all we are doing is sitting around talking." Leader: "You're feeling hopeless? When you feel hopeless do you ever think of suicide?"
13. Limit setting	13. Deciding when to restrict verbal expression or behavior that is not productive or is disruptive to group process	13. Don: "Since Monday is a holiday I think we should cancel group and just sleep in later." Leader: "If you are not getting enough sleep we can talk about ways to improve sleep. We will not cancel group on Monday morning." Another way to limit set is to let a group member know that what they are talking about or asking is off the group topic and offer to talk with them after group.
14. Making observations	14. Sharing observations can stimulate some group members to talk or respond; can also change the group's direction	14. "Don, you haven't contributed anything to the group's discussion, and we're almost out of time."

(continues)

Table 6-3	PMH Nurse Group Leader Communication and Intervention Techniques *(continued)*	
Techniques	**Descriptions**	**Examples**
15. Presenting reality	15. Listening to group member's perceptions, asking for perceptions of other group members, providing an opportunity for one member to compare their perceptions with others in the group, and stating facts	15. "Don has shared with the group that he used to work as an executive, but now he thinks that a future employer may think he is unstable. So far you have demonstrated your abilities to think logically. Does anyone else in the group think Don looks unstable?" -or- "You just stated that taking medications made you worse, but when you were taking medications you were able to work and have a relationship with your family."
16. Reassurance	16. Offering confidence about a positive outcome or confidence in the group member	16. Don: "I was afraid to come to the hospital; afraid my problems were too big." Leader: "That is a common fear, but we all are here to listen and help you work out those problems."
17. Support or understanding	17. Offering emotional support and communicating comprehension	17. Don: "I was up half the night because the night nurse wouldn't give me anything for my back pain." Leader: "That must have made you angry. Let's talk about some ways to deal with pain other than medication."

Sources: Keltner, Schwecke & Bostrom, 2007, pp. 149–150; Boyd, 2008, p. 195; Mohr, 2009, pp. 249–250.

GROUP MEMBER ROLES

Group member roles serve the purposes of completing tasks; continuing and enhancing group process; and meeting individual needs. Group member roles may be effective or ineffective regarding the group's progress towards meeting established goals.

Roles are classified as task, maintenance, or individual/personal. A healthy balance of task and maintenance roles is thought to be the most effective. Individual/personal roles are not viewed as helpful toward achievement of the group's goals. (Varcarolis, Carson, & Shoemaker, 2006, pp. 726–728; Arnold & Boggs, 2007, pp. 267–269; Keltner, Schwecke, & Bostrom, 2007, p. 166; Mohr, pp. 247–248; Townsend, 2009, p. 166).

1. Task roles—help identify problems and solutions that occur during group work.
    a. Coordinator—clarifies ideas and suggestions or shows how ideas may work; helps brings members together to pursue group goals.
    b. Elaborator—explains and expands on group ideas and plans.
    c. Energizer—motivates and encourages group members to fully participate and perform at their highest level.
    d. Evaluator—examines group performance and progress towards goals and adhering to standards.
    e. Information giver—shares relevant experiences, offers facts.
    f. Information seeker—asks for clarification of information received.
    g. Initiator—outlines tasks to be accomplished and offers ways to do so.
    h. Orientor—maintains group direction in moving towards target goals, helps keep focus.
2. Maintenance roles—help the overall functioning of the group by regulating, strengthening, and keeping the group going.
    a. Compromiser—assists in relieving conflict; assists to reach compromises acceptable to all group members.
    b. Encourager—recognizes and accepts contributions and ideas of other group members.
    c. Follower—acts as a passive audience listening attentively as other group members interact.
    d. Gatekeeper—assists in keeping communication open by encouraging participation and acceptance of all group members.
    e. Group observer—keeps track of and interprets what is happening in the group.
    f. Harmonizer—helps minimize tension by intervening when conflicts arise.
3. Individual/Personal roles—meet the individual group member's needs, but hinder the group's functioning and progress.
    a. Aggressor—negative; uses sarcasm and hostility when interacting with group members; blames, criticizes, or personally verbally attacks other members to degrade their status or the group's progress.
    b. Avoider—acts indifferent to group process, daydreams or doodles, distracts other members by whispering to others.

c. Blocker—argues or disagrees beyond reason, rejects possible solutions, is rigid, obstructs problem-solving/decision-making efforts, resists or impedes the group's efforts toward goal attainment.

d. Dominator—attempts to demonstrate superiority and assert authority by manipulating other members to gain control of the group.

e. Help-seeker—lacks true concern for the group; detracts from the group's focus by using the group to gain sympathy; tries to increase personal confidence by soliciting feedback from the group.

f. Know-it-all—gives everyone advice. When the group leader speaks, this person frequently interrupts. Sometimes the Know-it-all and the Monopolizer try to compete for the group members', or leader's attention.

g. Monopolizer—compulsively talks or dominates the conversation to decrease their own level of anxiety.

h. Play person/disruptor—lacks involvement, jokes or laughs.

i. Recognition seeker—boasts or points to their own achievements, expresses extreme ideas, or exhibits peculiar behavior for attention.

j. Scapegoat—is a disliked member who is blamed for any problems that occur in the group.

k. Self-confessor or Seducer—uses the group for inappropriate self-disclosure and feelings or thoughts not related to the group focus; inhibits group progress by premature self-disclosure or frightening of other group members.

l. Silent/mute member—avoids participating verbally possibly due to being uncomfortable disclosing personal information or trying to gain attention through remaining silent (Varcarolis, Carson, & Shoemaker, 2006, pp. 726–728; Arnold & Boggs, 2007, pp. 267–269; Keltner, Schwecke, & Bostrom, 2007, p. 166; Boyd, 2008, p. 197; Mohr, pp. 247–248; Townsend, 2009, p. 166).

COMMON PROBLEMS AFFECTING GROUPS

There are common problems that occur and can affect group progress and relationships (see **Table 6-4**). Problems usually occur in the working phase of the group and include resistance or testing behaviors (see Chapter 5) as well as when group members assume any of the individual/personal roles previously mentioned (Varcarolis, Carson, & Shoemaker, 2006, pp. 159–160; Mohr, 2009, p. 252).

Table 6-4 Common Problems Affecting Groups

Problems	PMH group leader intervention	Rationales
1. Demoralizing others	1.a. Listen to the content of what the client avoided.	1.a. While angry, self-centered or refusing to take responsibility for their own behavior and blaming others, the client may also be emotionally vulnerable and need support from the leader. The leader needs to maintain a balance between being therapeutically objective and caring.
	b. Share your interpretation and impressions of what is happening.	b. Sharing interpretations and impressions helps the leader decide what direction to pursue with this client and lets the client know the leader is listening.
2. Deviant behavior—behavior that does not conform to group norms or rules, undermines the group or meets personal needs	2.a. Attempt to identify the specific behavior.	2.a. It is important to deal directly with the behavior rather than ignore it and allow this client to disrupt the group. This also shows the leader's concern for the client.
	b. Ask if the individual group member is aware of their behavior and if they recognize the behavior as deviant.	b. It is therapeutic to assist the individual group member to acknowledge the behavior and possible underlying reasons or emotions.
	c. Explore how this behavior affects the rest of the group.	c. This provides an opportunity for the client to problem-solve and explore more effective, adaptive behaviors with the help of the group. If the group

(continues)

Table 6-4	Common Problems Affecting Groups *(continued)*	
Problems	**PMH group leader intervention**	**Rationales**
		member refuses help and insists on continuing the deviant behavior, the leader may as a last resort ask the client to leave the group and meet individually with the leader after the group has ended. Care must be taken to differentiate this type of behavior from bizarre behavior due to psychosis that may require prn medication, or medical problems including extremes of blood glucose levels or cardiac problems.
3. Fear of authority	3.a. Respond in an understanding manner regarding the group member's feelings even if the client is angry.	3.a. Acceptance of the individual group member's feelings allows them to acknowledge those feelings and lets the client know that the leader cares about the client. This also allows the rest of the group a chance to feel and acknowledge their own feelings.
	b. Reassure the client that you will not "punish" them.	b. This decreases the client's level of anxiety and fear of the leader and can help build trust.
	c. Listen attentively and allow the client to express themselves.	c. Group members need the leader to role model healthy communication and help convince the client experiencing a problem of the leader's genuine desire to help.

(continues)

Table 6-4 Common Problems Affecting Groups *(continued)*		
Problems	**PMH group leader intervention**	**Rationales**
	d. Use therapeutic communication to explore possible causes of feelings.	d. Exploring possible causes provides opportunities for increased self-awareness, personal growth, and encourages other group members who may have similar feelings to express them. Other group members may also have valuable input as to how to handle these feelings.
4. Initial anxiety	4.a. Explain that this is a common response to a new situation.	4.a. Explaining normal responses helps the client feel more comfortable and lets them know that this is not a symptom of increased illness; they are not alone in their feelings.
	b. Recognize any efforts made by the client to participate and provide positive feedback.	b. Recognizing and providing positive feedback lets the client know they are doing what is expected and rewards the type of behavior the leader wants the client to continue doing. It also increases the likelihood of the client continuing to participate.
	c. Assist the client to establish a member role.	c. The client will feel that they are an accepted member of the group as they assume a role rather than remaining more of an observer or silent participant versus an active participant. The client will also be more likely to work on both their own problems as well as the group goals.

(continues)

Table 6-4   Common Problems Affecting Groups *(continued)*

Problems	PMH group leader intervention	Rationales
5. Hidden agenda	5.a. Identify the source of the group member or members trying to accomplish an individual goal that interferes with group process and attaining group goals.	5.a. Identifying the source will help the leader and the other group members deal with the problem.
	b. Explore with the group how this hidden agenda is affecting the group's ability to function.	b. Hidden agendas can create anxiety in other group members and sabotage the group's progress. The person(s) involved may need referral for problems that cannot be dealt with in this particular group. In order to help both the person(s) propagating a hidden agenda and those who are not, the situation must be identified and dealt with. Appropriate referrals should be made.
	c. Limit set as needed with the person(s) directly involved in pursuing the hidden agenda.	c. Limit setting helps maintain and reinforce group rules, norms and therapeutic boundaries.
6. Rejecting help	6.a. Agree with the client, but remain therapeutically objective.	6.a. This pessimistic individual will continue to complain about and even take pride in problems that are perceived as unable to be solved and reject any solutions offered. The leader should avoid being drawn in emotionally by the client.

(continues)

Table 6-4 Common Problems Affecting Groups *(continued)*

Problems	PMH group leader intervention	Rationales
	b. Encourage the client to look at their behavior.	b. The leader attempts to reinforce reality, present facts, and help the client increase self-awareness as to how they may be contributing to the problems.
	c. Continue to reinforce the need for attending group.	c. If the client stays with the group long enough, they will begin to develop a sense of cohesion that may help them begin to at least think about some of the solutions the other group members suggest.
7. Resistance	7.a. Identify and confront the resistance behavior.	7.a. While some degree of resistance is to be expected initially, letting it continue is not therapeutic for the individual group member and can be disruptive to the group's progress.
	b. Explore the resistance behaviors with the individual group member (see Chapter 5).	b. Exploring will help both the leader and the individual group member find the source of the behavior and underlying issues that can be dealt with in one-to-one therapeutic interactions or with the client's therapist or psychiatrist. See previously identified task and maintenance roles in this chapter.

(continues)

Table 6-4   Common Problems Affecting Groups *(continued)*

Problems	PMH group leader intervention	Rationales
8. Silence	8.a. Be patient, but continue to encourage active participation. Give the individual group member time to think about what they want to say and tell them you will come back to them later during the group session for input.	8.a. Obviously the leader cannot force participation, but the individual member is not fully benefitting if not actively participating. Other group members may begin to resent this person for not participating. Encouraging active participation enforces group norms, and letting the client know you will come back to them shows patience, but that you still expect active participation.
9. Subgrouping	9.a. Clarify and reinforce the entire group's goals.	9.a. This intervention can help turn the subgroup's focus back to the entire group.
	b. Redirect the members of the subgroup back to the entire group's original goals.	b. This intervention can help turn the subgroup's focus back to the entire group.

Sources: Varcarolis, Carson & Shoemaker, 2006, pp. 159–160, 726–728; Boyd, 2008, p. 197; Mohr, 2009, pp. 252–253.

KEY ELEMENTS OF DOCUMENTATION

Documentation is important for many reasons, including providing proof that psychoeducation was offered and provided. Documentation must be done on all clients whether or not they attended. Clients have the right to refuse to attend group, but if they do it must also be documented. If a client does not attend, the reason for not attending should also be documented if known. For example, not all clients refuse, but may need to see a consulting physician who is only available during the time the group is scheduled to meet. This is not the client's fault and should be documented in a way that does not reflect negatively on the client's willingness to adhere to treatment. Some agencies or facilities have a specific education form that all disciplines use to document group as well as individual client teaching sessions; otherwise documentation is done using a narrative form. Key elements to include when documenting a psychoeducation group include:

1. Client's name
2. Date of hospitalization and diagnosis if the documentation is kept in a separate binder rather than in each individual client's medical record
3. Topic
4. Date, time and duration of the group
5. The name of the leader and coleader if more than one leader was present; having a coleader may be beneficial when there are clients who may need extra assistance with group tasks or physical assistance, who become ill and need to be taken out of group, or to handle disruptions.
6. Nonattendance and reason if known including refusal to attend
7. Individual and group goals
8. Progress toward attaining goals
9. Level of participation—active or attentive, but passive; attended, but refused to participate
10. Level of understanding, including verbalization of understanding or need for reinforcement of information; insightful comments or comments showing limited insight or judgment
11. Ability to accept support from group members or the leader or give support to other members
12. Bizarre, aggressive, or disruptive statements
13. Behavior—bizarre, disruptive, or aggressive behavior; need for redirection and acceptance or nonacceptance of redirection; ability to tolerate being in a group; ability to work with other members of the group
14. Reasons for needing to leave group early—pain, called out to see consulting physician, inability to tolerate the length/duration or the size of the group; behavior
15. If there is more than one session scheduled for this specific group or group topic, plans for the next session is documented
16. If this is a group attended by family members and friends, who attended and what their response was as well as interaction between clients and their family or friends

EXAMPLE OF A PSYCHOEDUCATION GROUP

The room has been prepared, chairs placed in a circle, and materials gathered prior to starting the group.

Leader: "Good morning. My name is Jackie, I am an RN, and this is a nursing psychoeducation group. For the next 45 minutes we will be talking about ways you can get a better night's sleep. Before we get started I want to assure you of confidentiality. Nothing said in group will be talked about off the unit. Anything said in group will only be shared with your psychiatrist and staff members involved in your care, including members of the treatment team. Also, I want to remind you of our general group rules: Please raise your hand if you have something to say. Please listen when other members are talking. If you need to use the bathroom, please do so before we start group. You do need to stay in group until it is finished. If you absolutely must leave, please do so quietly and not disturb the rest of the group members. Now let's go around the circle and introduce ourselves. Again, my name is Jackie," and turns to the group member to her right nodding her head to continue with the introductions. The group members introduce themselves and listen as Jackie continues.

Leader: "Many people in the United States have problems sleeping, including those who have mental health problems. Getting too little or too much sleep and not feeling rested no matter how much sleep you've had are symptoms of many mental health problems. What do you think are some causes of sleep problems other than being a symptom of mental health problems?"

Group member: "Drinking too much caffeine?"

Leader: "Yes, that's right. Very good. Can anyone name some sources of caffeine?"

Know-it-all: "Oh, I know every source of caffeine! Coffee, Mountain Dew, Coke, Red Bull . . ." and continues to talk.

Leader: "Thank you for sharing that information, but now I'd like to hear from someone else." The leader may wait for another group member to volunteer information or may call on someone by name.

Group member: "Doesn't tea also have caffeine in it?"

Aggressor: "Anybody knows that unless you're stupid."

Self-confessor: "Tea, which reminds me of this guy I had really great sex with. As a matter of fact it was just before I came in here (hospital)."

Leader: "First of all our group rules include treating each other with respect. We need to stay on our topic."

Monopolizer: "Yes, we certainly do need to be respectful of each other and not call people names. Yes, staying on topic is the right thing to do. We all need to listen to Nurse Jackie. I also know a lot of ways to help people sleep," looks directly at the Know-it-all, and continues without pausing "taking a warm bath before going to sleep, listening to soft music, and turning on a fan to block out other noises."

Know-it-all: "Well, if you'd let me finish I would have mentioned those ways and many more," looking back at the Monopolizer.

Leader: "Well, it seems that some group members have much knowledge to share with the group, but we are getting ahead of ourselves, and several of you haven't had a chance to speak. Let's hear from _____ (calls on a specific group member) about some other things that can interfere with getting a good night's sleep." The leader encourages this group member with a smile, eye contact, and a nod of her head.

Group member: "I have trouble sleeping when I have too much on my mind. I take sleeping pills, but am afraid of getting hooked on them."

Leader: "Thank you _____, for sharing your problem and your concern about taking sleeping pills. Does anyone else in the group have the same problem or concern?"

Aggressor: "What a baby! Afraid of getting hooked on sleeping pills."

Leader: Looks at the Aggressor and says, "You sound angry."

Aggressor: "You bet I'm angry being cooped up in here 24/7!"

Leader: "I understand you are here against your will. I think I'd be angry if I felt I was being forced to do something I didn't want to."

Aggressor: Makes a grunting sound and folds his arms across his chest.

Leader: "I'd like to spend some time talking more about this with you after group, but right now we are talking about problems sleeping. What keeps you awake at night?"

Aggressor: Looks at the floor for a minute and then replies, "My dad died a few months ago and I didn't go to the funeral. Now everyone's mad at me, but they don't know what I went through growing up with him."

Leader: With an empathetic facial expression, nods head, makes eye contact, and leaning forward responds, "It sounds like you are in a difficult position. Has anyone else in the group had a similar situation or experienced a loss or abuse?"

Some group members nod their heads.

Leader: "Does anyone have any advice or support to give?"

Two members talk briefly about their losses and offer to listen whenever this group member (Aggressor) needs them. The leader thanks them, goes back to discussing other problems interfering with sleep, and offers solutions other than taking medications. She encourages those who have concerns with taking sleeping medications to express their concerns to their psychiatrist.

Leader: "We have about 10 minutes, so let me summarize what we've been talking about . . ." She offers printed handouts with information on this topic for group members to keep. This helps remind and reinforce what was said in group. Printed materials may also be shared with family and friends. The leader reminds the group members of what break times and groups will be meeting next and the location according to the program schedule. While clients are expected to be responsible enough to follow the schedule, there are some clients experiencing psychosis, withdrawal from substances, or disorientation. These clients need additional assistance.

[The Leader may also demonstrate a relaxation technique and invite the group to try practicing the technique for use during hospitalization and after discharge.]

The Leader will document the group according to the agency's policy and follow up with individual group members as promised.

REFERENCES

American Psychological Association (2007). *APA dictionary of psychology*. Washington, DC: Author.

Arnold, E. C., & Boggs, K. U. (2007). *Interpersonal relationships: Professional communication skills for nurses* (5th ed.). St. Louis, MO: Saunders, Elsevier.

Boyd, M. A. (2008). *Psychiatric nursing: Contemporary practice* (4th ed.). Philadelphia, PA: Wolters/Kluwer/Lippincott, Williams, & Wilkins.

Fontaine, K. L. (2009). *Mental health nursing* (6th ed.). Upper Saddle River, NJ: Pearson Education Inc.

Keltner, N. L., Schwecke, L. H., & Bostrom, C. E. (2007). *Psychiatric nursing* (5th ed.). St. Louis, MO: Mosby, Elsevier.

Mohr, W. K. (2009). *Psychiatric-mental health nursing: Evidence based concepts, skills, and practice* (7th ed.). Philadelphia, PA: Wolters Kluwer/Lippincott, Williams, & Wilkins.

Tay, S. C. (2007). Compliance therapy: An intervention to improve inpatients' attitudes toward treatment. *Journal of Psychosocial Nursing, 45*(6), 29–37.

Townsend, M. C. (2009). *Essentials of psychiatric mental health nursing: Concepts of care in evidence based practice* (6th ed.). Philadelphia, PA: F. A. Davis Company.

Varcarolis, E. M., Carson, V. B., & Shoemaker, N. C. (2006). *Foundations of psychiatric mental health nursing: A clinical approach* (6th ed.). St. Louis, MO: Saunders, Elsevier.

Yalom, I. D. (2005). *The theory and practice of group therapy* (5th ed.). New York, NY: Basic Books.

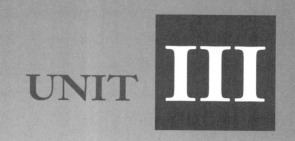

UNIT **III**

Psychiatric-Mental Health Nursing Skills for Assessment and Interventions

CHAPTER 7

Assessment and Interventions for the Client with Severe Anxiety

Sudha C. Patel

OBJECTIVES

The nursing student will be able to:

1. Differentiate between anxiety and anxiety disorders
2. Assess signs and symptoms of severe anxiety
3. Discuss proposed causes of severe anxiety
4. Discuss priority nursing interventions to reduce severe anxiety to moderate/mild level
5. Apply nursing process and critical thinking for severe anxiety
6. Explain types of nursing skills needed to deal with severe anxiety
7. Discuss the treatment modalities for the client who is exhibiting severe anxiety

KEY TERMS

Affect	Flashback
Anxiety	Fear
Anxiety disorders	Nursing process
Secondary gain	Posttraumatic stress disorder (PTSD)
Coping mechanisms	Severe anxiety
Defense mechanisms	Panic attack
Emotional numbing	Phobia

WHAT IS ANXIETY?

The term *anxiety* is derived from the Latin word *anxietus*. It means "to vex or trouble" (Antai-Otong, 2003). Anxiety is a natural and integral part of all living beings. It is a part of the human condition that plays an important part in the adaptation and home-ostasis process for adjustment and survival. Everybody experiences anxiety; it keeps human beings alive and able to feel fear. It is like a warning system built into the body to allow a human being in the face of danger to trigger the fight or flight response in order to survive. Anxiety is characterized by a diffused, unpleasant, vague sense of apprehension, often accompanied by autonomic symptoms such as headache, perspiration, palpitations, tightness in the chest, mild stomach ache, discomfort, and restlessness feelings (Sadock & Sadock, 2008). The National Institute of Mental Health (NIMH) states that anxiety is a normal reaction to stress. It helps one deal with a tense situation in the office, study harder for an exam, or keep focused on an important speech. In general, it helps one cope.

WHAT ARE ANXIETY DISORDERS?

When anxiety becomes an excessive, irrational dread of everyday situations, it turns into a disabling disorder (NIMH, 2009). The anxiety disorders are a group of related conditions rather than a single disorder and can look very different from person to person. The symptoms of anxiety disorders may vary among individuals; however, all anxiety disorders share one major symptom; persistent or severe fear or worry in situations in which most people would not feel threatened (Helpguide.org, 2010). It is important for the nurse to learn about anxiety and disorders related to anxiety. There is no exaggeration in saying that the 21st century is going from epidemic to pandemic stages in terms of anxiety and related disorders. In the United States over 40 million American adults age 18 years and older (about 18%) in any given year, along with millions of children, have anxiety disorders ranging from mild to severe, and these statistics are only on the reported cases to physicians. The disorders related to anxiety cause individuals to be filled with fearfulness and uncertainty. Unlike the relatively mild, brief anxiety caused by a stressful event (such as speaking in public or a first date), anxiety disorders last at least 6 months and can become worse if they are not treated. Anxiety disorders commonly occur along with other mental or physical illnesses, including alcohol or substance abuse, which may mask anxiety symptoms or make them worse. In some cases, these other illnesses need to be treated before a person will respond to treatment for the anxiety disorder (NIMH, 2009). *Anxiety disorder* as a term indicates the individual has an unrealistic, irrational, fear or anxiety of disabling intensity. The *Diagnostic and Statistical Manual of Mental Disorders* (DSM-IV-TR) (2007) recognizes the following seven types of anxiety disorders:

- Acute stress disorder—Anxiety lasts approximately 1 month following a traumatic experience. Posttraumatic stress disorder is similar, however, acute stress disorder subsides within that 1-month time period.

- Anxiety disorder due to medical condition—Some medical conditions such as asthma or cardiovascular disease may cause anxiety leading to panic attack, as well as obsessive compulsive behavior or severe anxiety.
- Obsessive-compulsive disorder (OCD)—The individual has recurrent distressing thoughts that manifest into an uncontrollable urge to engage in repetitive behavior to reduce the anxiety. The symptoms may last more than an hour and cause significant distress in the person's life, thus interfering with daily functioning.
- Panic disorder—Panic attack is the common feature in this disorder. In a panic attack, there is a sudden feeling of intense dread, fear of death, doom, or terror. The person is unable to name the source of their fear and may feel confused and have trouble in concentration. The physical symptoms experienced by the person are shortness of breath, palpitations, dizziness, chest pain, sweating, nausea or abdominal discomfort, and hot flashes. The person may have difficulty in speaking, memory impairment, and may ruminate. Panic attacks generally last for about 20 to 30 minutes. As per DSM-IV-TR, at least the first panic attack must be unexpected for the diagnosis of panic disorder.
- Posttraumatic stress disorder (PTSD)—Distressing thoughts, anger, and anxiety are the most common symptoms following a life-threatening or traumatic event in a person's life. The person experiences fear, feels helpless, relives the event, and tries to avoid being reminded of the event. DSM-IV-TR indicates that to diagnose PTSD, the symptoms must last for more than 1 month, and there must be significant impairment in the person's daily functioning level such as family, work, etc.
- Phobic disorders include agoraphobia, social phobia, and specific phobia. Agoraphobia involves a fear of open spaces. The individual feels anxiety about being in an open place or situation from which they think escape is impossible. The anxiety leads to avoidance of a variety of situations that leads to impairment of daily functioning. The person avoids situations and insists that somebody accompany them for outdoor activities. In social phobia anxiety occurs due to certain social situations or when performing in front of a group. In specific phobias, anxiety symptoms occur leading to a panic attack when the person is exposed to a specific single feared object or situation (e.g., flying, elevators, high places).
- Generalized anxiety disorder—In this disorder, there is excessive and persistent anxiety and worry lasting for at least 6 months (DSM-IV-TR, 2007, pp. 429–482).

PHYSIOLOGIC PROCESSES THAT ACTIVATE ANXIETY

Physiologic processes start within the brain. In order to understand the physiologic process of anxiety, it is important to know the functions of the brain. The limbic system is responsible for triggering human emotion, including fight or flight responses, as well as activating complex interactions between neurotransmitters and hormones. This process energizes or prepares the body and mind to deal with an actual or perceived threat. This is a normal and natural process in all living beings. There are four known physiologic factors that play an important role in producing anxiety in humans: (1) neurotransmitters, (2) hormones—the hypothalamic-pituitary-adrenal (HPA) axis, (3) sex hormones (estrogen, progesterone), and (4) nutrition and digestion (Pick, 2007).

Neurotransmitters

The first physiologic factor in anxiety is an imbalance between various neurotransmitter levels that can sensitize the brain for fear responses. A chronically high level of excitatory neurotransmitters such as norepinephrine and epinephrine, along with chronic low levels of calming, inhibitory neurotransmitters such as serotonin and gamma-amino butyric acid (GABA) will modify the brain chemistry to create clinical anxiety.

Hormones

Hormones are the second physiologic factor in producing anxiety. A hormonal system consists of an HPA axis that influences an individual's mood. Imbalances in hormone levels can lead to severe anxiety, panic attack, or chronic anxiety. The hypothalamus releases a hormone called corticotrophin-releasing factor (CRF). This factor triggers in a human a response for action. CRF activates the pituitary gland that in turn stimulates adrenocorticotropic hormone (ACTH), which triggers the adrenaline gland to release Cortisol. Cortisol opens the way for glucose, fat, and protein to reach to the body cells for energy and vigilance in the face of threat. In healthy individuals, the hormonal balances come back to normal levels once the actual or perceived threat or fear has dissipated. However, circumstances may disrupt this normal hormonal process and keep the adrenaline running and drive a person to the exhaustion stage. In this situation, levels of ACTH and Cortisol remain elevated causing anxiety, weight gain, speeding, aging, and disruption in the metabolic system. CRF also plays a vital role in anxiety. Persons with high anxiety also have high levels of CRF, which shows that in these individuals, their HPA axis is functioning at a high level all the time. Researchers reported that early emotional trauma may cause the CRF level to remain constantly high (Pick, 2007).

Sex Hormones

Sex hormones are the third factor contributing to anxiety. Estrogen and progesterone play a vital role in the production of anxiety. The levels of these hormones are directly impacted by the levels of adrenaline and Cortisol produced. When the level of these sex hormones falls, it impacts a person's mood and energy level. The frequency of feeling anxiety between women and men is 2:1; this difference is due to premenstrual syndrome (PMS), menopause, and the general hormonal ups and downs in reproductive age women (Pick, 2007).

Nutrition and Digestion

Food allergies and food sensitivities can cause anxiety symptoms. The research literature has identified a relationship between nutrition and a person's mood. The neurotransmitter serotonin also resides in the gut as well as in the brain and other parts of the body and is a major controller of mood. Thus the digestive system, neurotransmitters, hormones, brain chemistry, and mood all are interrelated and play a vital role as anxiety-producing factors (Pick, 2007).

PSYCHOLOGICAL PROCESSES THAT ACTIVATE ANXIETY

Some of the major schools of thought in psychology have played a major role in explaining the causes of anxiety. According to the psychoanalytical point of view, anxiety is generated from psychic conflicts among the id, ego, and superego. Behaviorists state that anxiety is a conditional response to a specific environmental or external stimulus; it is a learned response from observing the environment around the person (Sadock & Sadock, 2008). Thus, factors such as internal and external environmental conflicts generate inadequate coping capability and develop feelings of emptiness. A person views life as meaningless, aimless, and worthless; their ability to cope effectively in a given situation becomes ineffective. Ultimately ineffective coping skills generate anxiety (Antai-Otong, 2003).

NURSING ASSESSMENT

The following two tables explain the indicators used to observe and assess the physical, affective, cognitive, and behavioral signs and symptoms of an anxiety disorder, and to discern the how the level of anxiety affects signs and symptoms.

Physical and Psychological Signs and Symptoms

Cardiovascular	Neuromuscular	Gastrointestinal
Palpitations/pounding heart/heart racing	Increased reflexes	Loss of appetite
Elevated blood pressure	Startle reaction	Abdominal discomfort
Actual fainting	Eyelid twitching	Diarrhea
Lowered blood pressure	Insomnia	Abdominal pain
Decreased pulse rate	Tremors	Nausea
Respiratory problems:	Rigidity	Heartburn
• Shortness of breath	Spasm	Vomiting
• Difficulty getting air	Fidgeting	Urinary tract problems:
• Pressured chest	Pacing	• Pressure to urinate
• Shallow breath	Strained face	• Increased frequency of
• Lump in throat	Unsteadiness	urination
• Choking sensation	Generalized weakness	Skin problems:
• Gasping	Wobbly legs	• Flushed face
• Spasm of bronchi	Clumsy motions	• Pale face
		• Sweating
		• Hot or cold spells
		• Itching

Affective	Cognitive	Behavioral
Impatient	Anticipating worst	Restlessness
Uneasy	Fear of failure	Watching for signs of danger
Nervous	Irritability	Avoidance
Tense	Agitation	Impaired coordination
Anxious	Lack of focus	Hyperventilation
Fearful	Irrational thoughts	Speech difficulty
Apprehensive	Feeling like mind is going crazy	Postural collapse
Frightened	Hypervigilance	Momentary blindness
Alarmed	Inability to recall important	Hallucination
Terrified	things	Phobic behavior
Jittery	Confusion	

(continues)

Affective	Cognitive	Behavioral
Feeling tense and jumpy	Inability to control thinking Difficulty in concentration Difficulty in focusing Distractability Thought blocking Tunnel vision Lack of confidence in one's own skills and abilities Cognitive distortion	

Anxiety Levels and Their Effect on Physical, Affective,

Anxiety level	Physical	Emotional	Perceptual	Cognitive	Behavioral
Mild	Slightly elevated heart rate	Feels safe and comfortable	Slight widening of the perceptual field Observation is sharper than before.	Alert Attentive	Client is aware of the situation Grasping of understanding is better Client can recognize and name the anxiety. This is normal anxiety experience, that motivates client on daily basis. It also helps in the problem-solving process and learning.

(continues)

Anxiety level	Physical	Emotional	Perceptual	Cognitive	Behavioral
Moderate	Shortness of breath Mild gastric symptoms Facial twitches Trembling lips	Feeling uneasy Anxious	Narrowing of the perceptual field Does not notice what is going around unless attention is drawn by others	Selective inattention Can attend to task if directed to do so Able to sustain attention to a particular task Selectively inattentive to task outside of focal area	Sees, hears, and grasps less than before Learning can be facilitated by another individual's assistance. Client is able to state "I am feeling anxious now."
Severe	Frequent shortness of breath Increased heart rates Elevated blood pressure Dry mouth Upset stomach Anorexia Diarrhea Constipation	Fearful facial expression Anxiousness increased	Extreme narrowing of perceptual field Distorted inferences due to inability to observe the situation clearly	Difficulty in problem solving Difficulty in organization Attention is focused on small area of a given situation. Tendency to disassociate, unable to see what is going on outside of focus area. Unable to focus even if another suggests it.	Sees, hears, and grasps far less than previous level. Body trembling Tense muscles Exaggerated startle movement Inability to relax Difficulty in falling asleep Inability to name anxiety Problem-solving ability is greatly reduced.

(continues)

Panic	Shortness of breath	Feeling of losing control	Perceptual field completely disrupted	Fear of dying	Poor motor coordination
	Hyperventilation	Feeling of dying		Derealization	Agitation
	Choking, smothering sensation	Expression of terror		Depersonalization	Involuntary body movements
	Sweating	Fear of open spaces		Concern about having another panic attack	Trembling or shaking
	Hypotension			Disorganized thought process	Hyperactivity/Unsteadyness
	Dizziness				Inability to speak or act
	Fainting				Avoidance behavior
	Feeling of passing out; feeling dizzy, lightheaded, or faint				This is an extreme form of anxiety.
	Chest pain				Disorganized behavior and thinking
	Chest pressure				Can be dangerous to self or others due to distorted thought process
	Chills				
	Hot flashes				
	Nausea				
	Abdominal discomfort				
	Paresthesias, numbness, or tingling sensations				

Sources: Peplau, 1963; Fountain & Fletcher, 2003, p. 273; Boyd, 2008, p. 393.

Perceptual, and Cognitive Fields

Nursing diagnoses are formulated according to the identified client's problems and are based on the assessment and analysis of the data. Make sure while formulating the nursing diagnosis that you utilize the terminology according to the standard language recommended by the North American Nursing Diagnosis Association (1999) for development of nursing diagnosis. (Jakopac & Patel, 2009; O'Brien, Kennedy & Ballard, 2008)

NURSING INTERVENTIONS

Purpose: To reduce anxiety

Nursing interventions need to address the biologic, pharmacologic, psychological, sociological, and spiritual needs of the client by implementing therapeutic communication and therapeutic relationship building skills.

Client's needs	Nursing diagnosis/problem	Nursing interventions
Biological needs	Sleep deprivation	Monitor client's sleep pattern, and number of hours client sleeps during night or day.
		Discuss with the client the importance of bedtime routine.
		Educate client about foods and caffeinated beverages that may interfere with sleep; caffeine is a stimulant with a half-life of 8 to 14 hours depending upon amount and number of caffeinated beverages client consumed.
		Instruct client to avoid heavy foods at bedtime.
		Spend time with client, encouraging them to discuss the anxiety-producing situation and its relationship to sleep.
		Encourage client to attend support group to verbalize their feelings and thoughts about anxiety and how they deal with them. Attending support groups can assist client in learning new coping skills and in providing a ventilation opportunity to share and express feelings and thoughts to group.
		Decrease environmental stimuli for clients at bedtime such as dimming lights, lowering environmental noise in nurse's station, being consistent with unit rules for the turn-down time for TV and dayroom use at bedtime.
		Teach client importance of participating in relaxation activities before bedtime and be aware of overexertion as that can lead client to feel tired and restless, which can impair sleep.
		Provide sleeping medication if ordered as routine or prn if client asks for it.

REFERENCES

American Psychiatric Association (APA) (2007). *Diagnostic and statistical manual of mental disorders-IV-TR* (4th ed.). Arlington, VA: American Psychiatric Publishing Co.

Antai-Otong, D. (2003). *Psychiatric nursing clinical companion.* Clifton Park, NY: Delmar Learning.

Boyd, M. A. (2008). *Psychiatric nursing: Contemporary practice* (4th ed.). Philadelphia, PA: Lippincott, Williams, & Wilkins.

Fountain, K. L. (2003). *Mental health nursing* (5th ed.). Upper Saddle River, NJ: Pearson Education, Inc.

Helpguide (2010). *Understand, prevent and resolve life's challenges.* Retrieved from http://www.helpguide.org/

Jakopac, K. & Patel, S. (2009). *Psychiatric mental health case studies and care plans.* Sudbury, MA: Jones and Bartlett.

National Institute of Mental Health (NIMH) (2009). *The numbers count: Mental disorders in America.* Retrieved from http://www.nimh.nih.gov/health/publications/the-numbers-count-mental-disorders-in-america/index.shtml#Panic

North American Nursing Diagnosis Association (1999). *Nursing diagnosis: Definitions and classification, 1999–2000.* Philadelphia, PA: Author.

O'Brien, P. G., Kennedy, W. Z., & Ballard, K. A. (2008). *Psychiatric mental health nursing, An introduction to theory and practice.* Sudbury, MA: Jones and Bartlett.

Peplau, H. E. (1963). Level of anxiety. In M. Schultz & S. L. Vidbeck (2002), *Lippincott's manual of psychiatric nursing care plan* (6th ed.). Philadelphia, PA: Lippincott.

Pick, M. (2007). *Anxiety in women—causes, symptoms, and natural relief.* Retrieved from http://www.womentowomen.com/depressionanxietyandmood/anxiety.aspx

Sadock B. J., & Sadock V. A. (2008). *Concise textbook of clinical psychiatry* (3rd ed.). Philadelphia, PA: Wolters Kluwer/Lippincott, Williams, & Wilkins.

CHAPTER 8

Major Depression

Kim A. Jakopac

OBJECTIVES

The nursing student will be able to:

1. Recognize signs and symptoms that meet DSM-IV-TR criteria for major depression
2. Be familiar with common medical illnesses that can cause or exacerbate signs and symptoms of major depression
3. Perform a biopsychosocial nursing assessment or intake assessment of clients experiencing signs and symptoms of major depression
4. Identify and implement nursing interventions for clients experiencing signs and symptoms of major depression
5. Implement care for clients receiving electroconvulsant therapy (ECT)
6. Assess discharge planning needs of clients admitted with a diagnosis of major depression
7. Discuss special considerations regarding children/adolescents and elderly clients

KEY TERMS

Anergia
Anhedonia
Behavior modification
Bereavement
Cognitive behavioral therapy (CBT)
Electroconvulsant therapy (ECT)
Hypnosis
Interpersonal therapy (IPT)
Magical thinking
Major depression

Mood
Motivational enhancement therapy
Psychoanalysis
Psychodrama
Rational emotive behavioral therapy (REBT)
Reality therapy
Self-care
Supportive therapy
Unipolar

Major depression is an illness included in the American Psychiatric Association's (APA) *Diagnostic and Statistical Manual of Mental Disorders* (4th ed.), text revision (DSM-IV-TR) (APA, 2000, pp. 369–376, 404, 412–413). A large number of people worldwide experience symptoms of major depression, and there has been an increased effort to identify clients in primary care. See Chapter 9 for information related to bipolar disorders (hypomania) or mixed mood episodes.

SIGNS AND SYMPTOMS

At least four signs or symptoms of the APA criteria for major depression or unipolar depression must occur for a period of at least 2 weeks to meet the criteria for a diagnosis. The exception is suicidal or homicidal thoughts, which meet criteria for diagnosis without the 2-week qualifier. Signs and symptoms include:

- Suicidal or homicidal ideations (thoughts)
- Anhedonia
- Anergia
- Sleep disturbance
- Appetite disturbance
- Feelings of worthlessness or inappropriate guilt
- Decreased ability to concentrate
- Psychomotor retardation or agitation
- Somatic symptoms

Additional symptoms include feelings of hopelessness, helplessness, and powerlessness, as well as problems functioning on a day-to-day basis, problems with primary relationships or problems functioning at work or school (APA, 2000, pp. 369, 375, 376; Keltner, Schwecke, & Bostrom, 2007, pp. 369, 370). The client may feel a lack of control over their life, expect that the future will be as bad or even worse than it is at the present time (negativism), or feel angry or irritable (Varcarolis, Carson, & Shoemaker, 2006, pp. 335, 336). Clients may delay seeking treatment due to the stigma of mental illness until they have lost much time from work and are in danger of becoming unemployed or become suicidal. According to research by Halter (2004), many people think that the stigma regarding depression and the treatment of depression contributes to the "30,000 suicides" occurring in the United States each year (Varcarolis, Carson, & Shoemaker, 2006, p. 337). If a client experiences additional symptoms of psychosis, they are given a diagnosis of major depression with psychosis or psychotic features. Psychosis is not a sign of a typical diagnosis of depression (see Chapters 11 and 13).

Some clients develop depression as an adverse effect of medication (e.g., chemotherapy/antineoplastics) or as a reaction to severe losses, high levels of stress eliciting a greater than normal endocrine system response, chronic pain, or following the diagnosis of medical chronic or terminal medical illnesses (Kelly, 2007, pp. 1, 22; Keltner, Schwecke, & Bostrom, 2007, p. 380; Mohr, 2009, p. 856). Any client who has experienced severe losses, has acute or chronic pain, or has been diagnosed with chronic or terminal illnesses should be assessed for possible depression. Severe nutritional deficiencies can also cause symptoms of depression. Signs and symptoms of major depression are not due to other problems such as bereavement or illnesses such as chemical dependency, dementia, or medical illnesses. If symptoms are secondary to medical illnesses, the diagnosis will include the phrase "secondary to" as part of the entire diagnosis. According to the APA (2000), the average age of onset of major depression is the mid-20s (p. 372), although symptoms may be seen as early as late adolescence or even in childhood. Major depression occurs more often in women than men.

Pregnant women diagnosed with major depression have an increased risk of having an exacerbation of symptoms in the postpartum period, and nonpregnant women have an increased risk during their premenstrual period (O'Brien, Kennedy, & Ballard, 2008, p. 323). Postpartum depression occurs during the first 4 weeks following childbirth and is characterized by the symptoms of major depression. This condition affects the mother's ability to properly care for her infant and can interfere with normal parent–child bonding. In postpartum psychosis, psychotic symptoms are present along with mood symptoms, and there is increased danger for the infant's well-being. The mother should not be left alone with the infant while experiencing this condition. These conditions are much different than the postpartum "blues" that frequently occurs within the first 7 to 10 days following childbirth and includes symptoms of irritability, anxiety, and crying interspersed with periods of normalcy (Keltner, Schwecke, & Bostrom, 2007, p. 371).

According to Fontaine (2009), "The inheritability of major depression is 40 to 50%. The more severe the depression, the stronger the genetic link" (p. 303). For more information please refer to a general psychiatric-mental health nursing textbook for information on the various theoretical etiologies of major depression including neurobiologic or neurochemical, cognitive, psychosocial, intrapersonal, learning, and sociocultural (Keltner, Schwecke, & Bostrom, pp. 375–379; O'Brien, Kennedy, & Ballard, 2008, pp. 312–313; Fontaine, 2009, pp. 302–306).

Major depression is also different from a grief response, which is a subjective response elicited by the actual, perceived, or anticipated loss of anything of value, including relationships or retirement (see **Table 8-1**). A grieving response or mourning is adaptive unless it is delayed or unresolved. Research with terminally ill clients by

Table 8-1 Comparison of Grief and Depression	
Grief	**Depression**
Response to identified loss	Signs and symptoms occur for at least a 2-week period (except SI); not always an identified event/loss
Intact self-esteem	Disturbed self-esteem
More open expressions of anger	Suppression or indirect expressions of anger
"Good" days and "Bad" days	Persistent low, depressed mood
Able to experience moments of pleasure	Anhedonia
Responds to social contact	Burdened by social contact, prefer isolation
Time limited; improves with time	Persistent and can become worse
Not suicidal	Suicidal thoughts common; plan, attempts
May have transient somatic symptoms	Chronic somatic symptoms
Dreams about the deceased	Hallucinations, delusions if psychosis present
May experience poor concentration	Reports concentration and memory disturbances
Typically resolves without antidepressants	In most cases antidepressants needed to resolve
Maintains some feelings of hope	Prevalent hopelessness, helplessness, or powerlessness
Relates depressed feelings directly to the loss	Inappropriate guilt

Kübler-Ross identified five stages of behaviors and feelings experienced by clients responding to actual or perceived loss (Townsend, 2009, pp. 20–21). During the reaction to the death of a loved one (bereavement), a client may experience some symptoms similar to major depression, but a diagnosis of major depression is not given unless the symptoms are still present 2 months after the loss. Cultural differences must also be taken into account when the client is being diagnosed (APA, 2000, pp. 740–741).

COMMON MEDICAL ILLNESSES

As previously stated, some clients develop depression as a result of high levels of stress eliciting a greater than normal endocrine system response, as a reaction to chronic pain, or following the diagnosis of medical chronic or terminal medical illnesses or as adverse effects of medication (e.g., chemotherapy). Medical illnesses, nutritional deficiencies, and adverse effects of medications that are commonly associated with psychiatric-mental illnesses related to mood may be found in **Tables 8-2** and **8-3** (Varcarolis, Carson, & Shoemaker, 2006, pp. 328, 332; Keltner, Schwecke, & Bostrom, 2007, p. 380; O'Brien, Kennedy, & Ballard, 2008, pp. 254–255; Mohr, 2009, p. 856). Many substances/chemicals can cause signs and symptoms of depression, including alcohol, illegal drugs, misuse of prescription medications, or metal poisoning. The psychiatric-mental health (PMH) nurse should be aware of these other factors in order to obtain a holistic clinical picture of the client and thus provide high quality nursing care.

Table 8-2	**Common Medical Illnesses Causing or Exacerbating Signs and Symptoms of Depression**
Neurologic	Cerebrovascular accident (CVA)
	Head trauma
	Brain tumor
	Dementias
	Multiple sclerosis (MS)
	Huntington's chorea
	Parkinson's disease
	Seizure disorders
	CNS infections—encephalitis, HIV/AIDS
	Neurosyphilis
	Migraine headaches
Endocrine	Hypothyroidism
	Cushing's syndrome
	Addison's disease
	Diabetes mellitus (DM)
	Hypoglycemia
	Hyper- or hypoparathyroidism
	Pancreatic tumors
Cardiopulmonary/Hematologic	Myocardial infarction (MI)
	Congestive heart failure (CHF)
	Anemia
	Chronic obstructive pulmonary diseases (COPD)

(continues)

Table 8-2	**Common Medical Illnesses Causing or Exacerbating Signs and Symptoms of Depression (continued)**
Metabolic/Nutritional	Electrolyte imbalances Folate deficiency B12 deficiency Metal poisoning Uremia
Collagen Vascular/ Inflammatory	Systemic lupus erythematosus (SLE) Rheumatoid arthritis (RA) Polymyalgia rheumatica Temporal arteritis Sjogren's disease Ulcerative colitis
Infectious diseases	CNS infections—encephalitis, HIV/AIDS Tuberculosis (TB) Infectious mononucleosis Hepatitis C
Other	Cancers Sleep apnea Fibromyalgia—rheumatologic disorder Chronic fatigue syndrome Sexual dysfunction

Table 8-3	**Medications with Possible Adverse Affects on Mood/Depression**
Neurologic/Psychiatric	amantadine (Symmetrel), anticholinesterases—physostigmine (Antilirium), edrophonium (Tensilon), baclofen (Lioresal), barbiturates—phenobarbital (Luminal), mephobarbital (Mebaral), pentobartital (Nebutal), benzodiazepines—bromocriptine (Parlodel), chloral hydrate (Somnote), disulfiram (Antabuse), ethosuximide (Zarontin), levodopa (L-dopa), phenytoin (Dilantin)
Cardiovascular	clonidine (Catepres), digoxin/digitalis (Lanoxin), guanethidine (Ismelin), methyldopa (Aldomet), propranolol (Inderal), reserpine (Serpalan)

(continues)

Table 8-3	Medications with Possible Adverse Affects on Mood/Depression *(continued)*
Antibiotic/Antifungal	ampicillin (Polycillin), griseofluvin (Grisactin), metronidazole (Flagyl), nalidixic acid (NegGram), trimethoprim (TMP)
Analgesic/Anti-inflammatory	opiates, corticosteroids, indomethacin (Indocin), sulindac (Clinoril)
Antineoplastic	asparaginase (Elspar), azathioprine (Imuran), bleomycin (Blenoxane), hexamethylamine, vincristine (Oncovin), vinblastine (Velban)
Gastrointestinal	cimetadine (Tagamet), ranitidine (Zantac)
Other	alcohol, oral contraceptives, withdrawal from stimulants

(Adapted from Varcarolis, Carson, & Shoemaker, 2006, p. 328)

BIOPSYCHOSOCIAL NURSING ASSESSMENT

Information on the biopsychosocial nursing assessment or intake assessment is included in Chapter 4. In this chapter we will focus more on the specific assessment of a client who has already been diagnosed with major depression or is suspected of being depressed. As previously stated in Chapter 4, there are several screening tools that are frequently used to augment the assessment. The following screening tools may be used for a client with signs and symptoms of major depression. The signs and symptoms of bipolar disorders (see Chapter 10) may be missed and a more accurate diagnosis delayed if this information is not included.

- Hamilton Depression Scale (HDS)
- Beck Depression Inventory (BDI)
- Zung Self Rating Depression Scale
- Mood Disorder Questionnaire (MDQ)
- Edinburgh Postnatal Depression Scale (EPDS)
- SAD PERSONS Scale
- CAGE for Alcohol Abuse
- Holmes and Rahe Social Readjustment Scale
- The Hassles and Uplifts Scale
- Life Experiences Survey (LES)
- WHO Quality of Life Instrument
- Young Mania Rating Scale (YMRS)

Biopsychosocial Nursing Assessment Form

Section I

1. Vital signs
   a. Within normal limits (WNL)?
   b. If BP is elevated, is the client anxious, experiencing an adverse medication re-action, or is there a medical history of hypertension?
   c. If the BP is low, is the client dehydrated or experiencing a side-effect of med-ication? Is the client experiencing orthostatic hypotension?
   d. Is the client exhibiting tachycardia, and is it due to anxiety, adverse effects of medication, or a medical condition?
   e. Is the client exhibiting bradycardia, and is it due to adverse effects of medica-tion or is the client an athlete?
   f. If respirations are abnormal, is there a medical history of respiratory disease?
   g. Are any vital sign elevations due to drug or alcohol withdrawal?
   h. Do any vital sign abnormalities point to an infectious or inflammatory process?
2. Weight
   a. Is the client's weight appropriate for height? Underweight? Overweight/Obese?
   b. Does the client report any change in weight? How much and over what pe-riod of time? Unintended weight loss or gain of more than 5% of body weight in 1 month in adults or failure to attain expected weight gains in chil-dren is significant for problems.
   c. Any change in appetite?
3. Physical/mental disabilities/Physical deformities
   a. If physical/mental disabilities or physical deformities are present, what effect do these have on the client's mood and general outlook on life?
   b. Is the client coping with any disabilities/deformities, or are these disabilities/deformities hindering the client's ability to function on a day-to-day basis?
   c. Did the client bring all their sensory aids or prosthesis to the hospital?
4. Language/Education/Racial/Ethnic
   a. Is there a need to obtain an interpreter?
   b. Are there any barriers to learning? Typically a client who is depressed may re-port problems with concentration and memory. The client may need more time to think before answering questions, but should not be disoriented or confused. If symptoms of psychosis are present, the client will have more dif-ficulty learning (see also Section IV of this form).

5. Health insurance
   a. Does the client have sufficient health insurance for treatment needs?
   b. Is the client uninsured? Underinsured? Does the client have health insurance coverage for only physical problems, but lacks mental health benefits?
   c. Does the client need a social service referral?
6. Admission status
   a. Does the client understand their rights and whether they are on a voluntary or involuntary admission?
   b. Was the client given a copy of their rights?
   c. Is the client willing to allow family/friends to have information about them and sign the agency form indicating this?
7. Chief complaint
   a. Does the client understand the reason for hospitalization? The client's own words should be documented. If the client is too depressed to respond, this should be documented and include the reason provided by anyone who has accompanied the client or the psychiatrist.
   b. Does the client's understanding of the reason for hospitalization agree with the real reason for hospitalization or not? If the client is in denial of their need for hospitalization or is experiencing psychosis, the reason given may be very different, even bizarre, and will give the interviewer some information as to the client's mental state.

Section II

1. Symptom onset/duration/frequency/changes
   a. What specific symptoms does the client report, and when did they start? If the client reports suicidal thoughts or a history of a suicide attempt, refer to section V of the biopsychosocial nursing assessment in Chapter 4 and in this chapter. The client may have admitted to suicidal or homicidal thoughts in the emergency room, but may state that these no longer exist when you interview them. Many clients feel safe in the hospital and, therefore, are no longer suicidal at the time you are assessing them. It is still vitally important to continue to complete a full suicide assessment (include homicidal thoughts and plan) and obtain at least a verbal no-self-harm/harm to others contract, because the thoughts may return, and the client would be a danger to themselves or others. Depressed clients more typically report suicidal thoughts.
   b. Has the client experienced these symptoms the majority of at least a 2-week period? Is there a specific time of the day that the symptoms seem to be the most intense?

    c. Did a specific situation or event occur just prior to or around the same time the symptoms started?

    d. Do the symptoms seem to be worse related to different seasons of the year (e.g., late fall, winter, early spring)? Seasonal affective disorder (SAD) includes symptoms of major depression, but the symptoms worsen when there is less available sunlight during certain times of the year and improve when there is more available sunlight.

    e. Has the client noticed that anything makes the symptoms worse or helps relieve their symptoms? Have they tried anything to help relieve these symptoms including complementary/alternative methods?

    f. Does the client have any medical problems already listed on Axis III or any additional information that may not already be documented (see Tables 7-1 and 7-2)? Is there a new medical problem developing that will need further assessment (see sections VIII and X of the biopsychosocial nursing assessment in Chapter 4). There is a potential legal liability issue concerning psychiatric-mental health clients not receiving care for their existing medical problems or the identification and treatment of a new illness.

    g. List all allergies. Is the client working with any chemicals or potential neurotoxins in their work environment that could affect the CNS?

    h. Is anyone who has accompanied the client able to provide additional information? The client may be having difficulty concentrating and could have possibly forgotten important information that the accompanying family member, friend, or neighbor may be able to supply.

2. Cultural factors

    The PMH nurse should also be aware that the client's cultural group may have a different way of expressing psychiatric symptoms. The APA (2000) recognizes the importance of cultural factors and mentions recurring patterns of symptoms/behaviors that do not fit DSM-IV-TR criteria for specific diagnoses, cause distress for the person experiencing the symptoms, and a client's use of culturally specific language to describe their symptoms (APA, 2000, Appendix 1, pp. 897–903; Keltner, Schwecke, & Bostrom, 2007, pp. 168–169). Some clients may consult a shaman (traditional spiritual, folk healer) before seeking help from Western healthcare providers (e.g., Native Americans, African Americans). Identified cultural terms and symptoms related to feeling depressed include the following:

    a. Native American clients may describe depression as heart pain or feeling heart broken. They may also use the term "ghost sickness." Ghost sickness is described as a preoccupation with death, bad dreams, feelings of danger, loss of appetite, fear, anxiety, feeling worthless, feeling faint or losing consciousness, dizziness, confusion, or a sense of suffocation.

b. Hispanic clients may say they have lost their soul due to *mal ojo* (evil eye); report lethargy, sleep and appetite disturbances; and report somatic complaints.

c. Latino clients in the U.S. or Mexico may use the term *susto*, meaning fright or soul loss. Reported symptoms include appetite and sleep disturbance; low motivation, sadness, worthlessness, and problems with social and occupational roles.

d. Korean clients may describe a folk syndrome called *hwa-byung* or *wool-hwa-byung*, believed to be due to suppression of anger or "anger syndrome." Symptoms include insomnia, fatigue, panic, fear of impending death, depressed/sad affect, indigestion, anorexia, heart palpitations, generalized aches/pains, or the feeling of a mass around the stomach.

Section III

1. DSM-IV-TR admission diagnosis
   a. Does the client have more than one disorder on Axis I–III? Multiple problems will have an impact on the client's coping abilities, quality of life, ability to adhere to treatment regimens, and prognosis.
   b. Are there multiple psychosocial stressors on Axis IV?
   c. The GAF score is important for the information it provides related to the client's overall ability to function. Clients who are suicidal or homicidal will have much lower scores (i.e., range of 10–20/100)
   d. The client's prognosis will be affected by their insight, judgment, number of Axis I–III diagnoses, past ability to adhere to treatment, access to outpatient services, type of health insurance or lack of health insurance, coping abilities, knowledge of diagnoses and medications, and the availability of social support.
   e. Is the client taking medications regularly and as prescribed? If not, what reasons do they give? Sometimes clients cannot afford medications, but are too embarrassed to admit it. Transportation to obtain medications may be a problem if there is no pharmacy to deliver medications to clients who do not drive or have another way to pick up their medications. Clients may stop taking medications due to sexual side-effects and be too embarrassed to admit this. Also, occasionally some clients may experience adverse effects or "strange" thoughts, including suicidal thoughts or increased aggressive feelings, and stop taking medication rather than report this. Does the client temporarily stop taking medications to go out drinking with friends or family because they know they should not drink alcohol while taking their medications? It is *extremely important* to know what specific reasons clients have for stopping medications and address these reasons during the hospitalization and in discharge planning.

    f. Is the client taking medications that are contraindicated to be taken together?

    g. Has the client experienced adverse effects when taking psychiatric and medical medications together?

Section IV

1. Appearance
   a. Does the client appear to be their stated age, younger, or older? Clients who have chronic illnesses, experience chronic stress or abuse chemicals/substances may appear older than their stated age.
   b. Is there evidence of not attending to personal hygiene/ADLs? Casual, but clean clothing is perfectly acceptable, but soiled, foul smelling, or inappropriate clothing shows nonattendance to ADLs.
   c. Does the client admit to problems attending to personal hygiene/ADLs and what reason do they give? A client who is depressed may find it exhausting to perform ADLs/personal hygiene.

2. Attitude/psychomotor activity/eye contact
   a. Is the client cooperative, aware of their problem and seeking help voluntarily? This client will greatly benefit from being a partner in their treatment.
   b. Did the client agree to come into the hospital voluntarily only because they felt they did not have a choice and would otherwise be involuntarily committed? This client will be less trusting of the nurse and other mental health staff and possibly less cooperative. It may take longer to develop a therapeutic nurse–client relationship with them. This client is less aware of their problems, having some difficulty deciding what is in their best interest, and less aware of the need for treatment, but can receive the benefits of treatment if they accept what is offered. In time the client's attitude may become more positive and cooperative.
   c. Has the client been admitted on an involuntary commitment? This client may be aware that they are having problems, but refuses any help offered or may deny the existence of any problems or statements made to harm themselves or others. The client may deny that their actions were actually a suicide attempt. This client can still benefit from treatment and a therapeutic nurse–client relationship, but it may take much longer due to the client's denial of symptoms, trust issues, poor insight, poor judgment, possible uncooperativeness and refusal of treatment, and additional problems with thought processes if psychosis is also present.
   d. Is the client able to sit and calmly talk to the nurse? Displaying psychomotor retardation or agitation? Either extreme may be seen in clients with symp-

toms of major depression. Some clients may experience anxiety as part of their depressed mood. Other clients experience symptoms that meet DSM-IV-TR criteria for an anxiety disorder (see Chapter 7).

  e. Is the client able to maintain eye contact during the interview? Poor or fair eye contact would be a common sign in a client who is depressed. Is the client scanning the environment as if looking for someone or something; staring? The client may be experiencing paranoia or hallucinations.

3. Mood
  a. Does the client's stated mood match the affect you observe?
4. Affect
  a. Does the client's affect that you observe match the mood they report, or is it incongruent?
5. Cognition/orientation
  a. Is the client oriented in all spheres of orientation or only certain spheres? If disorientation is present, is there an Axis III diagnosis (e.g., head injury, cardiopulmonary illness, hypo/hyperglycemia) that it may be related to? Or is this a new symptom that needs to be reported?
  b. Is there any change in level of consciousness in the beginning of the assessment or at any time during the assessment? Is there an Axis III diagnosis (e.g., head injury, cardiopulmonary illness, hypo/hyperglycemia) that it may be related to? Or is this a new symptom that needs to be reported? Is the change due to alcohol intoxication, illegal drug use, or an unreported overdose?
  c. Is the client having difficulty completing a thought, following directions or repeating five digits forward and backward?
  d. Does the client display any problems with short-term or remote memory? Usually if the client is given additional time to think or cues before answering, their memory will be less impaired than initially reported. Does it seem as if the client is making up information? Did anyone accompany the client who can validate this information?
  e. Is the client having difficulty performing calculations, interpreting abstract proverbs, or identifying similarities/differences between common objects?
  f. Does the client know who the current president of the United States is?
6. Speech pattern
  a. A client who is depressed may speak softly, possibly in a monotone, at a slower rate than normal, and their responses may be delayed, but they should speak in a logical manner. If there is illogical, incoherent, or unintelligible speech, the client could be experiencing some psychosis, a medical problem, or be under the influence of drugs.

7. Thought processes
    a. The client may be indecisive, have decreased ability to solve problems, poor judgment related to difficulty concentrating, and decreased rate/speed of their thought processes as a result of major depression. A client who is experiencing a great deal of stress or psychotic thinking may demonstrate thought blocking.
    b. Preoccupations with unworthiness, guilt, or ruminations about past failings or current inability to meet obligations due to illness are not considered to be illogical unless they are of delusional proportion (e.g., thinks they are personally responsible for world poverty). For further assessment of psychosis, see Chapters 11 and 13.
    c. Has the client been using alcohol, illegal drugs, or misusing prescription medications?
8. Thought content
    a. A client who is depressed demonstrates themes of hopelessness, helplessness, powerlessness, worthlessness, unworthiness, inappropriate guilt, and negativism. They may have suicidal thoughts and plans and may have attempted suicide (see Chapter 9). They may also have feelings and thoughts of harming someone else due to focusing their feelings outwards rather than inwards. Refer to a general psychiatric-mental health nursing textbook for information on legal–ethical implications regarding "duty to warn" (*Tarosoff* v *The Regents of the University of California*).
    b. Many clients report somatic problems and minimize their feelings. They may even minimize previous statements of suicidal thinking or a suicide attempt. Clients should be assessed for passive suicidal thoughts and behaviors (see Chapter 9).
    c. If psychosis is present, see Chapters 11 and 13 for further assessment.
9. Insight/Judgment/Impulse control
    a. Is the client aware of their illness or do they deny or minimize symptoms?
    b. Is the client aware of their illness, but denies a need for treatment at this time?
    c. Does the client exhibit normal judgment in commonly encountered situations?
    d. Is the client making future plans? If yes, this is a positive indicator for a good prognosis.
    e. Does the client report impulse control problems?
10. Psychomotor function
    a. Disturbances need to be able to be observed by others.

b. Examples of psychomotor agitation include restlessness, pacing, or handwringing.

c. Examples of psychomotor retardation include slow body movements; increased pauses before answering questions; decreased volume, amount, or variety of the content of speech; muteness (see also item #6 in this section of the assessment).

d. Is there evidence of catatonia?

11. Motivation
   a. Has the client agreed to receive treatment voluntarily or do they feel forced into treatment?
   b. Does the client have a supportive family?
   c. Does the client have an understanding, supportive employer or are they being threatened with the loss of a job?
   d. Does the client have any pending legal charges or court hearings in the near future?
   e. Has the client been court-ordered into treatment?

Section V

1. Suicide/homicide/domestic violence risk
   a. Does the client currently admit to suicidal/homicidal thoughts or were they thinking of suicide/homicide prior to coming to the hospital?
   b. Does the client admit to passive suicidal thoughts or behavior if the answer was "no" to question "a"?
   c. Does the client have a plan and access to the means to carry out this plan? What is the degree of lethality if the client attempts to carry out this plan?
   d. If the client denies any thoughts or plans, does someone else (i.e., family, friends, neighbor, employer, coworker, etc.) have first-hand knowledge of the client's suicidal/homicidal threats?
   e. Does another member of the healthcare team have information related to any suicidal/homicidal thoughts or plans?
   f. Has the client attempted suicide prior to coming to the hospital? Is there a history of past attempts?
   g. Is the client able to at least verbally contract with staff to not harm themselves or others? Refer to the individual facility policy regarding verbal or written no-harm contracts.
   h. What level of observation should the client be placed on at this time? If able to contract at least verbally to not harm self or others, then safety checks

every 15 minutes should be adequate. If unable to contract, then the client will need to be placed on one-to-one or constant observation.

    i. What does the client do when they become angry? How do they express it? If in healthy, adaptive ways then there is no domestic violence risk; if in unhealthy, maladaptive ways, then there is an increased risk.

    j. Does the client currently have legal charges against them? Any history of legal charges?

    k. Has the client ever been on the receiving end of physical, verbal, or emotional violence? Is this currently happening to them?

    l. Does the client feel safe or unsafe in their current living situation? If no, is the client willing to speak to a social worker/case manger? If there are minor age children or elderly family members in the same living situation, the nurse will have to notify the social worker/case manager to be sure the situation is safe.

Section VI

1. Development
   a. What is the client's current stage of development according to Erickson, based on biologic age? Are they on the positive or negative side of the developmental task (e.g., intimacy versus isolation) (see also Appendix B)?
   b. Where is the client developmentally according to Freud? Piaget (see also Appendix C and Appendix D)?
   c. Has the client regressed to an earlier stage of development? Which one and according to what developmental theory?

Section VII

1. Psychiatric history/treatment
   a. Has the client ever been previously diagnosed with a psychiatric-mental illness and if so what was the diagnosis?
   b. Where and when did they receive treatment?
   c. Was the treatment inpatient, outpatient, or both? Was the treatment effective?
   d. Did the client ever receive ECT, and was it effective?
   e. Is the client aware of any problems their birth mother experienced during pregnancy or during labor and delivery? Anything that would affect oxygen supply, nutrition, or the physical safety of the fetus (e.g., trauma, accidents) during the prenatal and perinatal periods could affect brain development.

Section VIII

1. Medical-Surgical history/treatment
   a. Is the client currently being treated for a medical illness and by whom? Either the client's primary care provider (PCP) will continue to treat the client during the inpatient period or another medical physician on the hospital staff will do so.
   b. Has the client ever been hospitalized for any medical-surgical reason? Where and when?
   c. Any outpatient procedures? Where and when?

Section IX

1. Current/past chemical use/dependency
   a. Any current or past chemical use and age when started?
   b. Any current or past IV drug use?
   c. Preferred substance? What was the last substance the client used?
   d. Usual amount used? What was the last amount used and when? Try to obtain specific information related to amount used and time. Inform the client that you will be able to provide the best possible care if you know exactly what, how much, and when their last substance use was. The nurse also needs to be able to anticipate when the client will begin experiencing withdrawal symptoms.
   e. What type of symptoms does the client usually experience when they stop drinking/using? Has the client ever experienced delirium tremens (DTs)?
   f. What is the longest period of time the client has been chemical free? This shows the client has achieved this in the past and can do so again.
   g. Does the client have a sponsor they can call to let them know they are being hospitalized? The sponsor will be an ally in helping reinforce the need to continue treatment.

Section X

1. Review of systems
   a. Does the client report any problems?
   b. Is the client currently under the care of a physician for these problems and who is that physician? Many clients with psychiatric symptoms have comorbid illnesses including thyroid disorders, cardiac diseases including hypertension, diabetes mellitus, and seizure disorders.
   c. Are there new problems and is this the first time the client is reporting these?

d. Has the client lost or gained weight and during what amount of time has the weight change occurred?

e. Does the client report difficulty getting out of bed in the morning even when sleeping 8 or more hours? Difficulty falling asleep? Awakening in the middle of the night with difficulty getting back to sleep? Awakening too early and not being able to get back to sleep? Symptoms that would not be related to depression would include if the client gets up at night to use the bathroom due to drinking too much fluid before going to bed or do they have symptoms of an infection or, in males, an enlarged prostate?

f. Does the client have acute or chronic pain? How is it being treated?

g. If the client is a female within childbearing age, is there any possibility of her being pregnant? Has she had a tubal ligation or hysterectomy (when)? While some psychiatrists may cautiously prescribe some selective serotonin reuptake inhibitors (SSRIs), many medications prescribed for Axis I and III disorders have the potential to cause harm to a developing fetus (e.g., paroxetine (Paxil)) or the effects are unknown during the first trimester of pregnancy.

h. Has the client had an ECG/EKG? Clients age 40 years or older, or younger clients with a medical indication, usually are ordered an ECG/EKG on admission. Is there a previous one for comparison from a previous medical record or outpatient source?

i. Are there any abnormal findings on physical examination? Any abnormal cardiac or cranial nerve assessment should be reported and assessed further.

Section XI

1. Family history
   a. Is the client aware of their family's psychiatric, chemical dependency, or medical-surgical history?
   b. If there is a history of psychiatric, chemical dependency, thyroid, or neurologic problems in the family, who was affected?
   c. If a family member was treated with psychiatric medications or ECT, what specifically was effective and what was not? Because of genetics it is important not only to know if a family member has been ill, but also what treatment was effective because it may help decrease the amount of time it takes to find a medication that works well for the client.

Section XII

1. Social/occupation/legal/education

a. Does the client admit to any problems with relationships and if so with whom? Did the problems begin before they became aware of the symptoms of depression?

b. Is the client currently employed? If unemployed, what occupation(s) have they had? Do they have problems maintaining employment?

c. Does the client have a home to return to or are they currently homeless? Is the home safe?

e. Does the client have current legal charges pending? Does the client have a specific court date?

f. What was the highest grade or degree achieved by the client? This information will be important when choosing suitable teaching materials.

Section XIII

1. Ethnic/cultural/spiritual/coping/support

   a. Does the client have a specific ethnic/cultural/spiritual affiliation, and if so what is it?

   b. Are there certain rules or rituals related to health and spirituality that the client wishes to continue while hospitalized and can be accommodated within the safety regulations of the unit and hospital?

   c. Is the client aware of their stressors, and is their perception accurate? Do they minimize or exaggerate these stressors?

   d. What do they do to cope with these stressors?

   e. Who does the client turn to for support in times of stress?

   f. Does the client have a significant other or someone they feel close to?

   g. Does the client's significant other, family members, or close friends help or hinder the client?

   h. Is the client able to identify any of their own personal strengths? Hindrances? Clients who are depressed have low self-esteem and may have a poor self-concept, making it more difficult for them to identify personal strengths. They may focus more on what hinders them.

   i. Does the client seem to be a reliable historian, or do you doubt the information they provide?

Section XIV

1. Ego defense mechanisms—see Appendix A.

Section XV

1. Community resources/discharge planning

a. The community resources available will depend on the geographic location, amount of support available from family, friends, and religious or community organizations. Typically clients need food, housing, clothing, transportation, employment, medications, and outpatient treatment. The client may have both inpatient and outpatient health insurance benefits including mental health treatment, or they may not. If the client does not have health insurance to pay for outpatient mental health services and psychiatric medications (psychotropics), the nurse will have to refer the client to a social worker/case manager for possible sources of payment including Medicaid, United Way services, programs with sliding scale fees, prescription assistance programs, and other local community and religious organizations. The client's eligibility for assistance may depend on their income and monthly expenses. The process of applying for Medicaid may take time, and specific information is needed from the client. The number of providers who accept Medicaid or offer sliding scale fees is limited in many geographic areas, which decreases access to care. Also psychiatric medications can be very expensive and Medicaid may limit what medications are covered.

b. The client may be able to return to their regular employment and may have been receiving sick pay during hospitalization. However, if the client instead was required to file for temporary worker's compensation, it could take several weeks to receive any financial help. If this is the case, the client will also have to be evaluated before being allowed to return to work. The amount of money the client will receive from worker's compensation may or may not equal their regular salary, which could pose a problem paying for outpatient psychiatric-mental health treatment, medications, housing, food, utilities, transportation, clothing, and other basic needs. The client will need information regarding food banks, public transportation, Section 8 or other housing subsidy programs; programs to help pay for utilities, United Way agencies, and other local community and religious organizations. Some of this information is available on the hospital unit, and the client can also be referred to a social worker/case manager.

c. If the client is unemployed, but may meet criteria to be evaluated for vocational rehabilitation services to provide education and training for employment, the nurse would refer them to the social worker/case manager for information.

d. Unfortunately there are clients who have chronic mental health problems and may qualify for Social Security disability. Again, the nurse would refer them to the social worker/case manager for information. The process of applying for Social Security disability may take time, and specific information is needed from the client.

e. Discharge planning should include the following:

(1) Psychiatrist for monitoring symptoms and response to psychotropic medications, side-effects of psychotropics; reordering medications; ordering laboratory testing related to psychotropic medications

(2) Psychotherapy—individual, group, family with a psychologist, social worker, or APRN

(3) If unable to return to work immediately, day treatment/partial hospitalization program 5 days per week; if returning to work may attend an intensive outpatient (IOP) program 1–3 days per week for psychotherapy, monitoring of symptoms and side-effects of psychotropic medications

(4) Medical physician follow-up for monitoring and treatment of Axis III diagnoses; reordering medical medications and any laboratory tests related to those medications and illnesses

(5) Teaching—including diagnosis, medications, stress management, sleep promotion, coping skills, decision making, communication skills; relapse prevention including stopping medications being a major reason for relapse; keeping a schedule versus spending large amounts of time at home; keeping a list of people and hotline numbers to call when client becomes depressed or is having suicidal thoughts; balanced nutrition, regular exercise with a physician's approval, and other health promotion activities

(6) Support group information including resources from the American Foundation for Suicide Prevention: www.afsp.org, resources and support from the National Alliance on Mental Illness: www.nami.org, and a telephone hotline: National Suicide Emergency Hotline: 1-800-SUICIDE (1-800-784-2433) to call if experiencing suicidal thoughts

(7) Family—If the client has agreed to allow the family to receive information and be involved in their care, they will need information on the client's diagnosis; medications including common side-effects and what adverse effects to report immediately; family counseling (psychotherapy); and family support groups. The National Alliance on Mental Illness (NAMI) is a national organization with state and local chapters that provide support and education for family members and friends of clients as well as for the clients themselves. This organization also keeps families informed of legal issues affecting mental health clients.

Special Considerations

When assessing children/adolescents and the elderly, many of the same principles apply and similar information is needed as noted in the previous portion of this chapter. However, there are some special considerations when working with children/adolescents and the elderly.

Children/Adolescents

As with adults, children/adolescents may be diagnosed with more than one Axis I disorder. The signs and symptoms of major depression in children/adolescents are similar to those in adults, including suicidal thoughts, plans, or attempts. Even children/adolescents should be assessed for the possibility of suicide because children are not always able to express themselves verbally. Magical thinking and fantasy are normal in small children and may lead to feelings of inappropriate guilt or suicidal thoughts. Children may have homicidal thoughts or act on impulse when very angry, not realizing the impact of their actions and the permanence of death since in some fantasy animation, people come back to life. Anxiety and conduct disorders are frequently also diagnosed along with major depression (Sadock & Sadock, 2005, p. 3263). For information on anxiety and conduct disorders please refer to the DSM-IV-TR and a general psychiatric nursing textbook (APA, 2000, pp. 93–99, 429–430; Varcarolis, Carson, & Shoemaker, 2006, pp. 228–232, 634–635; O'Brien, Kennedy, & Ballard, 2008, pp. 218, 220–225, 336–340).

Adolescents are impulsive, emotional, and typically have difficulty seeing beyond tomorrow. They react strongly to experiencing losses of relationships, deaths, parental divorces, relocating, or being teased/rejected/bullied at school. The nurse should be alert to adolescent "Romeo & Juliet" type situations or suicide pacts. Adolescents who attempt suicide experience extreme irritability (Wozniak et al., 1996, p. 335). Some adolescents may imitate the suicidal behavior of others that they have read about, heard about, or seen (Sadock & Sadock, 2005, p. 3278). Even though parents and teachers are willing to listen to children/adolescents, their perception is not always accurate, and the child/adolescent may perceive that they have no one to talk to, which increases their feelings of loneliness and anger. Children/adolescents who currently or have a history of physical, sexual or emotional abuse, suffer from neglect, or have learning disabilities are more likely to develop major depression. Psychosis is less common in this age group, but if present, auditory hallucinations are more common than delusional thinking (Varcarolis, Carson, & Shoemaker, 2006, p. 648). The symptoms of major depression previously mentioned in this chapter still apply as well as some additional symptoms in this client population including:

- Thoughts of dying
- Preoccupation with death or illness
- Crying
- Irritability
- Anger and/or aggressiveness
- Nightmares
- Decreased academic performance
- Decreased interest in favorite toys, friends, or social activities
- Social isolation
- Boredom
- Somatic complaints
- Acting out in the form of risk taking, tantrums, sexual activity, alcohol/drug use, running away
- Preoccupation with morbid music, movies, artwork, poetry, books, websites, conversation topics
- Pessimism
- Brooding about a past experience
- Feelings of shame for letting the family down

As previously stated in Chapter 4, there are several screening tools that are frequently used to augment the assessment. The following screening tools may be used for children/adolescents with signs and symptoms of major depression:

- Behavior Assessment System for Children (BASC) for ages 4 to 18 years
- Child Behavior Checklist (CBDL) for ages 4 to 16 years
- Children's Depression Inventory (CDI) for ages 7 to 17 years
- Pediatric Anxiety Rating Scale (PARS) for ages 6 to 17 years
- Reynolds Adolescent Depression Scale (RADS)
- Children's Depression Rating Scale-Revised for ages 6 and older
- Diagnostic Interview Schedule for Children (DISC)
- Schedule for Affective Disorders and Schizophrenia for Children (K-SADS)
- Minnesota Multiphasic Personality Inventory-Adolescent (MMPI-A)
- Milton Adolescent Personality Inventory (MAPI)
- Milton Adolescent Clinical Inventory (MACI)

Teaching and psychotherapy in both the inpatient and outpatient settings should involve the family/caregivers. In addition to the teaching listed in **Table 8-4**, the family will be taught normal growth and development information. Community resource referrals and discharge planning will include emphasis on family counseling and

(continued on page 186)

Table 8-4   Nursing Interventions and Rationales for Major Depression

Problems	Interventions	Rationales
Suicidal or homicidal ideations/thinking	1. Begin to develop rapport and trust with the client (see Table 4-1): At admission, every 8 hours, and prn assess for suicidal ideations, plan, lethality of plan, access to the means to carry out plan, prior attempts, and chemical dependency.	1. Developing a rapport with the patient will assist in gaining the patient's trust and cooperation in the future and helps initiate the therapeutic nurse–client relationship. According to Render and Peplau (O'Brien, Kennedy, & Ballard, 2008, pp. 17–18), the therapeutic nurse–patient relationship is the foundation that must be established to initiate future work in the healing process.
		Suicidal ideations are more common than homicidal ideations, but both are extremely serious and must be assessed to protect the client and others. Clients with chemical abuse/dependency problems are at increased risk for committing suicide or homicide due to decreased inhibition. Suicidal/homicidal thoughts and urges are not always constant. They can be triggered by something another client says, a phone call, visitor, or something viewed on TV, therefore demonstrating a need for additional assessment and documentation.
	a. If the client reports homicidal thoughts toward a specific person, the nurse should obtain as much information as possible and report this to the psychiatrist, the immediate nursing supervisor and document this including who the information was reported to.	a. Obtaining information, passing it on and documenting are within the PMH nurse generalist's ethical–legal responsibilities and scope of practice. It will be up to the psychiatrist to decide if the information meets the "duty to warn" provisions of the Tarosoff ruling. The nurse does not notify the person potentially involved.

b. If the client is experiencing psychosis including hearing voices telling them to harm themselves or others, this needs to be reported and the client needs to be reassured of their own safety, and antipsychotic medication should be offered if ordered (see also Chapters 11 and 13).

2. Obtain at least a verbal no-self-harm or harm to others contract at admission, every 8 hours and prn.

3. Provide a safe, therapeutic milieu free from contraband/items that could be potential weapons (see also Chapter 3).

4. Use of self therapeutically and therapeutic communication techniques (see Table 4-1) are useful to assist client to verbalize feelings, precipitating events, reasons for attempting suicide, and what problems they think committing suicide will solve (see also Chapters 2, 4, and 5).

b. Some clients do experience psychosis, and this makes it more complicated to provide safety for the client and others. The psychiatrist needs to know that these symptoms are present to be able to treat all the client's problems. The client needs to feel safe, and antipsychotic medication can be very helpful for the psychotic symptoms (see also Chapters 11 and 13).

2. The PMH nurse will need to determine if the client is safe to leave on safety checks every 15 minutes or if they need to be placed on one-to-one or constant observation (COs). The ability to resist acting upon suicidal/homicidal thoughts and urges is not always possible. There is a need for additional assessment, obtaining at least a verbal no-self-harm or harm to others contract, and documentation.

3. This measure helps decrease the possibility of the client hurting themselves or others.

4. Assisting the client with verbalization of feelings, thoughts, concerns, or fears helps decrease the possibility of physically acting upon them. This also shows the client that the nurse is listening, is genuinely concerned, helps build rapport, trust, and the therapeutic nurse–client relationship.

(continues)

Table 8-4 Nursing Interventions and Rationales for Major Depression (continued)

Problems	Interventions	Rationales
	5. Reinforce that you are glad the client came and your willingness to help them.	5. This approach shows the client that the nurse believes that help is available, provides hope that the client can be helped, and that the client is a valuable human being worthy of help.
	6. Accept temporary emotional dependency needs and provide emotional support.	6. Normal reactions to loss, stress, anxiety, or crisis include temporary increased emotional dependency on others and psychological, even behavioral, regression to an earlier developmental stage. Accepting this and explaining this to patients helps increase their understanding of what is happening and that they are still valuable individuals worthy of help.
	7. Discuss the influence of any medical conditions or chronic pain on the client's perceptions, thoughts, and feelings. a. Encourage the client to discuss these conditions or chronic pain with the psychiatrist and medical physician, and offer to provide information on how medical illnesses and chronic pain affect mood.	7. This intervention acknowledges the presence of other factors, the reality of the influence of these factors on mood. a. Encouraging involvement and providing information helps provide the client with a sense of empowerment and hope that help is available.
	8. See Chapter 9 for more information related to working with suicidal clients.	8. See Chapter 9.
Anhedonia and anergia	1. Teach the client that anhedonia and anergia are symptoms of major depression.	1. The client needs to know that these are common symptoms of major depression. This provides hope that these symptoms will improve.

2. Teach the client that while the nurse and other mental health staff are available to help them, they will need to make an effort to attend to ADLs, including personal hygiene.

3. Encourage attendance at scheduled psychotherapy groups, psychoeducation groups, and activities before they actually feel better due to the time needed for the medication to take effect.

a. Remind the client of scheduled rest periods in the milieu program schedule.

4. Administer antidepressant or atypical antipsychotic medications (see Chapter 13) and other medication as ordered (e.g., pain medication, thyroid medications, DM medications).

2. The client may have been avoiding getting dressed or bathing as often due to decreased energy levels. The client does need to know that the nurse and other mental health staff will assist them as needed so that the client does not give into feelings of being overwhelmed and stop trying.

3. Clients think that they have to wait for the ability to experience pleasure to return and feel increased energy before being able to do anything, but this is not the case. Also, others around the client will notice improvement in affect and activities before the client is aware of the improvement.

The client will be taught about major depression, neurotransmitters, and medications individually and in psychoeducation groups.

a. This helps prevent the client from becoming overwhelmed with the level of expected activity they have been engaging in due to their symptoms. Also, elderly clients may need scheduled rest periods between groups/activities.

4. Antidepressant medications and most atypical/second generation atypical (SGA)/non traditional medications are used to treat major depression (see Chapter 13). Medications to treat other medical illnesses that can affect mood will also need to be administered to effectively treat the other illnesses, otherwise the client may still experience mood problems.

(continues)

Table 8-4 Nursing Interventions and Rationales for Major Depression (continued)

Problems	Interventions	Rationales
	5. Implement interventions that improve nutrition and sleep (see "Changes in appetite/weight" and "Sleep pattern disturbance" sections in this table.)	5. Poor nutrition and problems sleeping decrease available energy and influence mood.
Changes in appetite/weight	1. Obtain a baseline weight on admission, assess skin turgor and blood pressure. Assess laboratory glucose, total protein, albumin, RBCs, Hgb, Hct, MCV, and MCH values if ordered. Weigh at least once a week before breakfast on the same scale.	1. Obtaining a baseline weight and assessing skin turgor and blood pressure provide information to compare to normal height/weight charts and a general idea of fluid intake. Decreased glucose, total protein and albumin levels may indicate poor nutrition. Decreased RBCs, Hgb, and Hct may indicate nutrition-related anemias. Elevated MCV and MCH values may also indicate nutrition-related anemias. This information will be used to compare future assessment data to see if the client is improving.
	a. Clients who have been eating only once a day, who have fluid retention secondary to CHF or renal disease will need to be weighed daily.	a. Clients who have not been eating can actually die from starvation, malnutrition, and dehydration. Clients who have CHF or renal disease may accumulate excess fluid due to the disease processes and need to be more closely observed for fluid retention (e.g., abnormal lung sounds, dyspnea, 2–3 lb weight gain in 24 hours, edema of dependent areas (e.g., feet, ankles, sacrum; nocturia) and signs reported right away.
	2. Ask the client to complete a food/fluid intake diary for at least the past 3 days of food and fluid intake.	2. This will provide the nurse with information on how much the client is eating and drinking as well as if the client's dietary intake is nutritionally

balanced or not. The information can be correlated with the client's skin, weight, turgor, blood pressure, and laboratory values. Having the client perform this can also help the nurse assess the client's short-term/recent memory. See "Knowledge Deficits/Teaching Needs" section of this table.

3. Monitor intake and output every shift for at least the first 3 days of hospitalization.

3. This helps provide a more accurate account of what the patient is eating, drinking, and eliminating. For severely malnourished or elderly clients, the nurse may need to continue monitoring intake and output each shift.

4. Obtain information regarding the client's food preferences, food restrictions due to allergies or religious/cultural practices.

4. Including food preferences and restrictions will increase the client's cooperation and shows that they are seen as a person.

5. Assist clients with decreased appetite to choose small portions of foods higher in nutrient dense calories to increase nutritional content without overwhelming them by the amount of food at each meal. Also frequent snacks should be offered because initially they may not eat a normal amount at regular meal time. For clients with increased appetite the nurse will assist them to choose more vegetables and fruits that are lower in calories, provide nutrition, and help them feel full.

5. Clients who have not been eating well for some time may have difficulty eating a large meal at one sitting. However, they still need nutrients and calories to maintain body functions. These interventions can increase the likelihood of the client obtaining what they need. Clients who experience increased appetite as a symptom of major depression still need to eat, but in a way that satisfies their hunger without adding extra weight. This intervention will also help with the common side-effect of weight gain with many psychiatric medications.

(continues)

Table 8-4   Nursing Interventions and Rationales for Major Depression (continued)

Problems	Interventions	Rationales
	6. Encourage the client to eat in the dining room at a table with other clients rather than at a table all alone or in their room. a. Provide soft music during meal times.	6. and 6. a. Eating with others can stimulate the client to eat. The client will also imitate the behavior of other clients. Eating with others and listening to music makes the meal a social time that can lift mood and stimulate appetite. Most treatment program milieus do not allow clients to eat alone in their rooms, unless they are physically ill, to encourage clients to interact.
	7. Requesting a referral for a dietician consult may be necessary especially if dietary supplements are needed for diabetic or elderly clients.	7. The nurse will need to obtain an order from the psychiatrist for a dietary consult. Frequently, diabetic or elderly clients need temporary supplements until their appetite returns.
Sleep pattern disturbances	1. Assess the client's specific sleep pattern disturbance, number of total hours slept per night, whether or not the client feels rested, and whether or not the client naps during the day.	1. This establishes base line information. Sleep pattern disturbance is a symptom of major depression, and clients report difficulty falling asleep, waking up in the middle of the night with difficulty getting back to sleep or awakening early in the morning without being able to go back to sleep until their scheduled time to get up. Clients who are sleeping more hours than normal frequently report they do not feel rested. Also, daytime napping may have a negative effect on nighttime sleep pattern.
	2. Discuss with the client that this is a common symptom of major depression and the usual reasons people have difficulty sleeping even when they are not depressed.	2. The client may not be aware that sleep problems are a symptom of major depression, may assume it will eventually improve with time, or that some of their usual behavior may be contributing to the sleep problems.

3. Assist client in establishing a regular bedtime routine including a specific time to go to bed and awaken.

3. A regular bedtime routine promotes sleep by signaling the body and mind that it is time to prepare for sleep and later time to awaken. In the hospital the milieu program schedule includes a regular bedtime and awakening time, but the client will need to continue this strategy at home.

4. Discuss ways to eliminate distracting noise and light such as the use of dark window shades, heavier curtains, ear plugs, or a fan on low speed.

4. Noises and light can be irritating and cause mental stimulation with a body response of muscle tension, thus interfering with relaxation and falling asleep. Blocking out irritating noise with dark window shades, heavier curtains, ear plugs, or the use of fan at low speed ("white noise") is helpful. There are some people who listen to soft music at very low volume or use a night light, but many other people find these methods distracting. Interventions are tailored to the client's needs.

5. Teach the client to eliminate caffeinated beverages from the diet or at the very least refrain from drinking caffeinated beverages after the evening meal.

5. Caffeine is a stimulant, and the effects can be felt later when attempting to sleep. For example the effect of caffeine can be felt up to 4 hours after drinking a cup of coffee.

6. Suggest getting regular exercise (but avoid 2 hours before bedtime) with the client's physician's approval as to the type of exercise.

6. Regular exercise helps to release muscle tension, increase endorphins, decrease mental stress/anxiety, resulting in a more relaxed state.

7. Recommend eating a light snack while avoiding a heavy meal before bedtime.

7. This intervention works for some people especially if their blood glucose levels become too low during the night. Heavy meals do not improve sleep and can contribute to indigestion and weight gain.

(continues)

Table 8-4   Nursing Interventions and Rationales for Major Depression (continued)

Problems	Interventions	Rationales
	8. Recommend using relaxation exercises (e.g., deep breathing, progressive relaxation exercises) on a daily basis before bedtime.	8. Relaxation exercises help decrease muscle and mental tension producing a physical and mental relaxation response that promotes sleep.
	9. Recommend taking a warm bath/shower.	9. A warm bath/shower can also induce a physical and mental relaxation response to promote sleep. A hot bath/shower can cause vasodilation and result in a drop in blood pressure that could cause the client to feel faint and fall. Also a hot bath/shower can cause damage to tissue at the tips of toes and fingers, especially in clients who have cardiovascular diseases or DM.
	10. Recommend avoiding the use of sleep agents including herbals unless prescribed by psychiatrist. Exceptions include the use of herbals such as lavender, chamomile, or bergamot.	10. While sleeping agents may be useful as a short-term solution, some medications interfere with REM sleep. Not all herbal products are safe to use. Lavender has been helpful for promoting relaxation, and some clients find it helpful to spray it in the bedroom, use as bath salts or in massage oil/lotion. Bergamot is added to massage oil/lotion. Chamomile can be used in hot tea or added to massage oil/lotion. Caution should be taken by wearing gloves if using pure oils that may damage skin if not mixed in a massage oil or lotion. Pure oils should be added to a massage oil or lotion before applying to the skin or bath water. Some antidepressants can cause drowsiness as an expected side-effect, which may be used by the psychiatrist therapeutically

to help improve sleep. Sleep problems are a symptom of depression and when the depression improves the sleep pattern should also. For long-term solutions more natural methods are considered to be healthier.

	11. Recommend avoiding watching TV in the bedroom.	11. Even though some people say they fall asleep in front of the TV, having the TV on in the bedroom is too stimulating and actually interferes with falling asleep.
Helplessness/ hopelessness/ powerlessness	1. Provide emotional support and reassure the client that help is available.	1. This intervention shows the client that they are not alone, there is hope, and that the nurse cares about them.
	2. Assist the client to identify factors that they can control and focus on these. Discuss the importance of trying to be flexible with situations not within the client's control.	2. The client can be empowered by identifying and focusing on what they can control in the situation. Focusing on what can be controlled and attempting to be more flexible are better uses of the client's energy and resources.
	3. Explore with the client resources they have to work with, such as family members, friends, an understanding employer, or religious/spiritual contacts.	3. Clients may not be able to perceive how many resources or support they actually have due to being depressed. There is a tendency to focus on negative problems and what they lack to the exclusion of positive factors in their lives. Exploring resources increases their awareness and helps direct their focus on what resources they do have. This helps clients gain a sense of hope, increased control, and empowerment over their situation.

(continues)

Table 8-4   Nursing Interventions and Rationales for Major Depression (continued)

Problems	Interventions	Rationales
	4. Begin to assist the client to problem-solve.	4. Enlisting clients in problem solving helps direct their energy and focus on possible solutions and increasing their control over their situation.
	5. Encourage the client to attend all scheduled psychotherapy groups, psychoeducation groups, and activities.	5. According to Yalom, clients benefit from the curative factors of group including universality, instillation of hope, catharsis, and altruism. See Chapter 6.
Social isolation/ Withdrawn behavior	1. Encourage attendance at scheduled psychotherapy groups, psychoeducation groups, and activities before they actually feel better due to the time needed for the medication to take effect. a. Remind the client of scheduled rest periods in the milieu program.	1. Initially the client may want to isolate in their room rather than attend scheduled psychotherapy groups, psychoeducation groups, and activities. Encouraging the client to attend at least two groups on the first day of admission will be less overwhelming than insisting they attend everything on the program schedule.
	2. Inform the client the therapeutic milieu includes eating meals with other clients in a common dining room. If this is too overwhelming, the nurse may discuss with the psychiatrist and treatment team the possibility of initially placing the client with a few other clients in a smaller area, but not allowing the client to eat alone in their room. Then within a few days the client would be transitioned into the regular dining room.	2. The therapeutic milieu is designed to encourage social interaction. Clients who experience symptoms of major depression socially isolate and need an environment that discourages social isolation. Care should be taken when offering alternatives to the regular treatment milieu as other clients may view this as "special treatment" and resent clients they think are being allowed to behave differently.
	3. Spend brief, more frequent interaction one-on-one with the client and allow extra time for the client to respond to questions.	3. This intervention demonstrates the nurse cares about the client and helps decrease isolation, helps draw out the client, and is less overwhelming than being in a large group.

4. Arrange chairs in the day room in small groups of two or three and invite the client to sit, watch TV, talk, or play cards with the nurse or staff member and just a few other clients.

4. A smaller group is less overwhelming than being with all the clients on the unit at the same time. This type of setting encourages socialization even if initially the client is comfortable just sitting with others, but not interacting. Having a nurse or other staff member present provides emotional support and shows interest in the client as a person. This more relaxed setting may stimulate the client to ask questions or share information they may not feel comfortable doing in a larger group.

5. Provide positive reinforcement for any attempts made by the client to come out of their room and stay out on the unit.

5. Positive reinforcement helps increase the likelihood that the behavior will be repeated.

6. Point out areas on the unit where smaller groups of clients gather rather than being in the middle of the larger dayroom.

6. These areas may initially be more comfortable for the client until they adjust to the unit and symptoms begin to improve.

7. Provide smaller psychoeducation groups for clients who are severely socially withdrawn.
   a. Gently invite participation, but do not force the client to participate in group.

7. This also provides for a more relaxed setting and may stimulate more client participation while a larger group may make the client less comfortable.

8. Implement behavior modification if ordered.

8. Behavior modification is used to reinforce healthy, positive behavior. There are many types of behavior modification, but common systems include token economy systems and behavioral contracts. Behavior modification can be used for many reasons including encouraging clients to attend groups, perform ADLs, or practice more self-control.

(continues)

Table 8-4   Nursing Interventions and Rationales for Major Depression *(continued)*

Problems	Interventions	Rationales
Self-care deficits	1. Assist the client to obtain materials needed for bathing, grooming, and dressing.	1. This intervention prompts the client that it is time to attend to these needs. Due to anergia the client may procrastinate in attending to ADLs.
	2. Remind the client of the milieu schedule times provided for bathing and dressing while providing choices when possible.	2. See previous rationale item. Providing choices when possible between morning or evening bathing meets client's individual needs and increases comfort in an unfamiliar setting.
	a. Assist clients who are profoundly depressed with vegetative symptoms or have physical problems that prevent them from independently bathing, dressing, and remembering to use the bathroom. Offer the use of the bathroom every 2 hours while awake.	a. Clients experiencing profound depression or vegetative signs of depression may isolate in their bed, not eat, bathe, dress, use the bathroom regularly, or interact when approached. They may need to be physically assisted until there is improvement in the disorder. Also clients with physical problems will need assistance while encouraging independence as appropriate.
	3. Compliment efforts the client makes to bathe, dress, and improve appearance.	3. This intervention provides positive reinforcement and increases the possibility that the client will repeat the behavior.
	4. Assist profoundly depressed clients with vegetative symptoms with eating until these symptoms start improving. Offer frequent small portion nutrient dense, higher calorie snacks between meals. Encourage as much independence as possible.	4. Clients experiencing profound depression or vegetative signs of depression may isolate in their bed, not eat, bathe, dress, use the bathroom regularly, or interact when approached. Small portion nutrient dense, high calorie food provides high quality nutrition without overwhelming the client who may feel they have no energy to even eat or feed themselves.

	5. See "Changes in appetite/weight" section of this table.	5. See "Changes in appetite/weight" section of this table.
	6. See "Knowledge deficits/teaching needs" section of this table for other self-care activities.	6. See "Knowledge deficits/teaching needs" section of this table.
Ineffective coping	1. Identify and assess the client's current coping methods for adaptive and maladaptive methods.	1. This will establish a baseline, identify teaching needs, and provide a direction for further interventions. Adaptive methods are supported and teaching is provided on reasons why maladaptive methods can be harmful (e.g., alcohol, drugs, gambling, overeating, overspending, etc.)
	2. Share with the client personal strengths you have identified as well as factors that hinder the client. Include ways in which the client can use their strengths to help and counteract factors that hinder them.	2. Sharing this information and how the client can use it to help themselves will increase the client's sense of control and increase hope that will improve the ability to cope.
	3. Teach stress management techniques such as deep breathing, passive progressive relaxation exercises, simple meditation techniques, guided imagery (See Appendix F for specific exercises), benefits of massage therapy, aromatherapy, time management, problem-solving/decision-making strategies, journaling, and regular exercise with a physician's permission as to safe exercises.	3. Moderate to high levels of stress decrease the ability to cope and think clearly. Decreasing stress will improve the client's ability to cope and concentrate. Improved problem solving/decision making helps the client avoid mistakes that may be costly emotionally or financially and increase a sense of control over their life. Better time management helps relieve the pressure created by stress.
	4. Support the client's spirituality practices and needs including not only traditional religious practices, but also previously enjoyed hobbies, potential new hobbies, sports, music, inspirational readings, or gardening.	4. Clients who are depressed frequently experience spiritual distress or are unable to use their spirituality to cope as they normally would. Some clients may view their illness as a punishment from God and, therefore, may need to

(continues)

Table 8-4   Nursing Interventions and Rationales for Major Depression *(continued)*

Problems	Interventions	Rationales
		explore methods to increase their feeling of peace rather than forcing a return to traditional practices until they are ready to do so. Providing support and introducing new possibilities can help clients reconnect with their spirituality and use it to improve their coping ability. In many facilities not only are chaplains available, but also gymnasiums, swimming pools, horticulture areas, libraries, and enclosed outdoor areas to be closer to nature. Clients who are experiencing religious delusions may need to have contact with the chaplain and viewing of religious TV programs temporarily restricted to avoid worsening their symptoms.
	5. Identify people the client has turned to for support in the past and encourage the client in reaching out to these people now even if the client initially is doubtful they will be available this time.	5. Clients who are depressed frequently do not feel worthy of help or feel they are being a burden to others. They may need encouragement to reach out to others for help and support. Many times there are people all around them in their family, at church, at work, or in their neighborhood who would willingly help if asked. They may have tried to help the client, but their offers were refused because the client felt hopeless.
Low self-esteem	1. Review past accomplishments and successes, even seemingly small ones.	1. When clients are depressed they focus on and amplify any perceived failures and flaws. Everyone at some time in their life has succeeded at something, and they need to be reminded of this especially when they are experiencing symptoms of major depression.

2. Assist and teach the client to examine their negative thoughts with more realistic, logical thinking.

2. Perceptions are not always accurate especially when a person is depressed. When compared to realistic, logical thinking, it is easier to see inaccuracies in thinking. This is an important focus of Cognitive Behavior Therapy (CBT). The basic level PMH nurse can learn and teach clients basic concepts of CBT without practicing psychotherapy, which would be in the scope of practice of the APRN, psychologist, or social worker.

3. Discuss the unreality and destructiveness of perfectionism.

3. Unrealistic demands on ourselves increase a sense of failure, unworthiness, and inappropriate guilt that is not therapeutic.

4. Explore accepting mistakes and failures as part of being human, learning through these experiences, practicing forgiveness of ourselves, and moving forward.

4. Accepting, learning, forgiving, and moving forward are part of good self-esteem and mental health.

5. Teach and role play assertiveness skills.

5. People who lack assertiveness frequently have low self-esteem. Learning how to be assertive and practicing these skills can improve self-esteem. Role playing provides a way for clients to practice new skills in a safe, accepting atmosphere, accepting opportunities for feedback.

6. Ask the client to make a list of all their positive attributes and talents and refer to this list every day.

6. Clients who have low self-esteem have difficulty identifying positive attributes and talents or talking positively about themselves. With assistance they can experience increased awareness of their positive qualities and referring to the list every day can help reinforce and build up positive self-esteem.

(continues)

Table 8-4   Nursing Interventions and Rationales for Major Depression *(continued)*

Problems	Interventions	Rationales
	7. Teach the client to practice reciting positive affirmations every day.	7. Positive affirmations are statements that help build confidence. An example: "Every day in every way I am getting better and better." Some people post these in an area of their living space where they can see them and focus their attention in a positive direction.
Knowledge deficits/ teaching needs	The following areas are included in identifying knowledge deficits/teaching needs:	The more a client (and family if the client is willing) knows about their illness, medications, other treatment, and ways to help the self, the more control they will have over their illness and be better able to be involved in treatment decisions.
	1. Diagnosis, including that major depression is an illness that affects brain function and is a treatable illness; reasons why depression occurs, including the role of neurotransmitters, impact of genetic influence, signs and symptoms of major depression, and potential dangers of delaying treatment.	1. Most clients do not know that major depression is treatable, are unfamiliar with the signs and symptoms, yet know something is wrong, blame themselves for being ill, and do not realize what negative impacts and danger there is when delaying treatment.
	2. Medication—teaching includes the different classes/categories of medications used to treat major depression, including antidepressants and atypical antipsychotics; benefits, common side-effects, adverse effects to report and seek help for right away, food interactions, approximate amount of time it may take to feel the full effect, that it may take time to find the specific medication that helps their symptoms with the least	2. Since medication is a large part of treatment, it is very important that the client be informed about their medications. Providing information and reasons why it is important can help increase client adherence (compliance) with the medication regimen.

amount of side-effects, problems with suddenly stopping the medication, avoidance of alcohol/drugs or not taking anything including herbal supplements without the psychiatrist, APRN, or other physician's knowledge, importance of keeping their psychiatrist/APRN informed of problems or improvements (see also Chapter 13).

3. Other treatment—including individual and group psychotherapy; including therapies such as Cognitive Behavioral Therapy (CBT), Interpersonal Therapy (IPT), Motivational Enhancement Therapy, Rational Emotive Behavioral Therapy (REBT), Supportive Therapy, Client Centered Therapy, Reality Therapy, behavior modification, psychoanalysis, ECT, psychoeducation, hypnosis, psychodrama, nutrition, treatment of comorbid/co-occuring conditions that affect mood, treatment of chemical dependency, and family psychotherapy.

3. Medications are needed to regulate the balance of neurotransmitters, help improve the client's ability to concentrate and focus to be able to learn, but they will not help the client deal with interpersonal relationships, day-to-day problems/frustrations, improve social skills or change certain behaviors or provide insight. Medications do help the client cope to a degree, but they also need to learn other ways to cope. Adult clients who cannot tolerate side-/adverse effects of psychiatric medications, are taking other medications that interact with psychiatric medications, are elderly, or who are profoundly depressed, in danger of committing suicide and not responding to psychiatric medications may benefit from ECT and need to be informed that it is a procedure that is performed in a safe, humane manner, since it is likely the client has misconceptions from movies or has heard of past ECT practices.

(continues)

Table 8-4   Nursing Interventions and Rationales for Major Depression (continued)

Problems	Interventions	Rationales
	4. Self-care activities a. Physical exercise	4. & 4. a. Many clients do not realize that there is much they can do to help themselves in addition to taking medication and receiving psychotherapy. Research on the effects of physical exercise showed significant reduction in depression and decreased stress as well as having other health benefits in preventing cardiac diseases, diabetes, and obesity, which are comorbid/co-occuring conditions in many mental health clients. Most psychiatric medication side-effects include weight gain. Exercise combined with balanced nutrition can help offset these side-effects (Jensen, Decker, & Andersen, 2006, pp. 620-621; Frisch & Frisch, 2002, p. 267).
	b. Nutrition and hydration	b. Balanced nutrition is important for weight management, offsetting the medication side-effect of weight gain; the production of neurotransmitters, hormones, building and repair of body tissues; regulation of glucose levels, regulation of cholesterol levels, energy production, and regulation of bowel function (constipation may occur due to decreased physiologic processes during depressed episodes, side-effects of medications or lack of fiber in the diet). Adequate hydration is needed to prevent dehydration and consequences of electrolyte imbalance, low blood volume, urinary tract infections, or constipation (see also "Changes in appetite/weight" in this table).

c. Spirituality

    c. Many clients report that spirituality is central to their life because it provides them a reason to live. Many clients seek the counsel of clergy or other spiritual advisors to help deal with their symptoms of depression before seeking psychiatric treatment and as part of their discharge and relapse prevention plans. Many clients receive emotional/psychological benefits from spending time in natural surroundings (e.g., parks, beaches) that will be available when they are discharged from the hospital (see also "Ineffective coping" in this table).

d. Interpersonal relationships

    d. Social isolation, problems with interpersonal relationships, and loss of relationships are major problems for all clients who are depressed. Working with significant others, families, and friends of clients helps improve interpersonal relationships and provides much needed support that is important in healing and maintaining progress.

e. Stress management—teach client how alcohol and drugs actually can increase depressed feelings even though initially it seems that these substances relieve problems (see also Appendix F).

    e. Teaching self-care exercises provides clients with tools they can use on their own to give them more control and augment medications and psychotherapy. Many clients attempt to handle symptoms on their own by self-medicating with alcohol, illegal drugs, or prescription medications. Not only does self-medicating exacerbate depression, but clients also frequently end up with additional addiction problems that will also need to be treated (see also "Ineffective coping" in this table).

(continues)

Table 8-4 Nursing Interventions and Rationales for Major Depression *(continued)*

Problems	Interventions	Rationales
	f. Problem solving/decision making	f. Many clients do not have effective problem-solving/decision-making skills, but these can be taught to help prevent making the same mistakes over again.
	g. Healthy communication/assertiveness	g. Communication difficulties and nonassertiveness are common problems for depressed clients. Learning better methods can improve their interpersonal relationships and quality of life.
	h. Anger management	h. Many clients have difficulty expressing and managing anger. These skills are very useful and provide tools the client can use on their own to improve their relationships and decrease stress that comes from anger-related tension.
	i. Smoking cessation	i. Many clients with psychiatric-mental health problems smoke. It is very difficult for them to attempt to quit smoking or use of any tobacco products while their symptoms are not controlled. However, after their symptoms are more fully controlled, it may be easier for clients to begin a program to quit or at least decrease the amount of tobacco products they use. Clients should be warned about using the smoking cessation medication varenicline (Chantix) due to reports of increased feelings of depression and suicidal thoughts.

j. Maintaining a daily schedule including social activities and volunteering

k. Health responsibility involves keeping up with regular physical checkups, seeking medical attention when needed, adhering to medication and other treatment regimens, engaging in health promotion activities, and avoiding potentially harmful life-style behaviors.

l. Humor

m. Sexual concerns

j. Keeping busy or active and engaging in social activities is important for mental health. Clients who are depressed prefer to isolate and spend time inactive due to anergia and anhedonia. The client will need to maintain a schedule after regular work hours, on weekends, and holidays. This is even more important for clients who are not currently working. Volunteering helps both clients and recipients of the volunteer services.

k. Informing clients of their responsibility as partners in their healthcare increases their awareness and control over their health.

l. Clients who are depressed may have lost their appreciation for humor, but humor can contribute to a sense of well-being and help people cope with negative feelings or situations. Being able to laugh at ourselves is considered to be healthy.

m. Decreased interest in sexual activity is a symptom of depression. Also, some psychiatric medications have side-effects of impotence in males or decreased sexual desire in both males and females. Some clients stop taking medications because of sexual side-effects and experience a relapse in their symptoms. Clients may also be concerned

(continues)

Table 8-4   Nursing Interventions and Rationales for Major Depression (continued)

Problems	Interventions	Rationales
		that now that they have a "psychiatric diagnosis," current or potential sexual partners may no longer be interested in having relationships with them. These concerns need to be talked about, and many clients will not openly mention them until the nurse talks about them. Usually clients are relieved and appreciate being able to talk about these problems and ways to cope with them.
	5. Effective coping—see "Ineffective coping" and "Self-care activities" sections in this table.	5. Effective coping—the better clients are able to cope and the more they know about their illness, medications, and treatment the more likely they will adhere to treatment, the better their prognosis, the more likely they are to be involved in their healthcare decisions (see also "Ineffective coping" and "Self-care activities" sections of this table.)
Relapse prevention	1. Teach the client signs and symptoms to watch for that show they are starting to become depressed again and to report these to the psychiatrist/APRN (e.g., increase in symptoms, reemergence of symptoms previously absent, increased social isolation/withdrawal).	1. Early recognition and reporting of signs and symptoms leads to early treatment and avoidance of rehospitalizations or shorter hospitalization stays.
	2. Assist the client to realistically look at all the responsibilities and activities they have and decide how to prioritize responsibilities and ask for help to avoid feeling overwhelmed.	2. The client may feel they are a failure if not fulfilling many responsibilities, not realizing that they need time to recover. Many people do not have a realistic perception of how much they are logi-

cally capable of handling and cause themselves to be overwhelmed by stretching their time, energy, and resources too thin.

3. Teach the client the importance of maintaining structure in their life by keeping to a schedule, keeping up with social activities, and avoiding spending large amounts of time alone.

3. Many clients lack structure in their lives and need to learn how to obtain and maintain structure. Spending large amounts of time alone increases social isolation, dwelling on problems, and can lead to a relapse of depression.

4. Reinforce the need for the client to continue with the stress management including the positive/adaptive coping skills learned while in the inpatient setting.

4. It is necessary to make stress management including positive/adaptive coping skills a part of every day living to help prevent a relapse of depression and help maintain mental health.

5. Encourage the client to talk to someone when they first start feeling overwhelmed, depressed, anxious, or suicidal rather than waiting until they feel they cannot handle it anymore.
   a. Write a list of at least five people and their phone numbers who the client can call when they feel stressed, overwhelmed, depressed, or anxious. Have the client keep the list near the phone and programmed into their cell phone.
   b. Provide the client with the suicide hotline number 1-800-SUICIDE (1-800-784-2433).
   c. Reinforce the benefit of attending support groups regularly and provide contact information for appropriate groups.

5. Talking with others provides emotional support, decreases social isolation, and helps clarify perceptions.
   a. Having a list at hand versus having to look for phone numbers increases the chance that the client will actually place a call to someone. Also, the first person called may not be available, leading the client to give up and feel hopeless or give in to suicidal thinking.
   b. This provides an additional source of help for when the client is experiencing suicidal thoughts.
   c. Support groups led by lay persons provide opportunities to express feelings, obtain support, and learn from others who have similar problems.

(continues)

Table 8-4   Nursing Interventions and Rationales for Major Depression (continued)

Problems	Interventions	Rationales
	d. Suggest starting a journal of feelings, thoughts, reactions, and situations. The journal may be shared with their outpatient treatment team.	d. Journaling gives the client a method of keeping track of their own improvement and signs of impending relapse. The client can use it to help decide when and what they need to report to the psychiatrist and other members of the outpatient treatment team. It is another tool to help the client be an active part of their treatment. If the client feels comfortable with sharing the journal entries with the outpatient treatment team it can assist the team in keeping track of their improvement or impending relapse.
	6. Reinforce the need to continue practicing and using healthy communication and assertiveness techniques.	6. These techniques need to become a part of normal interaction for the client to improve and sustain good interpersonal relationships, handle conflict, and help the client obtain more of what they want in life.
	7. Use role play with a person the client trusts to rehearse potential overwhelming or stress-producing situations.	7. Role playing is an effective technique that can also be used outside of the inpatient setting.
	8. Reinforce the need to continue taking all medication exactly as prescribed while keeping the psychiatrist, APRN, and other physicians aware of problems rather than stopping medication suddenly.	8. It is imperative that the client adhere to the medication regimen to maintain neurotransmitter/neurochemical balance to help control signs and symptoms of major depression. Suddenly stopping medication can cause physical problems. The psychiatrist, APRN, and other physicians need to know of any side-effects or adverse effects to properly care for the client.

9. Reinforce the need to attend individual and group psychotherapy sessions regularly.

9. Psychotherapy is needed to help the client continue to deal with interpersonal relationships, day-to day problems/frustrations, improve social skills or change certain behaviors or provide insight. It takes time to learn new ways to deal with life's challenges.

10. Teach importance of including the client's significant other and other family members in their treatment unless there is a specific reason not to.

10. Significant others and family members can be very supportive and usually do not know much about major depression or psychiatric problems in general. Also, they may not realize that they may be contributing to the client's problems and need to learn new ways of relating to the client. However, there are situations where the client has valid reasons for not including these people in their treatment (e.g., abuse, violence, alcohol/drug use, refusal to believe the client needs treatment, etc.) that must be respected.

11. Teach the client of the need to inform all of their healthcare providers of their psychiatric medications.

11. The client may receive medications from other healthcare providers, even the dentist, that may interact with the psychiatric medications they have been prescribed. The client needs to keep all their healthcare providers informed to maintain medical safety.

education as well as services for the individual child/adolescent. Partial hospitalization or day treatment programs that focus on the needs of adolescents as well as after school programs would be included when needed.

Elderly

Elderly clients usually have experienced many losses in life including the deaths of family members and friends, experienced ageism (bias due to age), been forced to relinquish their driver's license or retire from employment. Even when choosing to retire, the life change can be difficult to cope with. Use of screening tools listed near the end of this section can help the nurse assess the amount of loss clients have sustained. During the normal aging process they may have experienced a gradual decline in skeletal-muscle flexibility, dexterity, physical stamina, slower reaction times, and slower retrieval of information from memory. Other elderly clients are very physically active and seem as if they have hardly aged at all. As previously mentioned in Chapter 4, many elderly clients have poor nutrition and may be dehydrated, which can lead to symptoms that may initially look like decreased mental function, fatigue, or dementia, but improve when normal nutrition and hydration needs are met. Deficiencies of certain B vitamins (B12 or B6) can lead to anemia, decreased energy, and depressed mood in some clients. Poor nutrition affects the body's ability to produce substances it needs for normal functioning including hormones and neurotransmitters. Some elderly clients who live alone may feel it is too much trouble to cook balanced meals for just one person. The nurse needs to carefully assess the nutrition status of elderly clients. The PMH nurse also needs to be alert to the possibility of alcohol abuse/ dependence as a way of coping with depression. Although unexplained accidents may be due to domestic violence or abuse, they may also be due to alcoholism. Elderly clients may not admit feeling depressed or seek help due to being used to handling problems on their own. It may be easier for them to talk about their physical symptoms and not make the connection between these symptoms and their feelings. The symptoms of major depression previously mentioned in this chapter still apply as well as some additional symptoms in this client population. Elderly clients may be deeply religious, but should still be assessed for suicidal thoughts, plans, and attempts (see Chapter 9). In a moment of extreme emotional distress or pain, clients may do anything to stop what they are feeling. Other clients may carefully plan a suicide attempt when they know family members will not be around.

Some of the signs and symptoms common to depressed elderly clients include:

- Increased concern with body functions
- Somatic complaints
- Anxiety or apprehension without specific reason

- Depressed mood
- Decreased appetite
- Insomnia
- Decreased interest and participation in social activities
- Low self-esteem, feeling insignificant

Elderly clients may also stop attending to not only ADLs, but care of medical problems by stopping taking medications and not keeping up with regular follow-up visits for monitoring of medical conditions. The symptoms of depression occur more slowly than delirium (from a few hours to a few days), but more quickly than dementia. Agitation, memory loss, and intellectual decline are associated with dementia (Varcarolis, Carson, & Shoemaker, 2006, pp. 425, 709). Elderly clients can be diagnosed with both depression and dementia, but they are separate disorders. As previously stated in Chapter 4, there are several screening tools that are frequently used to augment the assessment. The following screening tools may be used for elderly clients with signs and symptoms of major depression:

- Geriatric Depression Scale
- Holmes and Rahe Social Readjustment Scale
- The Hassles and Uplifts Scale
- Life Experiences Survey (LES)
- MiniMental State Examination (MMSE) or Folstein—if suspect dementia
- CAGE for Alcohol Abuse
- Michigan Alcoholism Screening Test-Geriatric Version (MAST-G)
- Wong-Baker FACES Pain Rating Scale
- Index of Independence in Activities of Daily Living
- Instrumental Activities of Daily Living
- Functional Activities Questionnaire

Community resource referrals and discharge planning may need to include more emphasis on mobility aids and medical equipment when working with elderly clients. Opportunities for elderly clients to volunteer or work part-time would be explored. Partial hospitalization or day treatment programs that focus on the needs of elderly clients as well as adult day care programs would be included when needed.

NURSING INTERVENTIONS AND RATIONALES

Nursing interventions are planned according to individual client needs, common signs and symptoms of major depression, age, education level, and cultural preferences. For specific nursing diagnoses, outcomes, and evaluation criteria, refer to a general psychiatric-mental health nursing textbook such as *Psychiatric Mental Health Nursing: An Introduction to Theory and Practice*, O'Brien, Kennedy & Ballard (2008); *Mental Health Nursing*, Fontaine (2009); *Psychiatric Nursing: Contemporary Practice*, Boyd (2008); *Psychiatric Mental Health Case Studies and Care Plans*, Jakopac & Patel (2009); and psychiatric care plan books such as *Psychiatric Nursing Care Plans*, Fortinash & Holoday-Worret or *Manual of Psychiatric Nursing Care Plans*, Varcarolis (2006). The interventions presented in Table 8-4 apply to the adult and elderly client with variations for the child/adolescent client as indicated.

Electroconvulsive Therapy (ECT)

ECT is defined by the APA (2007) as a controlled seizure induced by passing low-dose electric currents through one temporal (unilateral) or both (bilateral) temporal areas of the brain with the effects of potentially balancing neurotransmitters in the brain. In many states an adult client must be evaluated by two psychiatrists before being ordered to receive ECT (refer to your individual state practice guidelines). The client or the person the client has given medical power of attorney to must sign a written consent for this treatment after being provided information as to the benefits and risks of the procedure.

The client is prepared before the procedure in the same manner as any medical-surgical procedure, including completing a preoperative checklist and the administration of anesthesia and muscle relaxants. ECT must be performed in a surgical suite or outpatient surgery area with resuscitation equipment immediately available. The client is attached to EEG and telemetry machines for monitoring during the procedure, and oxygen is provided before the procedure as well as prn. The client's blood pressure, heart rate, respiratory rate, oxygen saturation, and temperature are closely monitored. A blood pressure cuff may be attached to one ankle so that the psychiatrist can observe muscle movements, because the client will have received muscle relaxants making it more difficult to observe movement. The client will be monitored in a postanesthesia recovery area until stable before returning to the psychiatric-mental health unit or if being done as an outpatient before being discharged to home. Initially, ECT is performed 3 times per week, not daily, in a series of 6 treatments. Another series of 6 treatments may be ordered, up to 18 treatments in a series of 6 per order. After the initial treatments have begun in the inpatient setting, the client may continue with ECT as an outpatient procedure to continue the initial 3 times per week treatments begun in the inpatient setting and for monthly maintenance treatment if needed. The client will need to have someone accompany them to provide transportation home. The client may be medically stable, but still too drowsy to drive, and anyone having any type of outpatient procedure will need to be released to an adult rather than discharged alone for safety and legal reasons (see **Table 8-5**).

Contraindications for ECT include the following:

- Recent cerebrovascular accident (CVA)
- Recent myocardial infarction (MI)
- Recent head trauma including subdural hematoma
- Intracranial mass/tumor
- Increased intracranial pressure
- Angina pectoris
- Congestive heart failure/heart failure (CHF/HF)
- Severe pulmonary disease
- Glaucoma
- Detached retina
- Major bone fractures
- Severe osteoporosis
- Thrombophlebitis
- High-risk pregnancies
- Extremely loose teeth (danger of aspiration)
- Current medications—monoamine oxidase inhibitors (MAOIs) may result in severe hypertension; atypical antipsychotic clozapine (Clozaril) may result in seizures or delirium (Keltner, Schwecke, & Bostrom, 2007, p. 575)

Table 8-5 Nursing Care of Clients Receiving ECT	
Pre-ECT care/interventions	**Rationales**
The following information must be on the client's medical record to be sent with the client to the procedure:	The client's information should be readily available for the accurate administration of anesthesia, medication, and in case of an emergency situation rather than having to totally rely on memory of the details for the client's safety.
• Order for ECT with accurate date/time/ psychiatrist signature	• The nurse cannot legally send a client from the unit for an unauthorized procedure.

(continues)

Table 8-5 Nursing Care of Clients Receiving ECT *(continued)*

Pre-ECT care/interventions	Rationales
• Informed consent	• The client or a person legally authorized to act on their behalf must legally give informed consent, meaning that the benefits of treatment and risks have been explained and the client or legally authorized person voices understanding of the information.
• NPO for at least 6 to 8 hours prior to ECT	• Any procedure requiring anesthesia or medications producing a muscle relaxant effect impair the client's ability to swallow, and there is a danger of aspiration. This danger is reduced by making the client NPO for a certain amount of time prior to the procedure.
• Complete Preoperative Checklist	• A Preoperative Checklist is a document completed before any medical-surgical procedure. This helps assure that certain information has been obtained and that the client has been properly prepared prior to the procedure, including the presence of an accurate identification armband, being placed in a hospital gown, the removal of dentures, recording of any dental implants/crowns/caps to prevent aspiration, removal of hair pins and nail polish. Hair pins could accidentally fall into the client's airway causing damage and obstruction; the client's oxygen saturation will be continuously monitored with a pulse oximeter. Nail polish can potentially block the signal and interfere with the accuracy of pulse oximetry readings.
• Labs/diagnostics—typically CBC, WBC, electrolytes, BUN, creatinine, urinalysis, chest x-ray, EKG/ECG, possibly C-spine and LS spine x-rays if there is a history of or suspected fractures	• Laboratory/diagnostic tests rule out current infections including pneumonia, which could present potential danger for the client and rule out any contraindications that were previously unknown or unreported. They also demonstrate the client's

(continues)

Table 8-5   Nursing Care of Clients Receiving ECT *(continued)*

Pre-ECT care/interventions	Rationales
	kidney function, including the ability to excrete anesthetic agents and medications. If the results of these tests are not on the medical record, the laboratory, x-ray, and other departments must be called and results obtained so that the nurse can notify the psychiatrist of any abnormal results and document this. If tests have not yet been ordered, the nurse will need to notify the psychiatrist and document whether or not they were ordered at the time of notification. ECT may be delayed due to lack of complete preoperative information or abnormal laboratory/diagnostic test results.
• History and physical	• A current history and physical must be on the chart. If it is not, the nurse should contact medical records in case it was dictated but has not been transcribed or placed on the chart.
• Accurate height and accurate current weight	• The client should be weighed the morning of the procedure and height verified. This information is used to identify the client and to determine accurate doses of anesthesia, muscle relaxant medications, and emergency medication if needed.
• Current vital signs and pulse oximetry	• Temperature, pulse, respirations, blood pressure and pulse oximetry should be taken in the morning before the client is sent for ECT. If ECT is delayed, they will need to be taken again. If they are abnormal, the psychiatrist should be notified and the client held on the unit until it is determined by the psychiatrist if ECT will be performed.
• Be sure the client empties their bladder.	• All of the client's muscles will be relaxed, and if the bladder is not empty the client will be incontinent of urine.

(continues)

Table 8-5   Nursing Care of Clients Receiving ECT *(continued)*

Post-ECT care/interventions	Rationales
The client's physical and mental status must be monitored closely upon return from post-anesthesia recovery:	The client has just been through a medical procedure and will require closer monitoring for physical and mental safety.
• Receive telephone report on the client's condition and care from the postanesthesia recovery nurse, record the report from the nurse in post-anesthesia recovery in the client's medical record, and place a copy of the post-anesthesia recovery room documentation on the medical record. Attention should be paid to any problems including side-effects of the procedure, anesthesia, medications, additional resuscitation efforts needed or medication administered for increased blood pressure.	• It is important to not only receive a telephone report, but also to record it to demonstrate the client's condition when the PMH nurse receives the client and assumes responsibility for their care. If there is any question of the client's medical stability, the client should remain in the postanesthesia recovery area until it is certain that they are stable enough to go back to the psychiatric-mental health unit for the client's physical safety. A copy of the client's condition and care provided in postanesthesia recovery provides documentation to compare the client's condition on the psychiatric-mental health unit and assist the nurse in assessing the client and noting problems early enough to start intervening to prevent complications.
• Take vital signs, pulse oximetry, and assess LOC and behavior upon return to the psychiatric-mental health unit and every 30 minutes times 2. Reorient the client to location and situation. If the vital signs, pulse oximetry, LOC are stable and behavior is normal, then continue taking vital signs and pulse oximetry every hour times 2. If the client continues to remain stable, continue with vital signs and pulse oximetry every 4 hours for 24 hours.	• These measures demonstrate if the client continues to be medically stable or if there is a need for further intervention. The client may experience respiratory depression from anesthesia and preoperative medications (e.g., succinylcholine (Anectine), methohexital (Brevital.) It is not unusual for the client to be drowsy, go to sleep, be temporarily disoriented or have facial flushing upon returning to the unit.
• Place the client on safety checks every 15 minutes for a 2-hour time frame.	• The client may already be on safety checks every 15 minutes, but if not then they will be placed on them for a 2-hour period for safety reasons. If the client is mentally stable at the end of the 2-hour period the nurse may place them back on safety checks every 30 minutes.

(continues)

Table 8-5 Nursing Care of Clients Receiving ECT *(continued)*	
Post-ECT care/interventions	**Rationales**
• Assess the client's gag reflex before administering medications that were previously held due to NPO status and before offering fluids and food.	• Due to anesthesia and preoperative/postoperative medications, the client's gag reflex may not have returned, and there is danger of aspiration until it does return.
• Assist the client with ambulation and toileting prn.	• Sometimes clients are unsteady on their feet upon returning to the unit.

Side-effects of ECT include the following:

- Drowsiness
- Headache
- Muscle aches
- Confusion and disorientation, which usually disappears within an hour
- Memory is often affected after ECT, but after a few months returns to normal (more severe memory problems if 20 or more treatments received)
- Hypertension
- Cardiac arrhythmias
- Respiratory depression r/t preoperative medications (Keltner, Schwecke, & Bostrom, 2007, p. 576)

Nursing Interventions Special Considerations

Children/Adolescents

When working with children/adolescents, the PMH nurse will need to tailor teaching information to the age and ability of the child/adolescent and also provide information for the parents or legal guardian. Additional teaching needs will include parenting skills, normal growth and development, and dealing with negative behavior. Children/adolescents and their parents or legal guardians will need emotional support, education, and explanations to deal with the limited visiting hours. Helping prevent children/adolescents from falling behind academically may be a challenge. Even when parents or legal guardians accept the need for medication for their children/adolescents, it may be difficult for children/adolescents to adhere to this type of treatment because of not wanting to seem different. Behavior modification techniques are frequently used with this client population. For example, token economy systems using plastic or rubber tokens/coins or a point system are effective to reward and reinforce positive behavior such as attending and participating in psychotherapy, psychoeducation, and activity groups; keeping their rooms clean/neat and beds made; attending to ADLs; completing homework assignments; sharing toys, computer equipment and games; helping each other; and refraining from physical or verbal aggression. Tokens or points can be exchanged for prizes or privileges such as extra TV, computer or game time, choosing movies for group viewing, or attendance at group outings. On the other hand, negative behaviors incur consequences such as losing tokens, points, or privileges. This type of behavior modification is extremely effective in this client population, but must be consistently applied for long-term improvement. Room searches for contraband may need to be performed more often with these clients.

Elderly

When working with elderly clients, the PMH nurse may need to provide more physical care than with other clients. These clients typically are ordered medications for medical diseases. Additional time for teaching may need to be allotted for, and spouses, children, or other caregivers will need information on diagnosis, medications, and other treatment. Reminiscence groups, social activities, and appropriate exercises including *tai chi* can help increase balance and muscle strength. Falls are a safety concern for this population not only due to age-related physical changes, but also due to the side-effects of psychiatric as well as other medications. These clients may need more assistance with ambulation and toileting. Incontinence of bladder or bowel may be a problem signaling a need for toileting every 2 hours while awake and more frequently changing while in bed. There may be a need for more meticulous skin care. Balanced nutrition, dehydration, and appetite can be a challenge when working with this population. Dentures may need repair or no longer fit properly due to weight loss. Eye glasses may need to be replaced. The client may benefit from hearing aids, but not have the money to purchase them or deny the need for such devices. Decreased vision and blindness due to cataracts or macular degeneration may present a problem when choosing teaching materials and leisure activities for these clients. Materials with larger type, magnifying lenses, and larger pieces are helpful as well as audiotapes. Talking book materials may be obtained through local libraries.

REFERENCES

American Psychiatric Association (2000). *Diagnostic and statistical manual of mental disorders* (4th ed.), text revision. Washington, DC: Author.

American Psychological Association (2007). *APA dictionary of psychology*. Washington, DC: Author.

Boyd, M. A. (2008). *Psychiatric nursing: Contemporary practice* (4th ed.). Philadelphia, PA: Wolters Kluwer/Lippincott, Williams, & Wilkins.

Fontaine, K. L. (2009). *Mental health nursing* (6th ed.). Upper Saddle River, NJ: Pearson Education Inc.

Fortinash, K. M., & Holoday-Worret, P. A. (2007). *Psychiatric nursing care plans* (5th ed.). St. Louis, MO: Mosby, Elsevier.

Frisch, N. C., & Frisch, L. E. (2002). *Psychiatric mental health nursing* (2nd ed.). Albany, NY: Delmar/Thomas Learning, Inc.

Halter, M. J. (2004). Stigma and help seeking related to depression: A study of nursing students. *Journal of Psychosocial Nursing and Mental Health, 42*(2), 42–51.

Jakopac, K. A. and Patel, S. C. (2009). *Psychiatric mental health case studies and care plans*. Sudbury, MA: Jones and Bartlett.

Jensen, L. W., Decker, L., & Andersen, M. M. (2006). Depression and health-promoting lifestyles of persons with chronic mental illness. *Issues in Mental Health Nursing, 27*, 617–634.

Kelly, J. (June, 2007). Genetic variation may impact response to antidepressants. *NeuroPsychiatry Reviews, 8*(1), 1, 26.

Kelly, J. (June, 2007). Pain compounds depression's impact for retired NFL players. *NeuroPsychiatry Reviews, 8*(6), 1, 22.

Keltner, N. L., Schwecke, L. H., & Bostrom, C. E. (2007). *Psychiatric nursing* (5th ed.). St. Louis, MO: Mosby, Elsevier.

Mohr, W. K. (2006). *Psychiatric-mental health nursing: Evidence based concepts, skills, and practices* (6th ed.). Philadelphia, PA: Wolters Kluwer/Lippincott, Williams & Wilkins.

O'Brien, P. G., Kennedy, W. Z., & Ballard, K. A. (2008). *Psychiatric mental health nursing: An introduction to theory and practice*. Sudbury, MA: Jones and Bartlett.

Sadock, B. J., & Sadock, V. A. (2005). *Kaplan & Sadock's comprehensive textbook of psychiatry* (8th ed.). Philadelphia, PA: Lippincott, Williams, & Wilkins.

Townsend, M. C. (2009). *Essentials of psychiatric mental health nursing: Concepts of care in evidence based practice* (6th ed.). Philadelphia, PA: F. A. Davis Company.

Varcarolis, E. M. (2006). *Manual of psychiatric nursing care plans* (3rd ed.). St. Louis, MO: Saunders, Elsevier.

Varcarolis, E. M., Carson, V. B., & Shoemaker, N. C. (2006). *Foundations of psychiatric mental health nursing: A clinical approach* (5th ed.). St. Louis, MO: Saunders/Elsevier.

Wozniak, J., Biederman, J., Kiely, K., Ablon, J. S., Faraone, S. V., Mundy, E. & Mennin, D. (1996). Part IV: Clinical issues. Mania-like symptoms suggestive of childhood-onset of bipolar disorder in clinically referred children. In *Annual progress in child psychiatry and child development: A selection of the year's outstanding contributions to the understanding and treatment of the normal and disturbed child*. London, UK: Psychology Press/Taylor & Francis Group.

SUGGESTED READINGS

Aho, A. L., Tarkka, M., Stedt-Kurki, P., & Kaunonen, M. (2006). Fathers' grief after the death of a child. *Issues in Mental Health Nursing, 27*, 647–663.

Bezchlibnyk-Butler, K. Z., & Jeffries, J. J. (2005). *Clinical handbook of psychotropic drugs* (15th ed.). Ashland, OH: Hogrefe & Huber.

Carpenito-Moyat, L. J. (2008). *Nursing diagnosis: Application to clinical practice* (12th ed.). Philadelphia, PA: Wolters Kluwer/Lippincott, Williams, & Wilkins.

College urges pregnant women to avoid paxil. (April, 2007). *The Journal for Nurse Practitioners-JNP,* 218.

Cox, L. L., Holden, J. M., & Sagovsky, R. (1987). Detection of postnatal depression: Development of the JO-item Edinburgh Postnatal Depression Scale. *British Journal of Psychiatry, 150,* 782–786.

Davis, J. M., & Gershtein, C. M. (2003). Screening for depression in patients with chronic illness: Why & how? *Disease Management and Health Outcomes, 11*(6), 375–378.

Falcone, T., & Franco, K. (Oct., 2006). Med/Psych update: Treating psychiatric reactions to medical illness. *Current Psychiatry, 5*(10), 105–119.

Fischbach, F. (2004). *A manual of laboratory and diagnostic tests* (7th ed.) Philadelphia, PA: Lippincott, Williams, & Wilkins.

Garzon, D. C. (2007). Childhood depression. *Advance for Nurse Practitioners, 15*(2), 35–44.

Hamrin, V., & Pachler, M. C. (2005). Child & adolescent depression: Review of the latest evidence-based treatments. *Journal of Psychosocial Nursing, 43*(1), 55–63.

Jarvis, C. (2004). *Physical examination & health assessment* (4th ed.). St. Louis, MO: Elsevier, Saunders.

Kupfer, D. J. (2004). Bipolar depression: The clinician's reference guide (BD-CRG). *Current Psychiatry,* June, 2004.

Lewis, S. L., Heitkemper, M. M., Dirksen, S. R., O'Brien, P. G., & Bucher, L. (2007). *Medical-surgical nursing: Assessment and management of clinical problems* (7th ed.). St. Louis, MO: Mosby/Elsevier.

Marcus, P. (2007). Understanding the use of genetics in psychiatry. Psychiatric Nursing Conference, New Orleans, LA.

McKenry, L., Tessier, E., & Hogan, M. (2006). *Mosby's pharmacology in nursing* (22nd ed.). St. Louis, MO: Mosby, Inc.

Mosby's medical, nursing, and allied health dictionary (6th ed.). (2002). St. Louis, MO: Mosby, Inc.

Muzina, D. J. (2007). Suicide intervention: How to recognize risk, focus on patient safety. *Current Psychiatry, 6*(9), 31–38, 45–46.

National Institute of Mental Health (NIMH) (September 23, 2010). Depression. Retrieved from: www.nimh.nih.gov/publicat/depression.cfm

Pinto-Foltz, M. D., & Logsdon, M. C. (2008). Stigma towards mental illness: A concept analysis using postpartum depression as an examplar. *Issues in Mental Health Nursing, 29,* 21–36.

Puskar, K. R., Sereika, S. M., Lamb, J., Tusaie-Mumford, K., & Guinness, T. (1999). Optimism and its relationship to depression, coping, anger, and life events in rural adolescents. *Issues in Mental Health Nursing, 20,* 115–130.

Risk factors and warning signs for suicide (2010). Retrieved from: American Foundation for Suicide Prevention: www.afsp.org

Saunders, J. C. (2008). Neuropsychiatric symptoms of hepatitis C. *Issues in Mental Health Nursing, 29,* 209–220.

Spittle, K. L. (Aug., 2005). Depression underdiagnosed in heart attack patients, associated with adverse outcomes. *NeuroPsychiatry Reviews, 6*(7), 14–15.

Stein, J. (Nov., 2007). Genes linked to suicidal thoughts during antidepressant therapy. *NeuroPsychiatry Reviews, 8*(11), 1, 16, 17.

Stevenson, M. (2007). Combination therapy effectively treats depressed adolescents. *NeuroPsychiatry Reviews, 8*(1), 11.

Stigsdotter Nyström, M. E., & Nyström, M. (2007). Patients' experiences of recurrent depression. *Issues in Mental Health Nursing, 28*, 673–690.

Stong, C. (Aug, 2006). Assessing suicide risk-separating attempts from ideation. *NeuroPsychiatry Reviews, 7*(8), 1, 19.

Sulton, L. L. (July, 2007). Brain injury: A primary-care perspective. *The Clinical Advisor*, 84–89.

Thomas, S. P (2003). From the editor: "Why did he do it?" Confronting issues of suicide and bereavement. *Issues in Mental Health Nursing, 24*, 1–3.

Townsend, M. C. (2005). *Essentials of psychiatric mental health nursing: Concepts of care in evidence based practice* (4th ed.). Philadelphia, PA: F. A. Davis Company.

Vannoy, S., Powers, D., & Unutzer, J. (2006). Making an impact on late-life depression: Partnering with primary care providers can double the effect of treatment. *Current Psychiatry, 5*(9), 85–92.

Wisner, K. L., Parry, B. L., & Piontek, E. M. (Jul., 2002). Postpartum depression. *New England Journal of Medicine, 347*(3), 194–199.

World Health Organization (WHO) (2010). Data and statistics: Suicide. Retrieved from http://www.who.int/research/en

Yigletu, H., Tucker, S., Harris, M., & Hatlevig, J. (2004). Assessing suicide ideation: Comparing self-report versus clinician report. *Journal of the American Psychiatric Nurses Association, 10*(1), 9–15.

CHAPTER 9

Assessment of Suicidal Ideations, Gestures, and Attempts

Kim A. Jakopac

OBJECTIVES

The nursing student will be able to:
1. Avoid inaccurate thinking patterns including myths related to suicide
2. Recognize risk factors for suicide
3. Perform a suicide risk assessment
4. Identify and implement nursing interventions for clients experiencing suicidal ideations, and those who have made suicidal gestures or have attempted suicide
5. Discuss special considerations regarding children/adolescents and elderly clients

KEY TERMS

Copycat suicide	Self-mutilation
Helplessness	Suicide attempt
Hope	Suicide gesture
Hopelessness	Suicidal ideation
Learned helplessness	Suicidal threats
Parasuicidal behavior	Suicide completed
Passive suicide	Suicide survivors

Suicide is defined by the American Psychological Association (APA) as the act of killing oneself (2007, p. 907) or the *intentional* act of killing oneself (Videbeck, 2008, p. 326). It is "the primary emergency for the mental health professional" (Sadock & Sadock, 2005, p. 2442).

INCIDENCE AND EPIDEMIOLOGY

Approximately one person dies every 16 minutes due to suicide. In the United States suicide remains the 3rd leading cause of death of people 15 to 24 years of age, the 2nd leading cause in ages 25 to 34, and the 11th leading cause of death for all ages (Varcarolis & Halter, 2010, pp. 547–549; Lynch, Howard, El-Mallakh, & Matthews, 2008, p. 46). In developing countries it is the 2nd leading cause of death for adolescents (Sadock & Sadock, 2005, p. 3266), and "worldwide suicide is the leading cause of violent death, outnumbering homicide and war-related deaths" (O'Brien, Kennedy, & Ballard, 2008, p. 330). "Suicide is the leading cause of death in psychiatric hospitals . . . 5 to 6% occur in inpatient units" (Lynch, Howard, El-Mallakh, & Matthews, 2008, pp. 47, 50). Depression and substance abuse are two of the greatest risk factors for suicide, but people who are extremely anxious, agitated, impulsive or in a manic state; feel overwhelmed; hear voices telling them to harm themselves (psychosis); have difficulty expressing feelings of anger; have terminal illnesses, declining health, or are in chronic pain also are at high risk (Varcarolis & Halter, 2010, pp. 548–549; APA, 2007, p. 907; Sadock & Sadock, 2005, p. 3268).

Many people who attempt suicide do not have a diagnosed psychiatric problem, but are in great emotional pain and just want the pain to end, similarly to people who suffer physical pain (Varcarolis & Halter, 2010, p. 548). Postmortem findings show a decreased amount of 5-HT, the neurotransmitter serotonin, in cerebrospinal fluid (CSF) and increased levels of corticotropin-releasing factor (CRF) in CSF as well as decreased binding sites for CRF in the frontal cortex. Alcohol lowers levels of 5-HT and also disinhibits activity, thereby adding to a tendency toward impulsivity in some individuals. According to Sadock and Sadock (2005), many people agree that less effective treatment of chronic pain is a major factor in patients' request for assistance with dying. "The current medical system does not adequately prepare new physicians to alleviate pain and suffering in the chronically ill," and the legal system "has prohibitive laws and regulations pertaining to narcotics, which too often results in physicians shunning such patients or treating them inadequately" (p. 2452). Some nurses also may have negative attitudes toward clients with chronic pain problems and label them as "drug seeking" when in reality they have legitimate chronic pain problems and need referral to a pain specialist who uses many modalities to address pain.

According to the Centers for Disease Control (CDC), "an estimated 50% or more of suicide completers have seen a primary care provider (PCP) in the month before their death," thus demonstrating a greater need for more screening for suicide risk (Sadock & Sadock, 2005, p. 2449). Thoughts of suicide are common in patients diagnosed with cancer. Some patients do not discuss their thoughts and feelings because of guilt related to their family members' possible reactions. The number of actual suicides is twice that of the general population, but the actual incidence may be underreported. A frequent cause is inadequate symptom control. It is therapeutic to acknowledge patients' thoughts and help them verbalize their feelings without supporting suicidal behavior. It is also important to remind family and friends that mentally competent, informed patients have the right to refuse medical treatment or stop current treatment (Sadock & Sadock, 2005, p. 2203).

Women attempt suicide more often, but men more often complete suicide due to the use of more lethal methods. The most common methods used to commit suicide include firearms, hanging, stabbing, jumping from high places, slashing wrists, and ingesting substances (e.g., overdoses of prescribed medications, illegal drugs, mixing medications or drugs with alcohol). Sometimes the method reflects the person's desire to act quickly while causing the least amount of pain or disfigurement. In other cases the method chosen may have a symbolic meaning (Sadock & Sadock, 2005, pp. 2449–2450). It is unknown how many vehicle accidents are actually suicide attempts. According to Fontaine (2009), lethality is determined by four factors: the degree of effort it takes to plan the suicide; how specific the plan is; how accessible the method or weapon is; and the chances of not being found or rescued in time (p. 565). Physicians may hesitate to document that a death was due to suicide to spare the family the effects of stigma and problems with life insurance policies. Then there are the highly publicized media cases of murder–suicide where a person kills others before ultimately killing themselves.

The Joint Commission (2008), NPSG.15.01.01, and NPSG.15.01.01 EP 3 requirements related to one of the national patient safety goals, suicide risk reduction, in psychiatric-mental health settings, general hospitals, emergency rooms, ambulatory clinics, and other settings. Information about the availability of a crisis hotline or other resources is also required for any patients identified as being at risk for suicide.

According to Sadock and Sadock (2005), the term *parasuicidal behavior* was developed by Kreitman to describe behaviors—including cutting the skin or ingestion of substances—that do not have a fatal outcome and may be used as a maladaptive coping mechanism to deal with strong emotions or disturbing thoughts. This term, along with the World Health Organization's (WHO) definition of a suicide attempt as being a deliberate, nonfatal act that will cause self-harm if there is no intervention from others, "conveys the view that some types of suicidal behavior are benign in nature," but this is far from the truth (pp. 3266–3267). Suicidal gestures and various acts of self-mutilation should not be taken lightly, because they have been associated with an increased risk of later completed suicides. Unintentional suicides may occur when gestures go wrong, or when people engage in reckless behavior such as drunk driving or children/adolescents playing "the choking game," a form of self-asphyxiation using belts, scarves, or even dog collars to a get "high" without drugs (Russell, Paulozzi, Gilchrist, & Toblin, 2008, p. 1418; Sadock & Sadock, 2005, p. 992).

CULTURAL FACTORS

In the United States, Caucasians of European descent still have the highest number of deaths by suicide, followed by Native Americans, Alaskan Natives, African-American men, Hispanic Americans and Asian Americans (Varcarolis & Halter, 2010, pp. 551–552; Townsend, 2009, pp. 266, 268). According to Fontaine (2009), "suicide pacts have become an increasing problem in Japan" (p. 567). Suicide rates increase with age in Asian-American populations, especially if there is a situation that is viewed as bringing shame to the family. Beliefs in reincarnation may also influence views of suicide. Otherwise suicide is viewed as being disrespectful to society or selfish. Students in India are believed to commit suicide over the high school exams necessary to qualify for university positions, and the suicide rate in China is higher for women than men. Rates for first-generation immigrants reflect suicide rates in their parents' country of origin.

Regarding religion, there are slightly higher rates of suicide among Protestants and Jews compared to Catholics in the United States, and Muslims reportedly have "much lower rates." The increase in suicide bombings most recently in the Middle East is contrary to Islamic beliefs, but some individuals believe that it is an honor to die in defense of their faith and is a direct route to heaven (Varcarolis & Halter, 2010, pp. 551–552; Townsend, 2009, p. 266; Varcarolis, Carson, & Shoemaker, 2006, p. 476; Sadock & Sadock, 2005, p. 2446). It is important to remember when assessing clients that even though they may state that they would not commit suicide because their religion prevents it, in a moment of extreme emotional pain, they may act impulsively and commit an act they normally would not.

MYTHS

Myths or misconceptions abound regarding suicide and suicidal people. Some common myths are listed in **Table 9-1** (Townsend, 2009, p. 265; Videbeck, 2008, p. 327).

Table 9-1   Myths and Facts Related to Suicide and Suicidal People

Myth	Fact
1. "If I mention the word suicide it will make the person start thinking about it, put it in their head."	1. People thinking of suicide are relieved to find someone they can talk to about their feelings.
2. "If a person attempts suicide once, they will not do it again."	2. The majority of people who die as a result of completed suicides have a history of a previous attempt.
3. "If the person's depression improves, the risk of committing suicide is over."	3. Many suicide attempts occur after there is a return of enough energy to carry out a plan and some improvement in mood has begun, but the depressed mood has not entirely been resolved. People just starting on medications or restarting medications are included in this group, making it extremely important to continue monitoring their mood and the presence or absence of suicidal ideations. With shorter hospital stays and more care being delivered in the community not only by psychiatrists, but by PCPs, the risk of missing crucial symptoms increases greatly.
4. "People who commit suicide are psychotic."	4. Although a large percentage of people who commit suicide have been diagnosed with a mental illness, many others have not been and find themselves in intolerable, overwhelming circumstances or great emotional pain and see no other alternative.
5. "People who talk about suicide do not actually commit suicide. Suicide happens without warning."	5. Most people who have completed suicide have given definite clues or warning signs about their intentions. Sometime the clues are subtle and consequently are ignored. At other times the warning signs were clear, but people around them did not know what to look for, and even if they did know would not have known what to do.

(continues)

Table 9-1 Myths and Facts Related to Suicide and Suicidal People *(continued)*	
Myth	**Fact**
6. "Suicidal threats or gestures are manipulative or done for attention and should be ignored."	6. All suicidal behavior is considered to be serious. There is always the potential of death. Any threats, gestures, or attempts should be viewed as a cry for help and treated accordingly.
7. "You cannot stop a suicidal person. He or she is fully intent on dying."	7. Most people who are suicidal are ambivalent about living or dying, which allows for the possibility of intervention and avoidance of death. If underlying psychiatric or medical conditions are treated, if circumstances improve or thinking patterns change with the help of psychotherapy, people can go on to live normal lives.

PROTECTIVE FACTORS

Protective factors are those that are thought to reduce a person's risk of committing suicide. The following items are considered to be protective factors (Varcarolis & Halter, 2010, p. 550; Fontaine, 2009, p. 564):

- Intact, positive social support system
- Intact reality testing
- Effective, healthy, adaptive coping skills including ability to problem-solve
- Access to healthcare
- Active participation in spiritual practices and activities
- Sense of responsibility to family members
- Pregnancy
- Satisfaction with life or acceptance of life as it is
- Absence of mental illness including substance abuse/chemical dependency
- Ongoing supportive relationship with a caregiver

RISK FACTORS

Risk factors for attempting suicide may be categorized as follows (see also **Table 9-2**).

Table 9-2	Risk Factors for Suicide
Psychiatric disorders	Major depression
	Depression accompanied by severe anxiety, agitation, or aggression
	Bipolar disorders
	Schizophrenia
	Dysthymia
	Adjustment disorder
	Conduct disorder
	Other psychotic disorders
Demographics	Male
	Elderly
	Caucasian
	Homosexual
	(In the past, living in urban areas, but currently no more so than in rural areas)
Family history	Suicide of a family member
Social factors	Socially isolated
	Divorced
	Widowed
	Living alone
	Problems with significant other/family
	Financial problems/low socioeconomic status/ downward social drift
	Professional occupation (e.g., physicians, dentists, architects, nurses, engineers, artists, policemen, lawyers, insurance agents)
	Previous suicide attempt
	Suicidal ideations
	Hopelessness
	Helplessness/Learned helplessness
	Lack of or decreased involvement in spiritual activities

(continues)

Table 9-2 Risk Factors for Suicide *(continued)*	
Co-occurring illnesses or disorders (Axis I or III)	Substance abuse/Chemical dependence
	Anxiety
	Panic disorder
	Medical problems/terminal illness/decline in health/chronic pain
Personality disorders (Axis II)	Borderline PD
	Narcissistic PD
	Antisocial PD
	Impulsive traits
Other factors (including crisis situations and Axis IV information)	Specific plan
	Access to means/means available
	Few reasons to live
	Lack of or limited social support
	Firearms in the residence/home
	History of child abuse
	Several adverse events
	Recent losses
	Fear of punishment, embarrassment or humiliation/loss of status/rejection
	Legal problems
	Anniversary time of previous loss/losses
	Severe insomnia
	Sudden change in behavior
	Giving away possessions, especially possessions with monetary or emotional significance
	Women in domestic violence and abuse situations

Sources: Varcarolis & Halter, 2010, pp. 548–549; Townsend, 2009, pp. 265–267; Lynch, Howard, El-Mallakh, & Matthews, 2008, pp. 46–48; Keltner, Schwecke, & Bostrom, 2007, p. 389; Sadock & Sadock, 2005, pp. 2448–2449, 2060.

- Psychiatric disorders (Axis I)
- Demographics
- Family history
- Social factors

- Co-occurring illnesses or disorders (Axis I or III)
- Personality disorders (Axis II)
- Other factors (including crisis situations)

SUICIDE ASSESSMENT

Assessing someone for suicidal ideations is not always comfortable, especially when the person conducting the assessment does not have much experience. The novice has many concerns including the possibility of saying something that will make the potentially suicidal person feel worse or failing to obtain important information that could save the person's life. The psychiatric-mental health (PMH) nurse must focus on the client rather than on personal anxiety and manage their own personal stress. When the nurse performing the suicide assessment is in a "neutral" emotional state, they are less likely to transfer energy in the form of anxiety to the client. Being in a neutral state also allows the PMH nurse to more easily listen to their own instincts and experience, which will lead to a more accurate assessment (Fortinash & Holoday-Worret, 2007, p. 96). "The development of a therapeutic alliance . . . may encourage patients to divulge information vital in determining suicidal risk factors" (Lynch, Howard, El-Mallakh, & Matthews, 2008, p. 49). The therapeutic use of self and therapeutic communication skills are essential to developing a therapeutic nurse–client relationship or therapeutic alliance (see chapters 2 and 4).

A client's mood state and mental status are important to know when preparing to conduct a suicide assessment (see also the biopsychosocial nursing assessment in Chapter 4). Standardized instruments may be used to augment the suicide assessment (Lynch, Howard, El-Mallakh, & Matthews, 2008, pp. 49–50). All of the following assessment instruments have been tested in research studies except for the Nurses' Global Assessment of Suicide Risk. Some of the following instruments may be used without having to obtain special permission, while for others permission must be obtained from the authors:

- Beck Suicide Intent Scale (SIS)
- Beck Hopelessness Scale (BHS)
- Resources for Living Inventory (RFL)
- Nurses' Global Assessment of Suicide Risk (NGASR)

When assessing clients for suicidal ideations, it is best to use specific terms and avoid placing the client in a position of having to contradict the nurse. For example, questions such as "You aren't thinking of killing yourself are you?" invite a "no" response when many times clients are thinking of suicide, but do not want to contradict the nurse who they view as being in a position of authority. This type of question is not empathetic and also implies that the topic of suicide is not open for discussion. The following are some examples of specific questions to ask when assessing clients for suicidal ideations (Varcarolis & Halter, 2010, p. 553; Fontaine, 2009, p. 564; Sadock & Sadock, 2005, pp. 2447–2448):

- "Are you afraid that you might actually kill or hurt yourself?"
- "Have you been thinking about harming yourself?"
- "Have you been thinking about death lately?"
- "Do you ever think about suicide?"
- "Have you ever attempted suicide?"
- "Do you have a plan for committing suicide? If so, what is your plan?"
- "Are you frightened you might actually carry out your plan?"
- "Have you ever felt that life wasn't worth living anymore?"
- "Have you ever wanted to just go to sleep and never wake up?"
- "Do you ever feel that no one would miss you if you were no longer alive?"

Case Example #1: Nurse–Client Interaction

Joan: "I've felt pretty down lately." Sits slumped in a chair with her hands clasped in her lap, looks down, sad affect, quiet voice.

Nurse: Sits down next to Joan, turns toward her with open body posture, leans forward, and in an empathetic tone of voice asks, "How down are you feeling?"

Joan: Briefly makes eye contact and makes an open gesture with her hands; then looks down again and says, "Oh, I don't know. Not much seems to matter to me. It's all so pointless."

Nurse: Studies Joan's face for a moment and uses silence for a minute. When Joan does not respond the nurse says, "What do you mean by pointless?"

Joan: Shrugs her shoulders, looks away, and replies, "The whole thing . . . life. Life is nothing, pointless, a bad joke."

Nurse: "Hmmm, are you saying your life isn't worth living?"

Joan: Looks up directly at the nurse as if searching her face and states, "Well . . . yes, I guess I am."

Nurse: Remains calm and in a caring tone asks, "Are you thinking of killing yourself, Joan?"

Joan: Lets out a sigh and replies, "Oh, I don't know, well sometimes. I don't think I'd ever go through with it though" and quickly looks away.

Nurse: Gently smiles and says, "We all care about you and want to help you. Let's talk more about how you are feeling and what you are thinking."

Joan: Looks up with tears in her eyes and nods her head (see **Table 9-3** and **Table 9-4**).

Note: The PMH nurse must remember to avoid agreeing to keep information secret from other staff members and the treatment team. It is unethical and in some cases could result in harm to the client.

Table 9-3   Examples of Overt vs Covert Statements of Suicidal Ideations and Nursing Responses

Type of statement	Example	Nursing responses
Overt (active)	"I just can't take it anymore."	"Are you thinking of hurting (killing) yourself?"
		"What can't you take anymore?"
	"Life isn't worth living."	"What do you mean by 'life isn't worth living'?"
		"Are you planning on ending your life?"
	"Everyone would be better off if I weren't around."	"How would people be better off if you weren't around?"
		"Who would be better off without you?"
	"I wish I were dead."	Silence to allow the client time to continue the thought.
		"Are you thinking of killing yourself?"
		"Tell me about the reasons you wish you were dead."

(continues)

	Table 9-3	Examples of Overt vs Covert Statements of Suicidal Ideations and Nursing Responses *(continued)*	

Type of statement	Example	Nursing responses
	"No one would miss me if I were gone."	"What do you mean by 'gone'?"
	"Will you miss me when I'm gone?"	Refer to previous response.
	"I won't be here when you come back tomorrow."	"Where will you be? Are you thinking of harming yourself?"
	"I can't stand the pain anymore."	"How do you plan to end the pain?"
		"Tell me about the pain."
		"Are you planning on committing suicide?"
		"Are you planning on ending your life?"
	"I want it to be all over."	"I wonder if you are thinking of suicide."
		"What exactly do you want to be 'over'?"
	"The voices are telling me to hurt/ kill myself."	"What are the voices telling you to do?"
		"Do you think you can resist doing what the voices are telling you to do?"
Covert (passive, hidden)	"My family won't have to worry about money problems much longer."	"What do you mean?"
		"Are you thinking of killing yourself?"
	"The pain will soon be over."	"How will the pain be over?"
		"How are you planning to end the pain?"
	"It won't matter much longer."	"What won't matter?"
	"It's okay now. Soon everything will be fine."	"It sounds like you've made a decision. Are you planning to commit suicide?"
	"You won't have to worry about me much longer."	Refer to previous response.

(continues)

Table 9-3   Examples of Overt vs Covert Statements of Suicidal Ideations and Nursing Responses *(continued)*

Type of statement	Example	Nursing responses
	"You have been nice to me. Remember me when I'm gone."	"We want to help you. I'm concerned that you may be thinking of killing yourself.
	"My life will never get any better."	"You sound depressed. Are you thinking of harming yourself?"
		"What makes you think your life 'will never get any better'?"
	"Nothing feels good to me anymore and probably never will."	Refer to previous response.
	"I just want to go to sleep and not think anymore."	"By 'sleep' do you mean 'die'?"
		"How are you planning to go to sleep and not think anymore?"
Nonverbal changes in behavior	Agitated to calm, peaceful	"You seem different today. What is the reason for the change?"
	Anxious to relaxed	
	Depressed to smiling	"I sense you've made a decision. Please share it with me."
	Problems focusing and making goals to more focused and goal directed	

Sources: Varcarolis & Halter, 2010, pp. 552–553; Fontaine, 2009, p. 565; Videbeck, 2008, p. 328.

Table 9-4   Suicide Assessment

	No	Yes	Comments
1. Ideation?			
a. Admits to suicidal ideation			
b. Overt or active statements			
c. Covert or passive statements (see examples in Table 9-3)			
2. Plan?			(Include description of plan)
a. Specific			
b. Vague			
c. Lethality			
d. Active (client will harm self)			

(continues)

Table 9-4 Suicide Assessment *(continued)*			
	No	**Yes**	**Comments**
e. Passive (client will allow others or circumstances to harm them)			
f. Has access to means/availability?			
3. Ability to form a verbal or written no-suicide/safety contract?			
4. Mental status (see also #7 & 8 in this table)			
a. Severe anxiety or panic level			
b. Agitation or aggression			
c. Hopelessness			
d. Helplessness, learned helplessness			
e. Confusion/disorientation			
f. Manic symptoms			
g. Psychotic symptoms			
5. Diagnosis			
a. Major depression			
b. Depression accompanied by severe anxiety, agitation, or aggression			
c. Bipolar disorder (I or II)			
d. Schizophrenia			
e. Dysthymia			
f. Adjustment disorder			
g. Conduct disorder			
h. Other psychotic disorders			
i. Substance abuse/Chemical dependence			
j. Anxiety			
k. Panic disorder			
l. Medical problems/terminal illness/ decline in health/chronic pain			
m. Borderline PD			
n. Narcissistic PD			
o. Antisocial PD			
p. Impulsive traits			

(continues)

Table 9-4   Suicide Assessment *(continued)*

	No	Yes	Comments
6. Past history of attempts (if yes, include methods; if rescued, interrupted by accident or sought medical attention on own?)			
a. Has an attempt been made while hospitalized in a medical-surgical setting or psychiatric setting?			
7. Current/Past use of substances?			
a. Is client currently under the influence of substances (if yes, what specifically)?			
b. Is the client withdrawing from substances (if yes, what specifically)?			
c. Type, amount, date & time last used			
8. Judgment			
a. Good			
b. Fair			
c. Poor			
9. Impulse control			
a. Good			
b. Fair			
c. Poor			
10. Circumstances (including Axis IV and V information)			
a. Firearms present in the residence			
b. Problems with significant others/ family			
c. Financial/employment problems			
d. Legal problems			
e. Few reasons to live			
f. Lack of or limited social support			
g. Several adverse events			
h. Recent losses			

(continues)

Table 9-4 **Suicide Assessment** *(continued)*			
	No	**Yes**	**Comments**
i. Anniversary time of previous loss/ losses			
j. Bereavement, grief issues			
k. Fear of punishment, embarrassment or humiliation/loss of status/ rejection			
l. Severe insomnia			
m. Decrease in/withdrawal from usual spiritual practices or activities			
n. Sudden change in behavior (e.g., becomes withdrawn, poor eye contact, increased anxiety, agitation, aggressiveness, or calmer, at peace)			
o. Giving away possessions especially possessions with monetary or emotional significance			

11. Ability to form a therapeutic alliance
   a. Agrees treatment is necessary?
   b. Accepts the nurse's presence?
   c. Agrees to work with the nurse?
   d. Expresses a wish to feel better?
   e. Able to verbalize feelings (also indicate if good, fair, or poor)?			

12. Person/Agency information reported to			
13. Recommendations/Referrals made (in an inpatient facility, indicate whether or not a change in level of observation and further precautions are needed)			

Special Considerations

When assessing children/adolescents and the elderly, many of the same principles apply and similar information is needed, as noted in the previous sections of this chapter. However, there are some special considerations when working with children/ adolescents and the elderly.

Children/Adolescents

According to Kaplan and Sadock (2005), rates of suicide are "extremely low before puberty" in all countries, but the reasons for this are unknown. Younger children do talk about suicide and some do attempt suicide, but the greatest risk factors, depression and substance abuse, occur less often before puberty (p. 3267). Prior adolescent suicide attempts are most common among females and those who have a mood disorder at the time of their deaths. Repeat attempts occur most commonly in adolescent males who present with hopelessness or have a history of depression, substance abuse, or psychosis. Most repeat attempts take place within 3 months of the initial suicide attempt. Repeat attempts are less common among those who have good peer relationships and live at home (Sadock & Sadock, 2005, p. 3269).

The underlying intent of an adolescent's suicidal behavior is difficult to determine. As many as 50% of adolescents seen in emergency rooms (ERs) report wanting to die, even though most did not take any precautions to avoid being discovered. Attempts may be planned in advance, but many are impulsive acts occurring shortly after a stressful event. A common precipitating event is the break-up of a love relationship or the anticipation of stressful events including punishment, ending of a relationship, taking a test, or relocation to a new neighborhood and entering a new school. The Youth Risk Behavior Survey results indicate that "three-fourths" of adolescents who thought about suicide had a plan even though many did not act upon it (Sadock & Sadock, 2005, pp. 3269, 3272). According to the results of "large, frequently repeated benchmark surveys," 30% of high school students have thought of suicide and 10% have made one or more attempts; however, only 2–3% received medical attention for their attempts. Unfortunately, many adolescent clients do not continue with care after discharge from ERs; therefore, it is strongly recommended that healthcare providers deal with factors directly related to the attempt (e.g., family strife, ending of relationships, fear of future events) while the adolescent is still in the ER. It is also strongly recommended that family teaching begin in the ER, including teaching about depression and other psychiatric disorders that may be involved, treatment of these disorders, the importance of follow-up care, scheduling the first appointment, how to remember follow-up appointments and how to handle missed appointments.

As with adults, suicide attempts occur more often in adolescent females, while suicide completions occur more often in adolescent males. Suicide is more common in Caucasian and Latino adolescents than in African Americans. Suicide is also more common in spring months with a secondary peak in fall months in both northern and southern hemispheres. "Epidemiologic studies indicate that across small areas in the

United States, the increase in SSRI prescriptions for teenagers has coincided with declines in the teenage suicide rate" (Sadock & Sadock, 2005, pp. 3268–3269).

Methods used to commit suicide are usually determined by availability and what others in the local area have used. These include firearms (legally, inadequately secured, or illegally obtained), hanging and jumping from a height; ingestion of substances, and self-asphyxiation including the use of carbon monoxide. Copycat suicides occur when adolescents identify with and imitate the behavior of a highly publicized suicide of a peer in the community, a teen idol, or other type of public figure (Varcarolis & Halter, pp. 2010, 551). When assessing children, play therapy and use of drawing may elicit more information due to decreased vocabulary and verbal expression of feelings when compared to adults. Favorite pastimes, games, TV shows, movies, music, peer relationships, and academic performance also provide more clues as to how children/adolescents are functioning, feeling, and thinking. Children/adolescents who have made a suicide attempt should not be discharged without a psychiatric evaluation and interviewing the parents (Sadock & Sadock, 2005, p. 3722) (see Chapters 8 and 10).

Elderly

Suicide rates increase with age. The highest rates of suicide are among those age 75 years and older. Many elderly clients use less noticeable or less easily identifiable methods such as taking more medication than prescribed, stopping taking medications prescribed for chronic medical illnesses, or stopping eating. They may give away possessions that have monetary or sentimental value. Older adults are also less likely to seek professional help for emotional problems or psychosis. When they do seek care, it is from their primary care physician (PCP) rather than from a psychiatrist (Sadock & Sadock, 2005, p. 3602). Elderly clients may not appear sad or tearful, but may be more socially withdrawn, apathetic, experience appetite and/or sleep disturbances, and easily dismiss their symptoms as signs of old age (Sadock & Sadock, 2005, pp. 2451–2452). It is much more difficult for healthcare providers to detect psychiatric problems in the elderly due to the presence of co-occurring medical problems (see Chapters 8 and 10).

Extra time should be scheduled when interviewing these clients to allow them sufficient opportunity to talk, allow for breaks or rest periods between information gathering sessions, and allow for family members to be involved according to clients' wishes and needs, especially when clients are cognitively impaired. Older clients expect to be respected, and more touching, including handshakes, is appropriate than when using the traditional psychiatric approach to client interaction (Sadock & Sadock, 2005, pp. 3603–3604). Also, direct or focused questioning may be more beneficial, and clear explanations should be given as with clients of any other age group.

NURSING INTERVENTIONS AND RATIONALES

Nursing interventions are planned according to individual clients needs. For specific nursing diagnoses, outcomes, and evaluation criteria, refer to a general psychiatric-mental health nursing textbook such as *Psychiatric Mental Health Nursing: An Introduction to Theory and Practice*, O'Brien, Kennedy & Ballard (2008); *Mental Health Nursing*, Fontaine (2009); *Psychiatric Nursing: Contemporary Practice*, Boyd (2008); *Psychiatric Mental Health Case Studies and Care Plans*, Jakopac and Patel (2009); and psychiatric care plan books such as *Psychiatric Nursing Care Plans*, Fortinash & Holoday-Worret (2007), or *Manual of Psychiatric Nursing Care Plans*, Varcarolis (2006). The interventions presented in **Table 9-5** apply to the adult and elderly client with variations for the child/adolescent client as indicated.

Discharge Planning

The community resources available will depend on the geographic location, and amount of support available from family, friends, and religious or community organizations. It is very important for the client to have as much social support as possible. The client will need follow-up care for psychiatric disorders including substance abuse and other medical diagnoses as appropriate. Refer to chapters 4, 8, and 9 for more information including psychotherapy, support groups, patient and family teaching. As previously stated in **Table 9-5**, the client should have the psychiatrist appointment in the next 24 hours if possible or as soon as is possible if being discharged from the ER or within 1 week if being discharged from a psychiatric-mental health unit. The client should be provided with the suicide hotline number (1-800-SUICIDE/ 1-800-784-2433) and should be assisted to write a list (placed in cell phone if possible) of at least three people they can call if thoughts of suicide return. Reassure the client that they will have an outpatient treatment team to work with, but can return to the ER if they feel suicidal and unable to reach their outpatient providers. Also reassure the client that it is normal to feel anxious when anticipating leaving the inpatient area, but they will have an outpatient treatment team and not be alone.

Table 9-5   Nursing Interventions and Rationales for the Suicidal Client

Problems	Nursing interventions	Rationales
Care for injuries sustained during suicide attempt/gesture	1. Assess the degree of physical injury sustained.	1. The client will need to be stabilized medically first before they will be able to be admitted to a psychiatric unit or meets criteria for admission to a medical-psychiatric unit.
	2. Provide care related to specific suicide attempt (e.g., gunshot wound, stabbing wound, airway occlusion, overdose, etc.).	2. Some clients require medical or surgical intervention and admission to an ICU or medical-surgical unit due to injuries sustained. If the client is on an involuntary commitment, the nurse must be aware of the time frame limitations depending on the state's mental health laws to avoid time lapse (end of the involuntary commitment) and legal problems regarding continuing to keep the client if the client insists on leaving the hospital AMA.
	3. Begin to develop rapport and trust with the client.	3. Developing a rapport with the patient will assist in gaining the patient's trust and cooperation in the future and helps initiate the therapeutic nurse–client relationship or therapeutic alliance. According to Render and Peplau (O'Brien, Kennedy, & Ballard, 2008, pp. 17–18), the therapeutic nurse–client relationship is the foundation that must be established to initiate future work in the healing process. The client may be more willing to divulge information if they feel they can trust the nurse. There are times when clients express anger that they have not been able to complete the suicide attempt and need the nurse to listen.

4. Request a full psychiatric evaluation.

4. The admitting physician/psychiatrist acting in the client's best interest will determine if the client meets criteria for admission, and which setting will best provide client safety regardless of the health insurance involved. Least restrictive alternatives must be explored as well as the client's current support system, resources, and history of treatment adherence (Kaplan & Sadock, 2005, p. 2450). Most states provide for a client's right to be hospitalized voluntarily unless they are unwilling to do so and meet criteria for involuntary admission (refer to your state's mental health laws). Careful documentation must be done of all care rendered and disposition of the client. For the suicidal client "The hospital milieu may be the most critical of early therapy in terms of safety and providing hope for recovery. Group experiences on the unit may also be helpful" (Kaplan & Sadock, 2005, p. 2451). The type of psychotherapy that is chosen is based on the client's diagnosis, underlying illness, and evidence of the effectiveness of treatment.

a. If the client is still suicidal they will need to be placed on 1:1 observation or COs.

a. Even before a client has had a psychiatric evaluation, if they are still thinking of suicide, a staff member, preferably someone with psychiatric-mental health experience, should be assigned to stay with the client at all times especially when they are in the ER, ICU or other medical-surgical areas of the hospital. Personal belongings should be removed from the immediate area after being searched by

(continues)

Table 9-5   Nursing Interventions and Rationales for the Suicidal Client (continued)

Problems	Nursing interventions	Rationales
		two staff members in the client's presence for legal reasons and given to family members/friends or locked in a secure area. Family members/friends may stay, but are not hospital employees and are not ultimately responsible for the client's safety.
	5. If the client is not hospitalized, appropriate referrals for outpatient treatment including a psychiatrist, psychologist/social worker or APRN for psychotherapy and other client needs should be made before the client leaves the ER. The help of family or friends should be enlisted to remove any firearms and other potential weapons from the home, and the client should not be left alone.	5. Unfortunately, if the client's suicide attempt is interpreted as a gesture/parasuicidal behavior or done for attention/manipulative, important assessment information and the opportunity to provide what treatment is in the client's best interest will be missed. The client may be referred for outpatient treatment when what they really need is inpatient treatment. The client may also interpret the outpatient referral as not being taken seriously and make another more life-threatening attempt. On the other hand, it is not appropriate for a client to continually use the ER or inpatient psychiatric setting in place of psychiatric-mental health care that is more appropriately obtained in the outpatient setting. Encouraging clients to be honest with their healthcare providers and to seek help before their symptoms become overwhelming is in their best interest and more easily allows care to be rendered in least restrictive settings.

a. The client should have the psychiatrist appointment in the next 24 hours if possible or as soon as possible.

a. In many areas of the country there are too few psychiatrists and other mental health professionals making it difficult to schedule appointments. However, someone who has been treated in an ER for a suicide attempt/gesture is a priority, high-risk client. Such a client should not be waiting weeks to be seen for the first time after being treated in an ER.

b. Provide the client with the suicide hotline number (1-800-SUICIDE/1-800-784-2433).

b. This information and planning ahead helps provide the client with some psychological, emotional comfort that they are not alone, have some control over their situation and can be empowered. It can also help prevent another suicide attempt.

c. Assist the client to write a list (place in cell phone) of at least three people they can call if thoughts of suicide return, especially if there is no one who can stay with the client.

c. See previous rationale.

d. Reassure the client that they can return to the ER or during office hours go to the outpatient healthcare provider for help if they still feel suicidal.

d. The client may experience increased anxiety at the thought of being discharged and not seeing a psychiatrist until at least the next day. Letting them know they can come back provides psychological, emotional comfort and can help prevent another suicide attempt.

e. Carefully document all referrals and instructions given to client including what to do if suicidal thoughts return and client's response.

e. Accurate documentation is a Joint Commission requirement and legal requirement. If in the unfortunate case where the client attempts suicide again, the record should show what steps the nurse took to ensure the client's safety. It should also show if the nurse was not comfortable discharging the client and what steps were taken to communicate this.

(continues)

Table 9-5   Nursing Interventions and Rationales for the Suicidal Client *(continued)*

Problems	Nursing interventions	Rationales
Suicidal ideations	1. Begin to develop rapport and trust with the client.	1. Again, developing a rapport with the patient will assist in gaining the patient's trust and cooperation in the future and helps initiate the therapeutic nurse–client relationship or therapeutic alliance. According to Render and Peplau (O'Brien, Kennedy & Ballard, 2008, pp. 17–18), the therapeutic nurse–client relationship is the foundation that must be established to initiate future work in the healing process (Boyd, 2008, p. 362). The client may be more willing to divulge information if they feel they can trust the nurse.
	a. Incorporate therapeutic use of self when performing a suicide risk assessment.	a. See previous rationale. The concept of the therapeutic use of self incorporates empathy, acceptance, positive regard, being open, being nonjudgmental and actively listening to the client as well as body posture indicating attentiveness. This will help the client know the nurse is truly listening and accepting the client at this moment in time, in this difficult situation, and genuinely wants to help the client. The client will be more willing to be completely honest with the nurse and provide information no matter how emotionally difficult it may be to discuss or hear.
	b. Refrain from looking shocked or making judgmental statements when assessing the client.	b. If the client perceives that the nurse is shocked, frightened, or disapproves of them, it is less likely that they will divulge important information that is crucial to providing care.

2. Assess for current or recent suicidal ideations every 8 hours and prn.

2. For client safety the nurse must establish if the client is thinking of committing suicide. Even though a client denies currently thinking about committing suicide it "does not automatically indicate the absence of risk because the patient may be so resigned to the idea of death that the prospect does not cause anxiety" (Kaplan & Sadock, 2005, p. 2448). Caution must also be taken with clients who are impulsive because one moment they may not be thinking of suicide, but may act impulsively without thinking.

a. If the client currently is not thinking of suicide, follow up with asking if the client will tell the nurse or staff member if they start thinking about suicide.

a. See the previous rationale.

b. Observe at least every 15 minutes for verbalizations and behavior that show the client is forming a plan.

b. See the previous rationale.

c. Assess for subtle as well as obvious changes in level of anxiety, agitation, energy or any behavior that contradicts the client's verbal responses.

c. "Severe overwhelming anxiety and agitation have been shown to be predictors of completed suicide" (Kaplan & Sadock, 2005, p. 1701). A client who previously was depressed, anxious or agitated and now is calm and more peaceful may no longer be ambivalent about ending their life because a decision and plan have been made.

3. Use therapeutic communication techniques to facilitate verbalization of feelings.

3. Therapeutic communication techniques are useful when facilitating client verbalization of feelings. It is very important for the client to verbalize feelings rather than act upon them or express feelings in maladaptive ways.

(continues)

Table 9-5   Nursing Interventions and Rationales for the Suicidal Client (continued)

Problems	Nursing interventions	Rationales
	a. Listen for themes in the client's verbalizations.	a. Identifying themes will help the nurse more fully assess the root cause of the client's emotional and spiritual distress.
	b. Suggest journaling or use of art supplies as other ways of expressing feelings.	b. Journal entries and art projects are also helpful ways of expressing feelings especially for clients who have difficulty verbally expressing feelings. The journal entries and art projects can be used to encourage clients to talk about their feelings more easily and gain insight.
Suicide plan	1. Determine if the client has a plan and whether it is specific or vague.	1. The presence of a plan, specificity, and lethality increase the risk of suicide. Again, caution must be used with clients who are impulsive because they may not be planning to commit suicide, but may act impulsively without thinking.
	2. Assess the degree of lethality of the method and availability/access to means.	2. Firearms are the most common method used, and many clients have them in their place of residence. Unfortunately, a client who is inpatient can still find ways to harm themselves if distraught, hopeless, helpless, extremely anxious, agitated, or aggressive.
	a. What methods were used if there is a history of previous suicide attempts?	a. A previous suicide attempt increases the risk of the client making another attempt.
	b. If the client has a plan, are they able to refrain from acting upon it?	b. If the client can refrain from acting upon the plan, it shows they are trying to help keep themselves safe and are participating in the therapeutic alliance.

Ability to contract for safety

1. Obtain a verbal or written no-suicide or safety contract with the client every 8 hours and pm (refer to specific facility or agency policies) (see also **Table 9-6**).

1. The PMH nurse will need to determine if the client is safe to leave on safety checks every 15 minutes or if they need to be placed on 1:1 or constant observation (COs). The ability to resist acting upon suicidal thoughts and urges is not always possible. There is a need for additional assessment, obtaining at least a verbal no-suicide or safety contract, and documentation. Some facilities require the client to be placed in a hospital gown with snaps (no ties) and shoe laces removed. Other facilities allow the client to remain in their own clothes minus the shoe laces and belts. Many facilities also allow only a heavy blanket and pillow without a pillowcase in place of bed linens (refer to the specific facility policies). Some questions have been raised regarding the value of obtaining a no-suicide or safety contract, but it is still common practice to do so and most facilities/agencies require staff to do so. However, the contract itself does *not* take the place of careful observation and assessment. A client may contract with the nurse, but for various reasons not abide by it (e.g., change in situation, change in mood, impulsivity, thought distortions, psychosis). Unfortunately, even in the inpatient setting suicide can occur with common objects such as the client's own socks, which on many psychiatric units the client may be allowed to have even on suicide precautions (Lynch, Howard, El-Mallakh, & Matthews, 2008, pp. 46–47; O'Brien, Kennedy, & Ballard, 2008, p. 331). Careful observation and

(continues)

Table 9-5   Nursing Interventions and Rationales for the Suicidal Client (continued)

Problems	Nursing interventions	Rationales
		assessment can identify if this is the case and result in closer observation and precautions for the client's safety (i.e., 1:1 or COs.). Contracts do help identify more quickly a client who cannot contract (Lynch et. al, 2008, p. 51; Kaplan & Sadock, 2005, p. 2451).
	a. Document whether or not the client is able to contract with the nurse. If unable to contract, document what action was taken and who the information was reported to.	a. Accurate documentation is a Joint Commission requirement and legal requirement.
	b. If the client currently is not thinking of suicide and does not have a plan, follow up with asking if the client will tell the nurse/staff member if they start thinking about suicide.	b. See previous rationales for "Suicidal ideations" in this table.
Milieu management	1. Provide a safe, therapeutic milieu free from contraband or items that could be potential weapons. This intervention, including more frequent observations (1:1 observation or COs) may be referred to as "suicide precautions" or "Level I or II suicide precautions/observations" depending on the agency/facility (see Chapter 3, Table 3-2).	1. This measure helps decrease the possibility of the client hurting themselves or others (see Chapter 3, Table 3-2). The milieu should feel safe to the client, and the nurse should refrain from thinking that a client who denies suicidal ideations now that they are on the psychiatric unit made statements earlier as a manipulation to obtain admission to the hospital. That is not to say that there are not times when a client may be looking for secondary gains and make statements to gain entry to the hospital to avoid legal entanglements, criminal elements, social/familial/occupational responsibilities, etc. More assessment information would be needed to make that type of judgment,

and it should be reported to the psychiatrist and treatment team. It is ultimately the responsibility and clinical judgment of the admitting physician/psychiatrist that determines whether or not a client meets criteria for inpatient admission.

a. If the client is in the ER, ICU or on a medical-surgical unit, personal belongings should be searched by two staff members in the presence of the client and removed from the immediate area or room, given to the family or friends to be taken home or placed in a locked area if support individuals are available.

a. A staff member, preferably someone with psychiatric-mental health experience, should be assigned to stay with the client at all times especially when they are in the ER, ICU, or other medical-surgical areas of the hospital. Personal belongings should be removed from the immediate area after being searched by two staff members in the client's presence for legal reasons and given to family members/friends or locked in a secure area. Family members/friends may stay, but are not hospital employees and are not ultimately responsible for the client's safety.

b. Document in the client's record what was done with the personal belongings.

c. If the client is able to form a verbal or written safety contract, place the client on safety observations every 15 minutes, notify the attending physician, and document the contract, observations, physician notification, and physician response.

b. This must be done for legal reasons and Joint Commission requirements.

c. The client must be observed more frequently because of the risk for suicide even if currently able to form a safety contract. The client should be assessed and another contract obtained every 8 hours and prn even if not currently on a psychiatric-mental health unit. The safety risks are even greater in other areas of the hospital. Documentation must be done for legal reasons and Joint Commission requirements.

Table 9-5   Nursing Interventions and Rationales for the Suicidal Client (*continued*)

Problems	Nursing interventions	Rationales
	d. If the client is not able to form a verbal or written safety contract, place the client on 1:1 observation or COs, and notify the attending physician (see Chapter 3, Table 3-2 and refer to individual agency policies).	d. This would be done if the client was currently on a psychiatric-mental health unit, and the safety risks are even greater in other areas of the hospital. Again, documentation must be done for legal reasons and Joint Commission requirements.
Mental status/ judgment/impulse control	1. Assess client's mental status, including judgment and impulse control.	1. A client with an abnormal mental status is at higher risk for harming themselves.
	a. Provide a calm environment.	a. A calm environment will help decrease anxiety, agitation, and reduce stress for a client experiencing psychosis. Hallucinations or delusional thinking can become worse when the client feels stressed.
	b. Reorient the client as needed.	b. A confused or disoriented client will misperceive what is happening in the environment or misperceive the words and actions of others. The client is at risk for harming themselves accidentally.
	c. Reinforce reality as needed.	c. A client experiencing psychosis or confusion has difficulty distinguishing reality from non-reality and may feel frightened or anxious, which can increase the risk of harming themselves.
	d. Assess the client's current ability to problem-solve and assist with problem solving as well as utilizing counseling and crisis intervention techniques (see Chapter 4, Table 4-3, Section IV, pp.64–69 (Unit I) and Chapter 18, Table 18-2, Phase 3, pp. 473–475 (Unit IV)).	d. A client who is suicidal has decreased problem-solving abilities at least temporarily and will need assistance. Counseling and crisis intervention techniques are used to help the client focus on the facts of their situation, people, and resources that can be helpful, and come to a more realistic assessment of the situation.

e. Assess the client's knowledge of relaxation techniques and teach new relaxation techniques.

f. Offer other distraction methods such as listening to soft music or opportunities to exercise within unit policies and the client's physical abilities.

g. Encourage/support spiritual practices and activities as much as possible.

h. Inform the client of the temporary nature of their feelings without belittling or downplaying current feelings (e.g., "I know you feel bad now, but you may not always feel this way"—Fortinash & Holoway-Worret, 2007, p. 97).

i. Administer scheduled medications and prn medication if appropriate less restrictive methods have not been effective or only partially effective or if the client is experiencing hallucinations or delusional thinking.

e. Increased stress levels cause increased anxiety. Increased anxiety levels have been associated with increased suicide completions as stated above

f. See the previous rationale.

g. Healthy spiritual practices and activities help the client find meaning in life's experiences, and provide comfort and support during emotionally difficult times.

h. Knowing that the feeling may be time limited may bring a sense of hope or relief. After the client has settled into the unit, teaching about a diagnosis or about crisis can begin.

i. Antipsychotic (for hallucinations/delusions/agitation) or anti-anxiety (for anxiety/agitation) medications may be needed depending on the client's symptoms and response to non-pharmacologic methods. Medications are also used in conjunction with nonpharmacologic methods to obtain a synergistic effect. The client's thoughts need to be clearer and more focused to allow for learning about their situation and how to cope, which is difficult when the client is dealing with depression, anxiety, racing thoughts, flight of ideas, confusion, disorientation, or psychosis.

Table 9-6   Example of a No-Suicide/No-Self-Harm/Safety Contract
"I, _____ (client name), agree to report to staff any time I have thoughts or feeling of harming myself, losing control, or destroying property."
Signature: _____
Witness: _____
Date/Time: _____
Note: The contract may be verbal or in writing and should be renewed every 8 hours and prn if the client's condition changes. The contract may also include other behavior the client agrees to engage in such as calling a suicide/crisis hotline, their psychiatrist or psychotherapist, and a list of support people to call when they feel depressed, anxious, or irritable in outpatient situations. The contract is documented in the client's record (refer to your individual agency policy).

Survivors of Suicide

A suicide survivor is a person who has lost a loved one or close friend to suicide rather than a person who has lived following a suicide attempt. Nurses and other healthcare professionals can also be included in the definition if a current or former client has committed suicide. Because the suicide victim cannot tell the survivors the reason why they committed suicide, the survivor is at the mercy of their own thoughts or conscience. Even when a note or letter was left, there are many unanswered questions. The survivor will need much support including support groups specific for suicide survivors and grief issues, education, and in some cases psychotherapy to deal with feelings of guilt, devastation, and loss (Sadock & Sadock, 2005, pp. 2452–2453).

Prevention

A 1984 study of PCPs and an education program in Sweden produced positive results, but education efforts needed to be repeated or reinforced every 3 years (Kaplan & Sadock, 2005, p. 2449). In 2001 the National Strategy for Suicide Prevention (NSSP) announced a massive effort to prevent suicide, including national goals of increasing public awareness that suicide is a public health problem, that it can in many cases be prevented, and support for more research (NY State OMH Policy Recommendations, 2005, p. 25). Goals of the National Strategy for Suicide Prevention include promoting awareness that suicide is a preventable problem; reducing stigma associated with mental illness and substance abuse; implementing training for recognizing people at risk and obtaining effective treatment; developing and implementing suicide prevention programs; improving access and community links with mental health and substance abuse services; and promoting research (Varcarolis & Halter, 2010, p. 556).

Primary Intervention

Primary intervention includes the prevention of suicide by providing support and education in hospitals as well as in a wide variety of community settings including schools, churches, community centers, and work settings (Varcarolis & Halter, 2010, p. 556). Refer to the Goals of the National Strategy for Suicide Prevention previously mentioned.

Secondary Intervention

Secondary intervention involves treatment of the actual suicidal gesture or attempt. This level of intervention requires good crisis intervention skills and also occurs in the hospital setting as well as in community settings including suicide–crisis telephone hotlines, clinics, schools, and jails (Varcarolis & Halter, 2010, p. 556).

Tertiary Intervention

Tertiary intervention, also referred to as "postvention," includes interventions with survivors of suicide. This level of intervention involves reducing the psychological and emotional trauma through providing support and education. Also referrals are made for community resources including support groups specific for suicide survivors and grief issues, and psychotherapy when appropriate (Varcarolis & Halter, 2010, p. 556).

REFERENCES

American Psychological Association (2007). *APA dictionary of psychology*. Washington, DC: Author.

Boyd, M. A. (2008). *Psychiatric nursing: Contemporary practice* (4th ed.). Philadelphia, PA: Wolters Kluwer/Lippincott, Williams, & Wilkins.

Fontaine, K. L. (2009). *Mental health nursing* (6th ed.). Upper Saddle River, NJ: Pearson Education Inc.

Fortinash, K. M., & Holoday-Worret, P. A. (2007). *Psychiatric nursing care plans* (5th ed.). St. Louis, MO: Mosby, Elsevier.

Jakopac, K. A., & Patel, S. C. (2009). *Psychiatric mental health case studies and care plans*. Sudbury, MA: Jones and Bartlett.

Joint Commission on Accreditation of Healthcare Organizations (JCAHO) (2008) NPSG.15.01.01 and NPSG.15.01.01 EP 3. *Suicide risk reduction*. Retrieved from: http://www.jointcommission. org/AccreditationPrograms/BehavioralHealthCare/Standards/09_FAQs/NPSG/Focused_risk_ assessment/NPSG.15.01.01/Suicide+risk+reduction.htm

Keltner, N. L., Schwecke, L. H., & Bostrom, C. E. (2007). *Psychiatric nursing* (5th ed.). St. Louis, MO: Mosby, Elsevier.

Lynch, M. A., Howard, P. B., El-Mallakh, P., & Matthews, J. M. (2008). Assessment and management of hospitalized suicidal patients. *Journal of Psychosocial Nursing*, *46*(7), 45–51.

O'Brien, P. G., Kennedy, W. Z., & Ballard, K. A. (2008). *Psychiatric mental health nursing: An introduction to theory and practice*. Sudbury, MA: Jones and Bartlett.

Russell, P., Paulozzi, L., Gilchrist, J., & Toblin, R. (2008). Unintentional strangulation deaths from the "choking game" among youths aged 6–19 years—United States 1995–2007. *JAMA: Journal of the American Medical Association*, *299*(12), 1418–1421.

Sadock, B. J., & Sadock, V. A. (2005). *Comprehensive textbook of psychiatry* (8th ed.). Philadelphia, PA: Lippincott, Williams, & Wilkins.

Townsend, M. C. (2009). *Psychiatric mental health nursing: Concepts of evidence-based practice* (6th ed.). Philadelphia, PA: F. A. Davis.

Varcarolis, E. M., Carson, V. B., & Shoemaker, N. C. (2006). *Foundations of psychiatric mental health nursing: A clinical approach* (5th ed.). St. Louis, MO: Saunders, Elsevier.

Varcarolis, E. M., & Halter, M. J. (2010). *Foundations of psychiatric mental health nursing: A clinical approach* (6th ed.). St. Louis, MO: Saunders, Elsevier.

Videbeck, S. L. (2008). *Psychiatric-mental health nursing* (4th ed.). Philadelphia, PA: Wolters Kluwer/Lippincott, Williams & Wilkins.

SUGGESTED READINGS

Carpinello, S. E. (2005). *Saving lives in New York: Suicide prevention and public health, volume 1: Challenge, strategy and policy recommendations*. New York State Office of Mental Health. Retrieved from http://www.omh.state.ny.us/omhweb/savinglives/Volume1/Vol1_pdfs/Vol1_Entire.pdf

CDC Morbidity and Mortality Weekly Report (MMWR) February 15, 2008. Retrieved from http://www.cdc.gov/mmwr/PDF/wk/mm5706.pdf

CDC podcast (2008): *The choking game can be deadly*. Retrieved from www2a.cdc.gov/podcasts/ player.asp?f=8058

Games Adolescents Shouldn't Play (GASP) Forum and community support (2008). Retrieved from www.deadlygameschildrenplay.com/en/home.asp. and GASP: Movie www.stop-the-choking-game.com/en/flash_vid.html

Joint Commission on Accreditation of Health Care Organizations (JCAHO) Behavioral Healthcare standards. Retrieved from http://www.jointcommission.org/AccreditationPrograms/Behavioral HealthCare/Standards/09AQs/default.htm

McAllister, M., Creedy, D., Moyle, W., & Ferrugia, C. (2002). Nurses' attitudes towards clients who self-harm. *Journal of Advanced Nursing*, *40*(5), 578–86.

McDonald, C. (Aug, 2006). Self mutilation in adolescents. *The Journal of School Nursing*, *22*(4), 193–200.

Mohr, W. K. (2006). *Psychiatric-mental health nursing: Evidence based concepts, skills, and practices* (6th ed.). Philadelphia, PA: Wolters Kluwer/Lippincott, Williams & Wilkins.

National Center for Injury Prevention and Control (NCIPC) (2008). Research Update for NCIPC. Retrieved from http://www.cdc.gov/ncipc/duip/research/choking_game.htm

Shives, L. R. (2005). *Basic concepts of psychiatric-mental health nursing* (6th ed.). Philadelphia, PA: Lippincott, Williams & Wilkins.

Thomas, S. P. (2003). From the editor—"Why did he do it?": Confronting issues of suicide and bereavement. *Issues in Mental Health Nursing, 24,* 1–2.

CHAPTER 10

Assessment of Bipolar Disorders: Acute Manic Phase

Kim A. Jakopac

OBJECTIVES

The nursing student will be able to:

1. Recognize signs and symptoms that meet DSM-IV-TR criteria for bipolar disorders
2. Be familiar with common medical illnesses that can cause or exacerbate signs and symptoms of bipolar disorders
3. Perform a biopsychosocial nursing assessment or intake assessment of clients experiencing signs and symptoms of bipolar disorders
4. Identify and implement nursing interventions for clients experiencing signs and symptoms of bipolar disorders
5. Assess discharge planning needs of clients admitted with a diagnosis of one of the bipolar disorders
6. Discuss special considerations regarding children/adolescents and elderly clients

KEY TERMS

Bipolar I
Bipolar II
Distractibility
Euphoria
Expansive/elevated mood
Flight of ideas

Grandiose
Hypomania
Labile
Mania
Mixed episode
Rapid cycling

*B*ipolar disorders are illnesses included in the American Psychiatric Association's (APA) *Diagnostic and Statistical Manual of Mental Disorders* (4th ed.), text revision (DSM-IV-TR) (APA, 2000, pp. 388–391, 394, 400–401, 413–417). A person who has been diagnosed with a bipolar disorder experiences symptoms of major depression at times and at other times experiences symptoms of mania. A large number of people experience signs and symptoms of bipolar disorders for several years before being accurately diagnosed due to usually seeking treatment for symptoms of depression. Refer to Chapter 8 for information related to major depression.

SIGNS AND SYMPTOMS

Bipolar I disorder consists of periods of depression and mania. Symptoms of mania occur for a period of 1 week (Bipolar II, previously termed "hypomania" symptoms last approximately 4 days and may be less intense than Bipolar I symptoms). These symptoms include:

- Persistently euphoric or expansive/elevated mood
- Irritable or labile mood

Also, during this time period of mood disturbance at least three of the following symptoms have persisted or four symptoms if the mood is only irritable:

- Decreased need for sleep
- Distractibility
- Excessive speech, more talkative than usual or pressure to keep talking
- Racing thoughts or flight of ideas
- Grandiose (delusional) thinking
- Religious preoccupation
- Increase in goal-directed activities
- Excessive involvement in pleasurable activities that will result in problems later on

(APA, 2000, pp. 388–389; Keltner, Schwecke, & Bostrom, 2007, pp. 396–398; Smith, 2009, p. 42)

In Bipolar I disorder, mixed episodes, and even in Bipolar II disorder, there are clients who feel and act extremely impulsively, which often results in physical injury; attempted suicide or homicide; experience of increased energy; experience of decreased appetite or forgetting to eat, which leads to weight loss; hypersexual feelings that can increase the risk of contracting sexually transmitted diseases; engaging in substance abuse; and creating financial hardship. Elevated vital signs may be present during the physical assessment. Additionally, the client has problems functioning on a day-to-day basis, problems with primary relationships, or problems functioning at work or school. Mixed episodes and rapid cycling presentations are more difficult to treat and have a poorer prognosis. Bipolar III or Spectrum and Bipolar disorder not otherwise specified (NOS) are terms used to describe situations where signs and symptoms similar to bipolar disorders are present, but where the degree of intensity and the amount of symptoms are not enough to qualify for diagnoses of Bipolar I, Bipolar II, or mixed episodes.

There are many etiologies of bipolar disorders, both biologic and psychological. "Bipolar disorder appears to run in families" (O'Brien, Kennedy, & Ballard, 2008, p. 323). According to Fontaine (2009), "Bipolar disorder has the greatest inheritability, where about 85% of the risk appears to be inherited" (p. 303). Refer to a general psychiatric-mental health nursing textbook for information on the various theoretical etiologies of bipolar disorders (Keltner, Schwecke, & Bostrom, 2007, pp. 394, 402–404; Boyd, 2008, pp. 369–370; O'Brien, Kennedy, & Ballard, 2008, p. 323; Fontaine, 2009, pp. 298, 302–305). Many people with mood disorders also have medical conditions that influence their mood and ability to think. Some medication side-effects may cause mood disturbances. However, the symptoms are not due to alcohol or substance abuse. Mixed episodes are more difficult to treat. Pregnant women diagnosed with bipolar disorders have an increased risk of having an exacerbation of symptoms in the postpartum period and nonpregnant women during their premenstrual period (O'Brien, Kennedy, & Ballard, 2008, p. 323). A large number of people experience signs and symptoms of bipolar disorders for several years before being accurately diagnosed due to usually seeking treatment for symptoms of depression.

COMMON MEDICAL ILLNESSES

As previously stated in Chapter 8, Tables 8-2 and 8-3, there are common medical illnesses and adverse effects of medications that cause signs and symptoms similar to mood disorders. If common medical illnesses are present or the client experiences adverse medication effects, the signs and symptoms due to primary bipolar disorders on Axis I can be exacerbated, making it necessary for the treatment of both the Axis I disorder and Axis III disorder to achieve full management of the client's symptoms. Common medical illnesses and adverse effects of medications related specifically to bipolar disorders are listed in **Tables 10-1** and **10-2**.

Table 10-1	Common Medical Illnesses Causing or Exacerbating Signs and Symptoms of Bipolar Disorders
Neurologic	Cerebrovascular accident (CVA)
	Head trauma
	Brain tumor
	Multiple sclerosis (MS)
	Huntington's chorea
	Seizure disorders—temporal lobe
	CNS infections—HIV/AIDS
Endocrine	Hyperthyroidism
	Any hyperactive state causing increased sympathetic nervous system stimulation and release of catecholamines (epinephrine, norepinephrine) by the adrenal medulla
Metabolic/Nutritional	Hypercalcemia
Infectious diseases	CNS infections—HIV/AIDS
	Lyme disease
Other	Anoxia
	Hemodialysis

Table 10-2	Medications with Possible Adverse Affects on Mood/Bipolar Disorders
Anti-inflammatory	Corticosteroids—prednisone (Deltasone), methylprednisolone (Solumedrol)
Antiviral	Interferon

Sources: McKenry, Tessier, & Hogan, 2006, pp. 852–855; Varcarolis, Carson, & Shoemaker, 2006, pp. 328, 332; Keltner, Schwecke, & Bostrom, 2007, p. 380; O'Brien, Kennedy, & Ballard, 2008, pp. 254–255; Mohr, 2009, p. 856.

BIOPSYCHOSOCIAL NURSING ASSESSMENT

Information on the biopsychosocial nursing assessment or intake assessment is included in Chapter 4. In this chapter we will focus more on specific assessment of a client who already has been diagnosed with a bipolar disorder or is suspected of having the signs and symptoms of a bipolar disorder. As previously stated in Chapter 4, there are several screening tools that are frequently used to augment the assessment. The following screening tools may be used for a client with signs and symptoms of bipolar disorders:

- Mood Disorder Questionnaire (MDQ)
- CAGE for Alcohol Abuse
- Holmes and Rahe Social Readjustment Scale
- The Hassles and Uplifts Scale
- Life Experiences Survey (LES)
- WHO Quality of Life Instrument
- Young Mania Rating Scale (YMRS)

Biopsychosocial Nursing Assessment Form

Section I

1. Vital signs (see also Chapter 8)
   a. If BP is elevated, is the client in a manic phase, anxious, experiencing an adverse medication reaction, or is there a medical history of hypertension?
   b. Is the client exhibiting tachycardia and is it due to a manic phase, anxiety, adverse effects of medication, or a medical condition?
2. Weight
   a. Is the client's weight appropriate for height? Underweight? Does the client report any change in weight? How much over what period of time? Unintended weight loss or gain of more than 5% of body weight in 1 month in adults or failure to attain expected weight gains in children is significant for problems.
   b. Does the client experience loss of appetite? Are they too busy to eat or forgetting to eat and is this related to symptoms of mania?
   c. Does the client eat, but eats less than is needed to meet the increased metabolic requirements secondary to the acute manic phase?
3. Physical/mental disabilities/physical deformities (see Chapter 8)
4. Health insurance (see Chapter 8)

5. Admission status (see Chapter 8)
6. Chief complaint (see also Chapter 8)
    a. Is the client's speech too rapid or pressured for the interviewer to understand? Is the client too excited or restless to communicate? If so, this needs to be documented.

Section II

1. Symptom onset/duration/frequency/changes
    a. What specific symptoms does the client report and when did they start? If the client reports suicidal thoughts or a history of a suicide attempt, see section V of the biopsychosocial nursing assessment in Chapter 4 and also Chapter 8. Bipolar clients may be suicidal or homicidal. The client in the manic phase may be extremely impulsive.
    b. Has the client experienced these symptoms for the majority of at least a 1-week period? If the time period is less, record how many days the client has experienced these symptoms and if there is a specific time of the day the symptoms seem to be the most intense.
    c. Refer to Chapter 8 for the remaining assessment information in this section related to the depressed phase of a bipolar disorder.
    d. Is anyone who has accompanied the client able to provide additional information? The client may be having difficulty concentrating, experiencing FOIs or rapid, pressured speech, and possibly forgetting important information that the accompanying family member, friend, or neighbor may be able to supply.
    e. Refer to Chapter 8 for the depression-related parts of this section of the biopsychosocial nursing assessment.
2. Cultural factors (see Chapter 8)

Section III

1. DSM-IV-TR admission diagnosis (see also Chapter 8)
    a. The client's prognosis will be affected by their insight, judgment, number of Axis I–III diagnoses, past ability to adhere to treatment, access to outpatient services, type of health insurance or lack of health insurance, coping abilities, knowledge of diagnoses and medications, and the availability of social support. A client diagnosed with a bipolar disorder will have problems with judgment and insight, and on medication will feel "slowed down" in thought, creativity or energy level, thus leading to nonadherence (noncompliance).

Prognosis will be significantly improved if there is social support and psychotherapy available.

Section IV

1. Appearance (see also Chapter 8)
   a. Is there evidence of not attending to personal hygiene/ADLs? Is the client wearing clothing that matches and is appropriate for the situation or are there mismatched articles of clothing, seductive clothing, unkempt hair, or smeared makeup (if a female client)? Has the client been noted to change clothes frequently or shower several times during the day or evening?
   b. Does the client admit to problems attending to personal hygiene/ADLs and what reason do they give? A client in a manic phase may be too busy, be moving too fast, or be too impatient to attend to ADLs.
2. Attitude/psychomotor activity/eye contact (see also Chapter 8)
   a. Has the client been admitted on an involuntary commitment? This client may be aware that they are having problems, but refuses any help offered or may deny the existence of any problems or statements made to harm themselves or others. The client may deny that their actions were actually a suicide attempt or homicide attempt. This client can still benefit from treatment and a therapeutic nurse–client relationship, but it may take much longer due to the client's denial of symptoms, trust issues, poor insight, poor judgment, possible uncooperativeness and refusal of treatment, and additional problems with thought processes if psychosis is also present.
   b. Is the client able to sit and calmly talk to the nurse? Displaying psychomotor retardation or agitation? Either extreme may be seen in clients with symptoms of a bipolar disorder depending on the phase of the illness. Does the client accept redirection if needed? Does the client respond well to limit setting?
3. Mood (see also Chapter 8)
   a. Is the client extremely happy or euphoric? Irritable? Is the mood labile? A euphoric client may make statements such as feeling "on top of the world" or talk about being invincible.
4. Affect (see also Chapter 8)
   a. Is the client's affect excessively bright or labile?
5. Cognition/orientation (see also Chapter 8)
   a. Does the client report having racing thoughts/FOIs, easy distractibility, or does the interviewer notice that the client jumps from topic to topic rather than completing an idea or sentence?

b. Does the client display any problems with short-term or remote memory? Are these problems related to easy distractibility or racing thoughts/FOIs?

c. Is the client having difficulty performing calculations, interpreting abstract proverbs, or identifying similarities/differences between common objects? Are these problems related to easy distractibility or racing thoughts/FOIs?

6. Speech pattern (see also Chapter 8)

a. A client who is experiencing a manic phase of a bipolar disorder may speak in a rapid, forceful or pressured rate and manner as if the words are being forced from their mouth. The volume may be loud and the speech difficult to keep up with or understand due to the rate, rambling content, or racing thoughts/FOIs. The interviewer may be unable to keep up with the client's speech, number of topics, and feel mentally exhausted after the interview process.

7. Thought processes (see also Chapter 8)

a. Is the client experiencing an increase in the speed of their thoughts or an increase in ideas? Is the client involved in a number of projects or a workload that is not practical for their situation? Does the client jump from topic to topic and have difficulty concentrating or completing a thought? The interviewer may have to frequently refocus the client back to the specific information needed due to the client's racing thoughts/FOIs or easy distractibility in a manic phase.

b. Has the client been using alcohol, illegal drugs, or misusing prescription medications? Clients diagnosed with bipolar disorders often experience and display impulsivity including substance or chemical abuse. They may also be using substances or chemicals to treat their symptoms (i.e., self-medicating).

c. Refer to Chapter 11 for further assessment if psychosis is present.

8. Thought content

a. Is the client experiencing an exaggerated sense of self-importance, grandiose delusions, religious preoccupation, or preoccupation with sex? A client in a manic phase would experience these symptoms.

b. Due to extreme impulsivity, clients should be assessed for active and passive suicidal thoughts, behaviors, plans, and access to means to attempt suicide or homicide (see Chapter 9). Refer to a general psychiatric-mental health nursing textbook for information on legal–ethical implications regarding "duty to warn" (*Tarosoff v The Regents of the University of California*).

c. Refer to Chapter 11 for further assessment if psychosis is present.

9. Insight/Judgment/Impulse control (see also Chapter 8)
   a. Does the client exhibit normal judgment in commonly encountered situations? Clients experiencing a manic phase overestimate their own talents and capabilities. They also may look at only the positive aspects of a situation and neglect to take into account any negative aspects.
   b. Is the client making future plans and are these plans realistic in their circumstances? If yes, this is a positive indicator for a good prognosis.
   c. Does the client report impulse control problems? If yes, this is a negative indicator for a good prognosis.
10. Psychomotor function (see also Chapter 8)
    a. Examples of psychomotor agitation include restlessness, pacing or hand-wringing when depressed. Other examples include exaggerated gestures, rapid, forceful movements, pacing quickly, or intruding into the personal space or conversation of another person when in a manic phase.
11. Motivation (see also Chapter 8)
    a. Does the client have a supportive family? Clients experiencing symptoms of bipolar disorders may have problems getting along with family members or friends.
    b. Does the client have an understanding, supportive employer or are they being threatened with the loss of a job? Clients experiencing symptoms of bipolar disorders may have problems getting along with coworkers or their bosses.
    c. Has the client been court-ordered into treatment? Clients experiencing symptoms of bipolar disorders may incur legal charges due to impulsivity, conflict with others, or using substances–chemicals.

Section V

1. Suicide/homicide/domestic violence risk (see also Joint Commission requirements for suicide risk reduction including "Primary prevention" in Chapter 9).
   a. See Chapter 8.
   b. What does the client do when they become angry? How do they express it? If in healthy, adaptive ways, then there is no domestic violence risk. If in unhealthy, maladaptive ways, then there is an increased risk.

Section VI

1. Development (see Chapter 8)

Section VII

1. Psychiatric history and treatment (see Chapter 8)

Section VIII

1. Medical-Surgical history and treatment (see Chapter 8)

Section IX

1. Current/past chemical use/dependency (see Chapter 8)

Section X

1. Review of systems (see Chapter 8)

Section XI

1. Family history (see Chapter 8)

Section XII

1. Social/occupation/legal/education (see Chapter 8)

Section XIII

1. Ethnic/cultural/spiritual/coping/support (see also Chapter 8)
   a. What does the client do to cope with these stressors? A client in a manic phase may engage in impulsive behavior to deal with stressors.
   b. Who does the client turn to for support in times of stress?
   c. Does the client have a significant other or someone they feel close to?
   d. Does the client's significant other, family members, or close friends help or hinder the client? Clients in a manic phase may have recently been arguing with their family members or friends.
   e. Is the client able to identify any of their own personal strengths? Hindrances? Clients in a manic phase have an inflated sense of self-esteem and may be able to identify many personal strengths or exaggerate their personal strengths.
   f. Does the client seem to be a reliable historian or do you doubt the information they provide? Clients in a manic phase may be grandiose to the point of being delusional.

Section XIV

1. Ego defense mechanisms (see Appendix A)

Section XV

1. Community resources/discharge planning (see Chapter 8)

SPECIAL CONSIDERATIONS

When assessing children/adolescents and the elderly, many of the same principles apply, and similar information is needed as noted in the previous portion of this chapter. However, there are some special considerations when working with children/adolescents and the elderly. Refer to Chapter 8 for information related to major depression that applies to the depressed phase of bipolar disorders.

Children/Adolescents

As with adults, children/adolescents may be diagnosed with more than one Axis I disorder. According to research conducted by Wozniak et al. (1996), "Mania may be relatively common among psychiatrically referred children. The clinical picture of childhood-onset mania is very severe and frequently comorbid with ADHD and other psychiatric disorders . . . more work is needed to clarify whether these children have ADHD, bipolar disorder, or both." (p. 323). It was also noted in this research that childhood-onset bipolar disorder was more insidious and chronic as well as also sharing comorbidity with anxiety disorders. Because of the insidious, chronic, and continuous nature of childhood-onset bipolar disorders, it may be difficult to determine exactly when the symptoms began. The symptoms may be atypical compared to an adult client's symptoms (Sadock & Sadock, 2005, pp. 3274–3275). Some symptoms of childhood-onset bipolar disorders overlap with Attention Deficit Hyperactivity Disorder (ADHD), and some children/adolescents are diagnosed with ADHD as a comorbid disorder. For information on ADHD, please refer to the DSM-IV-TR and a general psychiatric nursing textbook (APA, 2000, pp. 85–93; Varcarolis, Carson, & Shoemaker, 2006, pp. 644, 674–675; O'Brien, Kennedy, & Ballard, 2008, pp. 214–217). The signs and symptoms of bipolar disorders in children/adolescents are similar to those in adults including suicidal thoughts, plans, or attempts. Mood swings, emotional reactions, impulsivity, and fantasy may be exaggerated. Children and adolescents may have homicidal thoughts or act on impulse when very angry and not realize the impact of their actions and the permanence of death since in some fantasy animation people come back to life. The symptoms of bipolar disorders previously mentioned in this chapter still apply as well as some additional symptoms in this client population, including:

- Severe, persistent, often violently irritable mood more often than euphoria
- Rages–explosive temper with outbursts often including threatening or attempting to harm others
- Psychomotor agitation
- Aggressive behavior
- Oppositional behavior
- Crying
- Decreased academic performance
- Risk taking behavior
- Mixed episodes occur more often

(Read & Purse, 2009, p. 1; Wozniak et al., 1996, pp. 323–339; Sadock & Sadock, 2005, pp. 3274–3275).

As previously stated in Chapter 4, there are several screening tools that are frequently used to augment the assessment. The following screening tools may be used for children/adolescents with signs and symptoms of bipolar disorders:

- Diagnostic Interview Schedule for Children (DISC)
- Schedule for Affective Disorders and Schizophrenia for Children (K-SADS)
- Minnesota Multiphasic Personality Inventory-Adolescent (MMPI-A)
- Milton Adolescent Personality Inventory (MAPI)
- Milton Adolescent Clinical Inventory (MACI)

Teaching and psychotherapy in both the inpatient and outpatient settings should involve the family–caregivers. In addition to the teaching listed in Table 10-3, the family will be taught normal growth and development information. Community resource referrals and discharge planning will include emphasis on family counseling and education as well as services for the individual child/adolescent. Partial hospitalization or day treatment programs that focus on the needs of adolescents as well as after-school programs would be included when needed.

Elderly

The signs and symptoms of bipolar disorders in elderly clients are similar to those in younger adults. Elderly clients may have demonstrated some signs of bipolar disorders earlier in life, but family and friends may not have recognized the signs as symptoms of a psychiatric problem. See Chapter 8 for information related to major depression that applies to the depressed phase of bipolar disorders.

Sudden onset of symptoms, especially in the absence of a family history or any possible symptoms earlier in life may indicate a medical, Axis III condition that needs to be investigated (e.g., CVA, brain tumor) before assuming the symptoms are due to a bipolar disorder. For community resource referrals and discharge planning, see Chapter 8.

NURSING INTERVENTIONS AND RATIONALES

Nursing interventions are planned according to individual client needs, common signs and symptoms of bipolar disorders, age, education level, and cultural preferences. For specific nursing diagnoses, outcomes, and evaluation criteria, refer to a general psychiatric-mental health nursing textbook such as *Psychiatric Mental Health Nursing: An Introduction to Theory and Practice*, O'Brien, Kennedy, & Ballard (2008); *Mental Health Nursing*, Fontaine, (2009); *Psychiatric Nursing: Contemporary Practice*, Boyd, (2008); *Psychiatric Mental Health Case Studies and Care Plans*, Jakopac & Patel (2009); and psychiatric care plan books such as *Psychiatric Nursing Care Plans*, Fortinash & Holoday-Worret (2007) or *Manual of Psychiatric Nursing Care Plans*, Varcarolis (2006). The interventions presented in **Table 10-3** apply to the adult and elderly client with variations for the child/adolescent client as indicated. Refer to Chapter 8 for interventions dealing with the depressed phase of bipolar disorders.

Table 10-3   Nursing Interventions and Rationales for Bipolar Disorders

Problems	Interventions	Rationales
Suicidal or homicidal ideations/thinking	1. Begin to develop a rapport and a therapeutic nurse–patient alliance that is the beginning of the therapeutic nurse–client relationship. At admission, every 8 hours, and prn assess for suicidal ideations, plan, lethality of plan, access to the means to carry out plan, prior attempts, and chemical dependency (see also Chapter 4, Table 4-1 and Table 4-3, section V).	1. Developing a rapport with the patient will assist in gaining the patient's trust and cooperation in the future and helps initiate the therapeutic nurse–client relationship. According to Render and Peplau (O'Brien, Kennedy, & Ballard, 2008, pp. 17–18), the therapeutic nurse–client relationship is the foundation that must be established to initiate future work in the healing process. The client may also be more able to listen to and follow directions from a nurse they have a rapport and therapeutic relationship with. Potentially dangerous situations may be avoided or defused if the client has developed rapport and trust with nurses and staff members. Clients diagnosed with bipolar disorders are at risk for harming themselves or others due to extreme impulsivity, dramatic mood swings, irritability, psychomotor agitation, and excess energy. They may also be experiencing delusional thinking or hallucinations telling them to harm themselves or others. Clients with chemical abuse/dependency problems are at increased risk for committing suicide or homicide due decreased inhibition. This decreased inhibition added to extreme impulsivity, dramatic mood swings, and excess energy can cause a very dangerous situation.

Suicidal/homicidal thoughts and urges are not always constant. They can be triggered by something another client says, a phone call, visitor or something viewed on TV, thus demonstrating a need for additional assessment and documentation.

a. If the client reports homicidal thoughts toward a specific person, the nurse should obtain as much information as possible and report this to the psychiatrist and the immediate nursing supervisor, and document the information, including who the information was reported to.

a. Obtaining information, passing it on and documenting are within the PMH nurse generalist's ethical–legal responsibilities and scope of practice. It will be up to the psychiatrist to decide if the information meets the "duty to warn" provisions of the Tarosoff ruling. The nurse does not notify the person potentially involved.

b. If the client is experiencing psychosis including hearing voices telling them to harm themselves or others, this needs to be reported and the client needs to be reassured of their own safety, and antipsychotic medication should be offered if ordered (see also Chapter 13).

b. Some clients do experience psychosis and this makes it more complicated to provide safety for the client and others. The psychiatrist needs to know that these symptoms are present to be able to treat all the client's problems. The client needs to feel safe, and antipsychotic medication can be very helpful for the psychotic symptoms (see also Chapters 11 and 13).

2. Obtain at least a verbal no-self-harm or harm to others contract at admission, every 8 hours, and prn.

2. Clients with bipolar diagnoses are at high-risk for committing suicide due to extreme impulsivity, dramatic mood swings, psychomotor agitation, and excessive energy in the manic phase or the severity of depression in the depressed phase. A

(continues)

Table 10-3   Nursing Interventions and Rationales for Bipolar Disorders (continued)

Problems	Interventions	Rationales
		behavior contract actively engages the patient in their treatment and encourages personal responsibility for their behavior. It also demonstrates staff involvement. The client's condition may change, making it necessary to obtain another contract earlier than the next scheduled shift.
		The PMH nurse will need to determine if the client is safe to leave on safety checks every 15 minutes or if they need to be placed on 1:1 or constant observation (COs). The ability to resist acting upon suicidal/homicidal thoughts and urges is not always possible. There is a need for additional assessment, obtaining at least a verbal no-self-harm or harm to others contract, and documentation.
	3. Provide a safe therapeutic milieu free from contraband or items that could be potential weapons (see Chapter 3).	3. This decreases opportunities for the client to harm themselves or others.
	4. Use of self therapeutically and therapeutic communication techniques (see Table 4-1) to assist client to verbalize feelings, precipitating events, reasons for attempting suicide, and what problems they think committing suicide will solve (see Chapters 2, 4, and 5).	4. Assisting the client with verbalization of feelings, thoughts, concerns, or fears helps decrease the possibility of physical acting upon them. This also shows the client that the nurse is listening; is genuinely concerned; and helps build rapport, trust, and the therapeutic nurse relationship.
	5. Initiate and maintain safety rounds or checks every 15 minutes if the client is able to at least verbally contract not to harm themselves or others.	5. This measure ensures knowledge of the client's location and safety as well as the safety of other patients on the unit.

6. Decrease environmental stimuli (i.e., amount of people in area, noise, light).

7. Inform the client of unit rules regarding acceptable behavior and limit set when necessary.

8. Use a calm, matter-of-fact tone of voice when interacting with a client. Refrain from arguing or engaging in power struggles with the client.

9. Administer scheduled and prn medication as ordered. Reinforce need to take medication consistently no matter how the client feels. If the client has just been admitted, teaching may have to be delayed until the mood is more even and the thought processes less rapid.

6. A client diagnosed with a bipolar disorder is very sensitive to any environmental stimuli. A calm environment is less distracting or irritating and assists the patient to maintain control over impulsive or aggressive urges.

7. This lets the client know what is or is not acceptable and assists her to act in accordance with unit rules. This also gives the client a chance to attempt to regulate their own behavior as much as possible.

8. Because of labile mood, irritability, psychomotor agitation, and increased energy level it is not unusual for clients diagnosed with bipolar disorders in a manic phase, to argue with staff and engage in power struggles related to unit rules. Strong feelings, whether positive or negative, are transmitted as energy and can trigger increased emotion and aggression in an already emotionally labile client.

9. The client may be just starting on medication or having just stopped taking previously prescribed medication. In either situation there will not be a therapeutic blood level of medication needed to control symptoms. Most clients do not like to take medication due to the side-effects or do not believe they are ill and need medication. Failure to take medication or stopping medication on their own is a major cause of relapse

(continues)

Table 10-3   Nursing Interventions and Rationales for Bipolar Disorders (continued)

Problems	Interventions	Rationales
		and readmission. Also, when a client is first admitted, they may have much difficulty following conversations or learning new material due to their symptoms.
	10. When scheduling a client for group activities or therapies, keep the group size small and limit the amount of time the group meets.	10. This will provide the client with needed therapy and assist them to focus, but decrease the risk of becoming overwhelmed and agitated as a result of too many environmental stimuli.
	a. During the first few days of admission allow the client experiencing a manic phase to leave group early if unable to tolerate the size and duration of the group setting. Alert other staff members to monitor the client closely after leaving group to ensure their safety.	a. A client experiencing symptoms of a manic phase will have difficulty controlling their behavior, and if too stimulated by the size of the group and inability to focus on the topic, the situation could lead to the client physically acting out and causing danger to the others in the group. Therefore, for the first few days it may be safer to allow the client to leave group early. As the client's symptoms continue to improve and the hospital or program stay continues, the PMH nurse leading the psychoeducation group will require the client to stay in group for longer periods of time until they are able to tolerate being in group the entire time while being able to focus on the topic.
	11. For a client who attempts to hurt themselves or others, and all other interventions have not been effective, seclusion and restraint measures may need to be taken as a last resort (see Chapter 12).	11. Client safety is a priority, but needs to be balanced and guided by the legal principle of least restrictive treatment (Keltner, Schwecke, & Bostrom, 2007, pp. 54, 60). Seclusion can be used without restraints. The legal principle of beneficence guides the PMH nurse's duty to act for the benefit or good of the client (Guido, 2007, pp. 5–9, 71–72, 377–391).

| Disturbed thought processes | 1. Assess for changes in thought processes (e.g., racing thoughts or FOIs, delusions, hallucinations) and themes in thought content (e.g., grandiosity, religion, jealousy, special abilities, aggression, violence, vulnerability, inferiority). | 1. This intervention provides baseline assessment information and helps the PMH nurse plan and prioritize nursing care. This intervention allows you to monitor if the client's condition is improving, worsening, or remaining the same. It also helps determine if there was a specific trigger that preceded the deterioration of their condition. Themes in delusional thinking not only help you identify triggers that initiate this type of thinking, but also help you identify problematic issues the client is dealing with. A client with religious preoccupation may think of themselves as an agent of God, hear the voice of God or another higher power, think of themselves as having a spiritual message to deliver or having to perform an action directed by God/higher power. |
| | 2. When interacting with a client experiencing a manic phase, keep the time frame brief and use simple, short sentences. | 2. A client in a manic phase is euphoric or irritable, has dramatic mood swings, is easily distracted, experiences racing thoughts or FOIs, and psychomotor agitation. This makes is very difficult for them to concentrate on any conversation, information, or directions they are being given. Brief, more frequent interactions using simple, short sentences help make it easier for the client to pay attention and tolerate the presence of the nurse. |

(continues)

Table 10-3   Nursing Interventions and Rationales for Bipolar Disorders (continued)

Problems	Interventions	Rationales
	3. Assist the client to differentiate between delusional thinking, hallucinations, and reality-based thinking by reorienting them to place, person, and time and presenting factual information.	3. Initially the client will have difficulty determining which thoughts are real and which are delusion or hallucinations. This may be frightening and frustrating to the client. The nurse can help the client with this process while providing understanding and emotional support.
	4. Avoid arguing with the client while reinforcing reality by using therapeutic communication techniques and providing factual information as to what the nurse actually hears, sees, or has proof of in a calm, nonjudgmental manner. (e.g., In response to the client stating he is the King of France, the nurse may respond "In your record the case manager documented that you are a janitor at a high school.").	4. The client will insist more strongly that the delusion or hallucination is actually true. They may become upset and agitated, and escalate into physically acting out behaviors. This approach avoids upsetting or provoking the client while assisting to reorient them to reality.
	5. Decrease environmental stimulation (i.e., amount of people in area, noise, light).	5. Since a client experiencing a manic phase is overly sensitive to environmental stimuli, they experience increased stress and this can trigger delusional thinking or hallucinations.
	6. Assess and document the client's mental status every shift.	6. Areas such as mood, affect, thought processes, thought content including suicidal/homicidal ideations, speech, psychomotor activity, appearance, cognition, judgment, and insight provide a clinical picture of the client's mental stability and are very important to assess. The PMH nurse plans nursing care, evaluates progress toward planned outcomes, and changes plans depending on the client's progress.

Intervention	Rationale
7. Administer mood stabilizer and antipsychotic medications as ordered.	7. There are many mood stabilizers available for the treatment of bipolar disorders. Atypical SGAs and novel antipsychotics have been approved for monotherapy (i.e., used alone without mood stabilizers). Older antipsychotics may also be used with mood stabilizers for delusional thinking if other medications are not effective.
8. Spend time 1:1 with patient in diversional activities such as listening to quiet music, a relaxation exercise, or playing cards. a. Gradually add a few other clients to form a small group to engage in diversional activities.	8. This will help distract the client, keep them focused in reality, and provide role modeling of social skills. a. Gradually adding more clients and forming a small group helps the client in a manic phase more easily tolerate the presence of others and reinforce not only the use of diversional activities, but also appropriate social skills. While clients in a manic phase are very social, they may become very irritable due to their labile mood and not be able to tolerate the presence of very many other people at a time.
9. When the client is more able to focus and be still, teach them to go to a quiet place and use diversional activities to cope when beginning to feel irritable, agitated, or restless.	9. Teaching the client ways to help themselves cope in appropriate activities helps engage the client in their own treatment and promotes independence.
Sleep pattern disturbances	1. Assess the client's sleep pattern, including if they take naps during the day.	1. Establishes base line information. Daytime napping may have a negative effect on nighttime sleep pattern.

(continues)

Table 10-3   Nursing Interventions and Rationales for Bipolar Disorders (continued)

Problems	Interventions	Rationales
	2. Schedule a balance of activity and rest periods when the client is in a manic phase.	2. During manic episodes the body expends a great amount of energy, and the client risks becoming extremely fatigued physically without being able to stop activity on their own and will need assistance with balance.
	3. Assist client in establishing a regular bedtime routine including a specific time to go to bed and awaken.	3. A regular bedtime routine promotes sleep by signaling the body and mind that it is time to prepare for sleep.
	4. Eliminate distracting noise.	4. A client in a manic phase is easily distracted and experiences racing thoughts. Noise will increase this tendency, making it even more difficult to fall asleep.
	5. Use the initially expected side-effects of medications as a therapeutic effect for insomnia.	5. Mood stabilizers and antipsychotics cause drowsiness as an expected side-effect. As the client's body adjusts to the medication, this side-effect will decrease, but by that time their sleep pattern should be more normal. Sleeping agents may not be ordered unless it is necessary, and then it should be for a short amount of time or only prn to avoid disrupting REM stage sleep. Also, many sleep agents may be habit forming.
	6. When the client is less easily distracted and not as affected by racing thoughts or FOIs, teach them the importance of getting enough sleep to avoid triggering another manic episode.	6. Sleep is restorative for body, mind, and spirit. Also, too little or inconsistent sleep may trigger a manic episode for many clients with bipolar disorders.

7. When the client's mood is more stable, and they are experiencing fewer delusional and racing thoughts, teach ways to promote sleep after discharge, including:
   - Eliminating noise or using "white noise" (low-speed fan)
   - Eliminating light in the bedroom and caffeinated beverages from the diet
   - Getting regular exercise (avoid 2 hours before bedtime)
   - Eating a light snack while avoiding a heavy meal before bedtime
   - Using relaxation exercises (e.g., deep breathing, progressive relaxation exercises) on a daily basis before bedtime
   - Taking a warm bath
   - Avoiding the use of sleep agents including herbals unless prescribed by psychiatrist
   - Establishing and continuing a regular bedtime routine
   - Going to bed and awakening around the same time on a consistent basis
   - Using the bedroom for sleep only rather than for watching TV

8. Explore complementary therapies with the client such as aromatherapy and meditation when mood is more stable. Caution the client to use only calming scents such as lavender, chamomile, or bergamot rather than rosemary or sage that can be more stimulating.

7. The client should be as involved in their care as possible to promote collaboration, provide more control over their condition, and promote independence.

8. Simple meditation techniques are easy to learn and along with aromatherapy, promote relaxation of body, mind, and spirit. Research shows that people who practice transcendental meditation have been able to lower their levels of catecholamines. Epinephrine and norepinephrine

(continues)

Table 10-3   Nursing Interventions and Rationales for Bipolar Disorders (continued)

Problems	Interventions	Rationales
		are catecholamines that are released by the adrenal medulla during sympathetic nervous system stimulation that occurs during hyperactive states including manic episodes. Catecholamines also act as neurotransmitters, and an excess would contribute to the symptoms of a manic phase.
Nutrition and hydration	1. Obtain a baseline weight on admission; assess skin turgor, and blood pressure. Assess laboratory glucose, total protein, albumin, RBCs, Hgb, Hct, MCV, and MCH values if ordered. Weigh at least once a week before breakfast on the same scale.	1. Obtaining a baseline weight and assessing skin turgor and blood pressure provide information to compare to normal height/weight charts and provide a general idea of fluid intake. Decreased glucose, total protein, and albumin levels may indicate poor nutrition. Decreased RBCs, Hgb, and Hct may indicate nutrition-related anemias. Elevated MCV and MCH values may also indicate nutrition-related anemias. This information will be used to compare future assessment data to see if the client is improving.
	a. Clients who have been eating only once a day, or have fluid retention secondary to CHF or renal disease, will need to be weighed daily.	a. Clients who have not been eating can actually die from starvation, malnutrition, and dehydration. Clients who have CHF or renal disease may accumulate excess fluid due to the disease processes and need to be more closely observed for fluid retention (e.g., abnormal lung sounds, dyspnea, 2–3 lb weight gain in 24 hours, edema of dependent areas such as feet and ankles, sacrum, nocturia) and signs reported right away.

2. Monitor intake and output every shift for at least the first 3 days of hospitalization.

2. This helps provide a more accurate account of what the patient is eating, drinking, and eliminating. For severely malnourished or elderly clients, the nurse may need to continue monitoring intake and output each shift.

3. Assist the client to complete a food/fluid intake diary for at least the past 3 days.

3. The client may not be able to complete a food diary even with assistance due to the symptoms of a manic phase. The food intake diary may need to be postponed until the client's symptoms have begun to subside. In this situation information would be obtained for what the client can remember "typically" eating.

4. Obtain information regarding the client's food preferences, food restrictions due to allergies, or religious–cultural practices.

4. Again, obtaining complete information may need to be delayed until the symptoms of a manic phase begin to subside or family members can provide the information (the client will have to give permission for any contact with family or friends). Including food preferences and restrictions will increase the client's cooperation and show that they are seen as a person.

5. Provide nutrient dense finger foods (e.g., cheese, hard boiled eggs, sandwiches, fruit, raw vegetables, yogurt).

5. Due to easy distractibility, impulsivity, excess energy, and psychomotor agitation in a manic phase, it is difficult for a client to sit still long enough to eat an entire meal. Finger foods can be eaten while the client is pacing or moving about the unit. The client needs protein as well as other nutrients.

(continues)

Table 10-3   Nursing Interventions and Rationales for Bipolar Disorders *(continued)*

Problems	Interventions	Rationales
	6. Requesting a referral for a dietician consult may be necessary, especially if the client has lost a considerable amount of weight due to not eating, or has decreased appetite or increased metabolism. Dietary supplements are needed for diabetic or elderly clients.	6. The nurse will need to obtain an order from the psychiatrist for a dietary consult. Frequently, diabetic or elderly clients need temporary supplements until their appetite returns.
Labile mood	1. Use a calm, matter-of-fact, and consistent approach when dealing with a client experiencing labile mood.	1. A client experiencing labile mood is very sensitive to what is happening in the environment, including the activities of nurses and other mental health staff. The client's reaction to nurses and other mental health staff frequently is stronger than normal.
	2. Meet with the client more often, but keep each interaction brief.	2. This intervention assures the client that you are there to help them, but avoids causing increased frustration and irritability for the client.
	3. Administer mood stabilizer and antipsychotic medications as ordered.	3. Medications used to treat bipolar disorders include mood stabilizers, atypical SGAs, and novel antipsychotics that have been approved for monotherapy (i.e., used alone without mood stabilizers).
	4. Teach the client to remove themselves from the area if they feel that they cannot control their mood.	4. This intervention gives the client some measure of control. Later on after the client's symptoms have become more controlled, the client will be taught to try to ignore their frustration in an effort to build tolerance and assume responsibility rather than just leave the area.

	Interventions	Rationales
	5. Maintain a quiet environment.	5. The client's heightened sensitivity to environmental stimuli will cause them to overreact, and a noisy, overcrowded environment can intensify mood swings.
Easy distractibility	1. Provide a quiet environment when teaching the client new information.	1. A quiet environment will help the client focus on the information being taught.
	2. Use simple, short sentences and clear directions when interacting and teaching the client.	2. Simple, short sentences and clear directions are easier to understand and help the client focus on the information being taught.
	3. Keep interaction and teaching time short (i.e., 10 to 20 minutes) and end the interaction or teaching session if the client still has problems focusing.	3. Shorter interaction and teaching times will help the client focus. Insisting that the client stay the entire time when they are unable to focus can cause or increase frustration. Not only is the client easily distracted, but also easily frustrated, irritable, and experiencing labile mood. This can lead to escalation of emotions and physical acting out.
	4. Use teaching materials that are concise and clear.	4. Teaching materials that are concise and clear are more likely to hold the client's attention.
	5. Administer mood stabilizer and antipsychotic medications as ordered.	5. Medication is given to bring the client's neurotransmitters into balance and to control symptoms of bipolar disorders.
	6. When scheduling a client for group activities or therapies, keep the group size small and limit the amount of time the group meets.	6. This will provide the client with needed therapy and assist them to focus, but decrease the risk of becoming overwhelmed and agitated as a result of too much environmental stimuli.

(continues)

Table 10-3   Nursing Interventions and Rationales for Bipolar Disorders (continued)

Problems	Interventions	Rationales
Risk for injury/ impulsivity	1. Maintain a physically safe environment (see Chapter 3). a. Remind the client to wear proper fitting, nonskid footwear.	1. and 1a. A client experiencing a manic phase will have poor judgment, impulse control problems, psychomotor agitation, excess energy, and racing thought/FOIs. They can easily trip or fall. They can also impulsively pick up an object and hurt others or themselves. Also, euphoria can cause the client to misjudge any potential danger in a situation, resulting in an increased risk to the client.
	2. Verbally redirect the client, reinforce appropriate social behavior, and limit set as needed.	2. Frequently clients intrude into the personal space or conversations of others. This intrusiveness can irritate or increase other clients' fears, anger, or paranoia. As a result of this, a physical altercation may erupt causing injury. Also, clients' who exhibit loud speech and euphoria can irritate other clients.
	3. Teach the client to walk away and seek out staff to talk to when feeling impulsive urges.	3. Initially the client will need assistance to walk away, but as the medication reaches a therapeutic blood level and symptoms subside, it will be easier for them to do so. Until then, nurses and other mental health staff will need to continue to verbally redirect the client, reinforce appropriate social behavior, and limit set as needed.
Psychomotor agitation/ Excess energy	1. Provide appropriate physical outlets such as exercise.	1. Physical activity helps release excess energy and tension.
	2. Provide a schedule of activities balanced with rest periods.	2. Balancing activity and rest helps prevent the client from becoming exhausted. A client in a manic phase will continue to engage in activity and not be aware of normal fatigue.

3. Teach relaxation techniques such as deep breathing, guided imagery, or simple meditation.

4. Administer mood stabilizer and antipsychotic medications as ordered.

   a. If the client reports feeling anxious and they have anti-anxiety medication ordered, they may need to be offered the anti-anxiety medication.

   b. Stay with the client and encourage them to use relaxation techniques.

   c. If the client is overstimulated during visiting hours, take the client to a quieter area of the unit or to their room.

3. Relaxation techniques help activate a parasympathetic nervous system response and help give the client some control over their symptoms. Initially the client may only be able to try deep breathing due to symptoms of mania. As the symptoms begin to subside, the client will be able to learn other techniques.

4. Medication is given to bring the client's neurotransmitters into balance and to control symptoms of bipolar disorders.

   a. Psychomotor agitation can be triggered by anxiety.

   b. The nurse's presence can be calming, and the use of relaxation techniques helps the client control their own symptoms.

   c. Removing the client from an overly stimulating environment will help them gain control and is a less restrictive approach.

Religious preoccupation

1. Closely monitor and limit the client's reading materials and TV programs–movies that contain religious topics.

1. A client who is religiously preoccupied will obsessively read, watch, and talk about religious topics. If the client also is experiencing psychosis, they will focus on the religious delusion or hallucinations and may act upon them.

(continues)

Table 10-3	Nursing Interventions and Rationales for Bipolar Disorders *(continued)*	
Problems	**Interventions**	**Rationales**
	2. Provide leisure reading materials and TV programs–movies that do not contain religious material.	2. The client will need something to take the place of the religious materials and programs they have been interested in. Spirituality is an important component of health and well-being. There are other ways to address the client's spirituality without referring to organized religious materials (e.g, music, poetry, drawing, painting).
	3. Use therapeutic communication techniques to refocus the client's conversation when their verbalizations are filled with religious content.	3. The client is preoccupied and will need help to focus on other topics.
	4. After the symptoms have become more controlled, a limited amount of religious material may be slowly reintroduced, and contact with the client's religious advisor reinstated, but it will depend upon the individual client's progress and mental state.	4. Since spirituality is an important component of health and well-being it cannot be totally ignored, but care must be taken with a client experiencing extremes in thought and behavior or psychosis.
Hypersexuality/ Sexual promiscuity	1. Limit set when the client makes inappropriate sexual comments or displays inappropriate sexual behavior.	1. A client in a manic phase is impulsive and frequently makes sexual comments or jokes, and may display inappropriate sexual behavior toward the nurse, other mental health staff, or other clients. Limit setting can help control some of this behavior until the client's symptoms become more controlled.
	2. Model appropriate social behavior.	2. Modeling of socially appropriate behavior helps the client learn what is acceptable.
	3. Reinforce the unit rules regarding appropriate social behavior and expectations.	3. This intervention helps control some of this behavior until the client's symptoms become more controlled.

4. Closely monitor the client's reading materials and TV programs–movies.

4. Inappropriate materials or programs–movies will trigger inappropriate behavior in a client who is impulsive.

5. Reinforce safe sex practices.

5. The client needs to protect themselves when unable to control sexual impulses that cause high risk for contracting and spreading STDs including HIV/AIDS and hepatitis. This also helps protect the community the client lives in.

6. When the client is less distracted and more able to focus, teach and reinforce information on STDs, including HIV/AIDS and hepatitis.

   a. If the client wishes to be tested for STDs, including HIV/AIDS or hepatitis, notify the client's psychiatrist.

6. It is best not to assume that all clients know about the risk of diseases related to unsafe sex practices.

   a. A client experiencing hypersexuality or sexual promiscuity is at high risk for contracting and spreading STDs including HIV/AIDS and hepatitis.

Knowledge deficit/ Teaching needs

The following areas are included in identified knowledge deficits/teaching needs:

The more a client (and the family) knows about their illness, medications, other treatment, and ways to help the self, the more control they will have over their illness and be better able to be involved in treatment decisions. Providing education for the client (and the family if the client is willing) is a critical part of the PMH nurse's role (Tugrul, 2003, p. 184).

1. Diagnosis including that bipolar disorders are illnesses that affect brain function and are treatable; reasons why bipolar disorders occur including the role of neurotransmitters, impact

1. Diagnosis–most clients do not know that bipolar disorders are treatable, are unfamiliar with the signs & symptoms and yet know something is wrong, blame themselves for being ill, and do

(continues)

Table 10-3   Nursing Interventions and Rationales for Bipolar Disorders (continued)

Problems	Interventions	Rationales
	of genetic influence, impact of psychosocial stressors, signs & symptoms of bipolar disorders, and potential dangers of delaying treatment	not realize what negative impacts and danger there is when delaying treatment.
	2. Medication—teaching includes the different classes–categories of medications used to treat bipolar disorders including mood stabilizers and atypical antipsychotics; benefits, common side-effects and adverse effects to report and seek help for right away; food interactions; approximate amount of time it may take to feel the full effect; that it may take time to find the specific medication that helps their symptoms with the lowest number and level of side-effects; problems with suddenly stopping the medication; need to avoid alcohol or drugs or not taking anything including herbal supplements without the psychiatrist, APRN or other physician's knowledge; importance of keeping their psychiatrist/APRN informed of problems or improvements (see also Chapter 13).	2. Since medication is a large part of treatment it is very important that the client be informed about their medications. Providing information and reasons why it is important can help increase client adherence (compliance) with medication.
	3. Other treatment—including individual and group psychotherapy, including therapies such as CBT, IPT, motivational enhancement therapy, REBT, supportive therapy, client centered therapy, reality therapy, behavior modification, psychoanalysis, ECT (for the depressed phase only), psychoeducation, hypnosis, psychodrama, nutrition, treatment of comorbid/co-occuring conditions that affect mood, treatment of chemical dependency, and family psychotherapy.	3. Medications are needed to regulate the balance of neurotransmitters and help improve the client's ability to concentrate and focus to be able to learn, but they will not help the client deal with interpersonal relationships, day-to-day problems and frustrations, improve social skills or change certain behaviors or provide insight. Medications do help the client cope to a degree, but they will still need to learn other ways to cope.

4. Self-care activities

   a. Sleep promotion/sleep hygiene activities—see "Sleep pattern disturbances" section in this table.

   b. Physical exercise

   c. Nutrition and hydration—including drinking at least six 8-ounce glasses of water per day.

4. Many clients do not realize that there is much they can do to help themselves in addition to taking medication and receiving psychotherapy.

   a. Disruption in sleep patterns can help trigger symptoms of mania.

   b. Physical exercise can help release tension, dissipate excess energy, and improve sleep, schedule of regular meal times and drinking as well as providing health benefits for cardiac diseases, diabetes, and obesity that are comorbid/co-occuring conditions in many mental health clients. Most psychiatric medication side-effects include weight gain. Exercise combined with balanced nutrition can help offset these side-effects (Jensen, Decker, & Andersen, 2006, pp. 620–621; Frisch & Frisch, 2002, p. 267).

   c. Balanced nutrition is important for weight management; offsetting the medication side-effect of weight gain; the production of neurotransmitters, hormones, building & repair of body tissues; regulation of glucose and cholesterol levels; energy production; and regulation of bowel function (constipation may occur due to decreased physiologic processes during depressed episodes, side-effects of medications or lack of fiber in the diet). Adequate hydration is needed to pre-

(continues)

Table 10-3   Nursing Interventions and Rationales for Bipolar Disorders (continued)

Problems	Interventions	Rationales
		vent dehydration and consequences of electrolyte imbalance, low blood volume urinary tract infections or constipation. A 2500 to 3000 ml daily fluid intake is recommended for clients being stabilized on lithium carbonate (Eskalith) as well as avoiding caffeinated beverages that have a diuretic affect (McKenry, Tessier, & Hogan, 2006, p. 410). Male clients taking topiramate (Topamax) need to increase their fluid intake to offset the risk of developing kidney stones.
	d. Coping skills—teach stress management techniques such as deep breathing, passive progressive relaxation exercises, simple meditation techniques, guided imagery (see Appendix F), massage therapy, aromatherapy, time management, problem-solving/decision-making strategies, anger management, journaling, and regular exercise with a physician's permission as to safe exercises.	d. Moderate-to-high levels of stress negatively impact clients and can trigger or exacerbate symptoms as well as decreasing the ability to cope and think clearly. Decreased stress will improve the client's ability to cope and concentrate. Improved problem solving/decision making helps the client avoid mistakes that may be costly emotionally or financially and increase a sense of control over their life. Better time management helps relieve the pressure created by stress.
	e. Relaxation—see previous intervention	e. See previous rationale
	f. Practicing appropriate social & communication skills	f. Clients experiencing symptoms of a manic phase are extremely social, but can be physically intrusive and verbally aggressive. They need to practice appropriate social and communication skills.
	g. Smoking cessation	g. Many clients with psychiatric-mental health problems smoke. It is very difficult for them to attempt to quit smoking or use of any tobacco products while their symptoms are not

controlled. However, after their symptoms are more fully controlled, it may be easier for clients to begin a program to quit or at least decrease the amount of tobacco products they use. Clients should be warned about using the smoking cessation medication varenicline (Chantix) due to reports of increased feeling of depression and suicidal thoughts.

h. Informing clients of their responsibility as partners in their healthcare increases their awareness and control over their health.

h. Health responsibility—keeping up with regular physical checkups, seeking medical attention when needed, adhering to medication and other treatment regimens, engaging in health promotion activities, and avoiding potentially harmful life-style behaviors

i. Interpersonal relationships

i. Social isolation may result from problems with interpersonal relationships due to symptoms of a manic phase or choosing to isolate due to symptoms of a depressed phase. Loss of relationships is a major problem for all clients experiencing psychiatric illnesses. Clients diagnosed with bipolar disorders frequently divorce and have problems with coworkers and employers. Working with significant others, families, friends, and employers of clients helps improve interpersonal relationships and provides much needed support that is important in healing and maintaining progress.

(continues)

Table 10-3   Nursing Interventions and Rationales for Bipolar Disorders (continued)

Problems	Interventions	Rationales
Relapse prevention	1. Teach the client signs and symptoms to watch for that show they are starting to exhibit manic symptoms or symptoms of depression again and to report these to the psychiatrist/APRN. a. Teach the client to listen to comments made by others around them (e.g., that they are acting unusual or don't seem to be themselves lately).	1. Early recognition and reporting of signs and symptoms leads to early treatment and avoidance of rehospitalizations or shorter hospitalization stays. a. Clients do not like to hear from others if they are not doing well, but in order to prevent a full blown relapse and potential hospital admission, it is important that they do so. Other people may also notice signs of medication side-effects that clients either are unaware of or are afraid to mention.
	2. Assist the client to realistically look at all the responsibilities and activities they have and decide what a normal amount is versus signs of a manic phase.	2. Many people do not have a realistic perception of how much they are logically capable of handling and overestimate their abilities, time, and resources when experiencing a manic phase. Being too busy to obtain enough sleep and attend to nutritional/hydration needs will cause problems later on.
	3. Teach the client the importance of keeping good sleep habits including going to bed and awakening about the same time every day.	3. Changes in not only the amount of sleep, but the usual time can have an effect that leads to possibly triggering of a manic phase.
	4. Reinforce the need for the client to continue with stress management and relaxation techniques including the positive–adaptive coping skills learned while in the inpatient setting.	4. It is necessary to make stress management and relaxation techniques including positive–adaptive coping skills a part of everyday living to help prevent a relapse of depression and help maintain mental health.

5. Reinforce the need to continue taking all medication exactly as prescribed while keeping the psychiatrist, APRN, and other physicians aware of problems rather than stopping medication suddenly.

6. Reinforce the need to attend individual and group psychotherapy sessions regularly.

7. Teach importance of including their significant other and other family members in the client's treatment unless there is a specific reason not to.

5. It is imperative that the client adhere to the medication regimen to maintain neurotransmitter/neurochemical balance to help control signs and symptoms of bipolar disorders. Suddenly stopping medication can cause physical problems.

   The psychiatrist, APRN, and other physicians need to know of any side-effects or adverse effects to properly care for the client.

6. Psychotherapy is needed to help the client continue to deal with interpersonal relationships, day-to-day problems and frustrations, maintain balance, improve social skills or change certain behaviors or provide insight. It takes time to learn new ways to deal with life's challenges.

7. Significant others and family members can be very supportive in helping the client adhere to their treatment regimen. They usually do not know much about bipolar disorders or psychiatric problems in general. Also, they may not realize that they may be contributing to the client's problems and need to learn new ways of relating to the client. However, there are situations where the client has valid reasons for not including these people in their treatment (e.g., abuse, violence, alcohol/drug use, refusal to believe the client needs treatment, etc.), which must be respected.

(continues)

Table 10-3   Nursing Interventions and Rationales for Bipolar Disorders (continued)

Problems	Interventions	Rationales
	8. Teach the client of the need to inform all of their healthcare providers of their psychiatric medications.	8. The client may receive medications from other healthcare providers—even the dentist—that may interact with the psychiatric medications they have been prescribed. The client needs to keep all their healthcare providers informed to maintain medical safety.
	9. Reinforce the benefit of attending support groups regularly and provide contact information for appropriate groups. a. Provide information on family support groups.	9. Support groups led by lay persons provide opportunities to express feelings, obtain support, and learn from others who have similar problems. a. Families need much support dealing with the client's symptoms and their own reactions to the client's illness.

	10. Suggest starting a journal of feelings, thoughts, reactions, and situations. The journal may be shared with the client's outpatient treatment team.	10. Journaling gives the client a method of keeping track of their own improvement and signs of impending relapse.
		    The client can use it to help decide when and what they need to report to the psychiatrist and other members of the outpatient treatment team. It is another tool to help the client be an active part of their treatment.
		    If the client feels comfortable with sharing the journal entries with the outpatient treatment team, it can assist the team in keeping track of the client's improvement or impending relapse.

11. Use role play with a person the client trusts to rehearse potential overwhelming, stress, or anger-producing situations.

12. Encourage appropriate practice and use of spiritual practices.

11. Role play is an effective technique that can also be used outside of the inpatient setting.

12. Many clients report that spirituality is central to their life because it provides them a reason to live. Many clients seek the counsel of clergy or other spiritual advisors to help deal with their symptoms in a depressed phase of bipolar disorders before seeking psychiatric treatment and as part of their discharge and relapse prevention plans. Clients with religious preoccupation may have to take it slower. Many clients receive emotional/psychological benefits from spending time in natural surroundings (e.g., parks, beaches) that will be available when they are discharged from the hospital.

REFERENCES

American Psychiatric Association (2000). *Diagnostic and statistical manual of mental disorders* (4th ed., text revision). Washington, DC: Author.

Boyd, M. A. (2008). *Psychiatric nursing: Contemporary practice* (4th ed.) Philadelphia, PA: Wolters Kluwer/Lippincott, Williams, & Wilkins.

Fontaine, K. L. (2009). *Mental health nursing* (6th ed.). Upper Saddle River, NJ: Pearson Education Inc.

Fortinash, K. M., & Holoday-Worret, P. A. (2003*). Psychiatric nursing care plans* (4th ed.). St. Louis, MO: Mosby.

Fortinash, K. M., & Holoday-Worret, P. A. (2007*). Psychiatric nursing care plans* (5th ed.). St. Louis, MO: Mosby, Elsevier.

Frisch, N. C., & Frisch, L. E. (2002). *Psychiatric mental health nursing* (2nd ed.). Albany, NY: Delmar/Thomson Learning, Inc.

Guido, G. W. (2007). *Legal & ethical issues in nursing* (4th ed.). Upper Saddle River, NJ: Pearson/Prentice Hall.

Jakopac, K. A. and Patel, S. C. (2009). *Psychiatric mental health case studies and care plans.* Sudbury, MA: Jones and Bartlett.

Jensen, L. W., Decker, L., & Andersen, M. M. (2006). Depression and health-promoting lifestyles of persons with chronic mental illness. *Issues in Mental Health Nursing, 27,* 617–634.

Keltner, N. L., Schwecke, L. H., & Bostrom, C. E. (2007). *Psychiatric nursing* (5th ed.). St. Louis, MO: Mosby, Elsevier.

McKenry, L., Tessier, E., & Hogan, M. (2006). *Mosby's pharmacology in nursing* (22nd ed.). St. Louis, MO: Mosby, Inc.

Mohr, W. K. (2009). *Psychiatric-mental health nursing: Evidence based concepts, skills, and practices* (7th ed.). Philadelphia, PA: Wolters Kluwer/Lippincott, Williams, & Wilkins.

O'Brien, P. G., Kennedy, W. Z., & Ballard, K. A. (2008). *Psychiatric mental health nursing: An introduction to theory and practice.* Sudbury, MA: Jones and Bartlett.

Read, K., & Purse, M. (2009). Red flags: Symptoms of bipolar disorder in children. Retrieved from http://www.bipolar.about.com

Sadock, B. J., & Sadock, V. A. (2005). *Kaplan & Sadock's comprehensive textbook of psychiatry* (8th ed.). Philadelphia, PA: Lippincott, Williams, & Wilkins.

Smith, D. J. (2009). How to recognize and treat bipolar II disorder. *Current Psychiatry, 8*(7), 41–48.

Tugrul, K. (Dec., 2003). The nurse's role in the assessment and treatment of bipolar disorder. *Journal of the American Psychiatric Nurses Association, 9*(6), 180–186.

Varcarolis, E. M. (2006). *Manual of psychiatric nursing care plans* (3rd ed.). St. Louis, MO: Saunders, Elsevier.

Varcarolis, E. M., Carson, V. B., & Shoemaker, N. C. (2006). *Foundations of psychiatric mental health nursing: A clinical approach* (6th ed.). St. Louis, MO: Saunders, Elsevier.

Wozniak, J., Biederman, J., Kiely, K., Ablon, S., Faraone, S., Mundy, E., & Mennin, D. (1995a): Mania-like symptoms suggestive of childhood onset bipolar disorder in clinically referred children. *Journal of the American Academy of Child Adolescent Psychiatry 34,* 867–876.

SUGGESTED READINGS

Antai-Otong, D. (June, 2007). Psychopharmacology of bipolar disorders. Psychiatric Nursing Conference, New Orleans, LA.

Arce, A. (2009). Family-focused therapy may benefit bipolar children. *NeuroPsychiatry Reviews*, *10*(1), 1, 16.

Cain, N. N., Davidson, P. W., Burhan, A. M., Andolsek, M. E., Baxter, J. T., Sullivan, L., Florescue, H., List, A., & Deutsch, L. (Jan., 2003). Identifying bipolar disorders in individuals with intellectual disability. *Journal of Intellectual Disability Research*, *47*(1), 31–38.

Carpenito-Moyat, L. J. (2008). *Nursing diagnosis: Application to clinical practice* (12th ed.). Philadelphia, PA: Wolters Kluwer, Lippincott, Williams, & Wilkins.

Chung, H., Culpepper, L., De Wester, J. N., Grieco, R. L., Kaye, N. S., Lipkin, M., Rosen, S. J., & Ross, R. (Nov., 2007). Part 3: Clinical management of bipolar disorder: Achieving best outcomes through a collaborative care model. *Supplement to Current Psychiatry*, S11–18.

Chung, H., Culpepper, L., De Wester, J. N., Grieco, R. L., Kaye, N. S., Lipkin, M., Rosen, S. J., & Ross, R. (Nov., 2007). Part 4: Treatment by phase: Pharmacologic management of bipolar disorder. *Supplement to Current Psychiatry*, S19–32.

Dunn, K., Elsom, S., & Cross, W. (Feb., 2007). Self-efficacy and locus of control affect management of aggression by mental health nurses. *Issues in Mental Health Nursing*, *28*(2), 201–217.

Fontaine, K. L., & Fletcher, J. S. (2003). *Mental health nursing* (5th ed.). Upper Saddle River, NJ: Pearson Education, Inc.

Geracioti, Jr., T. D. (2006). Identifying hyperthyroidism's psychiatric presentations. *Current Psychiatry*, *5*(12), 84–92.

Gonzales, R., & Suppes, T. (2008). Stimulants for adult bipolar disorder. *Current Psychiatry*, *4*(11), 33–45.

Joint Commission on Accreditation of Healthcare Organizations (JCAHO). (Dec., 2008) NPSG.15.01.01 and NPSG.15.01.01 EP 3. Suicide risk reduction. Retrieved from http://www.jointcommission.org/AccreditationPrograms/BehavioralHealthCare/Standards/09_FAQs/NPSG/Focused_risk_assessment/NPSG.15.01.01/Suicide+risk+reduction.htm

Krakowski, M. (2007). Violent behavior: Choosing antipsychotics and other agents. *Current Psychiatry*, *6*(4), 63–70.

Kupfer, D. J. (2004). Bipolar depression: The clinician's reference guide (BD-CRG). Continuing education supplement by *Current Psychiatry and Lilly*, 1-84.

La Torre, M. A. (Jan.–Mar., 2002). Integrated perspectives: Enhancing therapeutic presence. *Perspectives in Psychiatric Care*, *38*(1), 34–36.

Lewis, S. M., Heitkemper, M. M., & Dirksen, S. R. (2004). *Medical-Surgical nursing: Assessment strategies and management of clinical problems* (6th ed.). St. Louis, MO: Mosby.

Literature Monitor: Delay in childhood bipolar disorder treatment may result in adverse outcomes. (June, 2007). *NeuroPsychiatry Reviews*, *8*(6), 25, 27.

Macneil, J. S. (Aug., 2005). Psychotherapy can reduce mood disorder relapse. *Clinical Psychiatry News*, *33*(8), 23.

Marcus, P. (June, 2007). Suicidal ideation: Assessment and prevention. Psychiatric Nursing Conference, New Orleans, LA.

Merriman, J. (2007). Clock gene disruption may produce mania symptoms in patients with bipolar disorder. *NeuroPsychiatry Reviews*, *8*(6), 18.

Mosby's medical, nursing, and allied health dictionary (6th ed.). (2002). St. Louis, MO: Mosby, Inc.

Mullen, J., Endicott, J., Hirschfeld, R. M., Yonkers, K., Tarcum, S., & Bullinger, A. L. (Eds.). (2004). *Manual of rating scales: For the assessment of mood disorders.* Wilmington, DE: Astrazeneca Pharmaceuticals LP.

National Alliance on Mental Illness: http://www.nami.org

Neu, J. E., & DeNisco, S. (2007). Practical approaches to treating patients with bipolar disorder. *The American Journal For Nurse Practitioners, 11*(1), 1–24.

Pollack, L. E., & Cramer, R. D. (2000). Perceptions of problems in people hospitalized for bipolar disorder: Implications for patient education. *Issues in Mental Health Nursing, 21,* 765–778.

Sachs, G. et al. (2007). Study sheds light on medication treatment options for bipolar disorder. *New England Journal of Medicine NIH News Release.* Retrieved from http://www.nih.gov/news/pr/mar2007/nimh-28.htm

Sadock, B. J., & Sadock, V. A. (2003). *Kaplan & Sadock's synopsis of psychiatry: Behavioral sciences/ clinical psychiatry* (9th ed.). Philadelphia, PA: Lippincott, Williams, & Wilkins.

Saunders, J. C. (2008). Neuropsychiatric symptoms of hepatitis C. *Issues in Mental Health Nursing, 29,* 209–220.

Schultz, J. M., & Videbeck, S. L. (2005). *Lippincott's manual of psychiatric nursing care plans* (7th ed.). Philadelphia, PA: Lippincott, Williams & Wilkins.

Sirven, J. I. (July, 2007). Dangerous duo: Anti-epileptics plus herbals. *Current Psychiatry, 6*(7), 116.

Stein, J. (Nov., 2007). Genes linked to suicidal thoughts during antidepressant therapy. *NeuroPsychiatry Reviews, 8*(11), 1, 16, 17.

Stong, C. (Aug., 2006). Assessing suicide risk—separating attempts from ideation. *NeuroPsychiatry Reviews, 7*(8), 1, 19.

Stong, C. (June, 2007). Bipolar disorder: Underrecognized, poorly treated. *NeuroPsychiatry Reviews, 8*(6), 1, 18.

Stuart, G. W., & Laraia, M. T. (2005). *Principles and practice of psychiatric nursing* (8th ed.). St. Louis, MO: Mosby, Elsevier.

Thompson, J., McFarland, G. K., Hirsch, J. E., & Tucker, S. M. (2002). *Mosby's clinical nursing* (5th ed.). St. Louis, MO: Mosby.

Townsend, M. C. (2008). *Nursing diagnoses in psychiatric nursing* (7th ed.). Philadelphia, PA: F. A. Davis.

Umlaaf, M. G., & Shattell, M. (2005). The ecology of bipolar disorder: The importance of sleep. *Issues in Mental Health Nursing, 26,* 699–720.

US Department of Health and Human Services National Institutes of Health: NIH News National Institute of Mental Health. (Sept., 2006). Bipolar disorder exacts twice depression's toll in workplace: Productivity lags even after mood lifts. Retrieved from http://www.nih.gov/news/pr/sep2006/nimh-01.htm

US Department of Health and Human Services National Institutes of Health: NIH News National Institute of Mental Health. (March, 2006). Study sheds light on medication treatment options for bipolar disorder. Retrieved from http://www.nih.gov/news/pr/mar2007/nimh-28.htm

Wagner, D. L. (June, 2007). Flighty patients a clue to hypomania. *Current Psychiatry, 6*(6), 116.

Yigletu, H., Tucker, S., Harris, M., & Hatlevig, J. (2004). Assessing suicidal ideation: Comparing self-report versus clinician report. *American Psychiatric Nurses Association, 10*(1), 9–15.

CHAPTER 11

Assessment of Schizophrenia

Sudha C. Patel

OBJECTIVES _____

The nursing student will be able to:
1. Recognize positive and negative signs and symptoms that meet DSM-IV-TR criteria for schizophrenia
2. Be familiar with common medical illnesses that can cause or exacerbate signs and symptoms of schizophrenia
3. Perform a biopsychosocial nursing assessment or intake assessment of clients experiencing signs and symptoms of schizophrenia
4. Identify and implement nursing interventions for clients experiencing signs and symptoms of schizophrenia
5. Implement care for clients receiving psychotropic medications
6. Assess discharge planning needs of clients admitted with a diagnosis of schizophrenia

KEY TERMS _____

Alogia	Hallucination
Avolition	Negative symptoms
Delusion	Positive symptoms
Flat/blunted affect	Psychosis

Schizophrenia is one of the psychotic disorders included in the American Psychiatric Association's (APA) *Diagnostic and Statistical Manual of Mental Disorders* (4th ed.), text revision (DSM-IV-TR) (APA, 2000, pp. 297–3230). In the United States, this disorder affects approximately 1% of the population over a lifetime (Sadock & Sadock, 2008, p. 157). This disorder usually begins prior to age 25 years and lasts throughout life. Both patient and family suffer due to social stigma and ignorance of the disorder.

DIAGNOSIS

There is no single characteristic that is pathognomonic in schizophrenia; the disease can produce a wide spectrum clinical picture that is chronic and debilitating. According to DSM-IV-TR, in schizophrenia there are specific groups of signs and symptoms. At least two or more of the following signs and symptoms must exist for at least 1 month to indicate a diagnosis of schizophrenia:

- Hallucinations
- Delusions
- Disorganized speech
- Grossly disorganized behavior
- Negative symptoms such as flat affect, alogia, and avolition as per DSM-IV-TR criteria for schizophrenia must occur for a period of at least 1 month and duration of illness for at least 6 months to meet the criteria for a diagnosis.
- There must be impairment in functioning and absence of diagnosis of schizoaffective and mood disorders.

No laboratory tests so far have been identified that are diagnostic for schizophrenia (APA, 2000, p. 305). The major feature of the schizophrenia is a break from reality; that is, a person with schizophrenia exhibits delusions, perceptual disturbances, and/or disorganized thinking among other symptoms, and these symptoms are not due to medical conditions or substance use. The subtypes of schizophrenia include paranoid, disorganized, catatonic, undifferentiated, and residual, all of which are based on clinical symptomology (APA, p. 315–316).

SIGNS AND SYMPTOMS

In general, the symptoms of schizophrenia are divided into two broad categories: positive and negative (APA, 2000, p. 299). Positive symptoms occur when there is an excess or distortion of normal functioning level, whereas negative symptoms occur when there is a diminishing or loss of normal functioning level (APA, 2000, p. 299).

Positive symptoms include hallucinations or perceptual disturbances, delusions or disorganized thought content and speech, and bizarre behavior.

Negative symptoms include restriction in range and intensity in expression of feeling or affect, exhibiting flat to blunted affect, apathy and inattentiveness, and distortion in language and thought process or disorganized speech. These negative symptoms are less dramatic then positive symptoms, although they are considered by some to be at the core of the schizophrenic disorder (O'Brien, Kennedy, & Ballard, 2008, p. 291).

PATHOPHYSIOLOGY

Dopamine Hypothesis

The exact cause of schizophrenia is not known; however, it is hypothesized that it is partly related to an increased level of dopamine in the central neural tract. To substantiate this hypothesis, the antipsychotic drugs that are most successful in treating schizophrenia are dopamine receptor antagonists. Some stimulant drugs such as cocaine and amphetamine excite dopaminergic pathways, which then mimic the schizophrenic symptoms in the person (Sadock & Sadock, 2008, p. 159). The dopamine hypothesis also identifies the two specific affected dopamine pathways in the brain: (1) prefrontal cortical—responsible for negative symptoms, and (2) mesolimbic—responsible for positive symptoms.

Other Neurotransmitter Abnormality

Levels of some neurotransmitters are affected, such as increased levels of serotonin and norepinephrine, and decreased levels of gamma-aminobutyric acid (GABA) (Sadock & Sadock, 2008, p. 159).

BIOPSYCHOSOCIAL NURSING ASSESSMENT

The nursing assessment includes a holistic approach, covering the biopsychosocial status of the patient.

Biologic Assessment

It is vital for the nurse to take a detailed history with the client and/or family members and conduct a complete physical examination and screening for the existence of any medical problem and/or use or abuse of any substance that can mimic the signs and symptoms of schizophrenia. Clients with schizophrenia have higher mortality rates and rates of comorbid medical illnesses such as diabetes, hypertension, and cardiopulmonary illnesses.

The psychiatric-mental health (PMH) nurse needs to screen for the physical health status of the patient. The patient with schizophrenia exhibiting positive and negative symptoms usually exhibits a self-care deficit and has sleep and nutritional deprivation. It is important to do a nutrition assessment since psychotropic medication can alter the nutritional status of the patient. The client's weight may need to be taken daily or weekly to keep track of any loss or gain of weight. The client also may develop a metabolic syndrome such as diabetes due to an antipsychotic medication (e.g., ziprasidone HCL [Geodone]). Assess patient's water intake. Assess for polyurea or polydipsia. Conduct an assessment for hyponatremia, hypervolemia, excessive urination, incontinence, or increased blood pressure (Boyd, 2008, p. 329).

It is also vital to obtain baseline data about physical and psychological functioning of the patient before starting psychotropic or other medications. Clients need to be screened as per agency protocol using an available standardized assessment instrument before starting antipsychotic medications. Some examples of commonly used scales in the psychiatric setting are: (1) Abnormal Involuntary Movement Scale (AIMS) and (2) Dyskinesia Identification System: Condensed User Scale (DISCUS).

Psychosocial Assessment

History of Illness

The psychosocial assessment includes taking a history of illness from the client or a family member and conducting a mental status examination. There are several standardized assessment scales available in a hand book of psychiatric measures published by American Psychiatric Publishing Company (2000). Depending upon the agency protocol, the PMH nurse may use the appropriate scale to collect data on symptoms.

It is important to note that some clients with schizophrenia are unable to recognize that they have a mental illness. This may be due to the symptoms of alteration in thoughts, perceptions, and behavior common to schizophrenia. At some time during the taking of the history, the client may deny having a mental illness or need for the treatment.

Nursing Assessment of Mental Status

Appearance

A patient with schizophrenia may vary in appearance from completely disheveled with poor hygiene and bizarre dress, and be irritable and agitated, to appearing obsessively groomed, quiet and possibly immobile, in a stupor, or lethargic. Some clients may be excessively talkative, use bizarre postures and be likely to become violent without any provocation; these symptoms could be in response to hallucination or internal stimulation (i.e., disorder of perceptions). The PMH nurse may find some odd behavior in the client, such as tics and atypical mannerisms, as well as echopraxia, in which the client mimics the posture of the examiner (Sadock & Sadock, 2008, p. 168).

Alteration in Mood and Affect

In clients with schizophrenia, there is an alteration in mood–affect status. Clients commonly display two ranges of affective symptoms: (1) from no emotional response or flat affect to a reduced emotional responsiveness or blunted affect, or (2) excessive and inappropriate emotional outbursts ranging from rage to happiness to anxiety. Clients also can exhibit feelings of isolation, ambivalence, or depression and apathy.

Perceptions—Hallucinations

In schizophrenia, there is an alteration in one or more of the five senses, causing hallucinations. These are considered positive symptoms. Most common are visual or auditory (hearing voices) hallucinations. These types of hallucinations are not based on real images or sounds. The heard voices are usually threatening, insulting, and are accusing the client. There may be two or more heard voices talking to each other, or they may give derogatory remarks to the client about their life or behavior. Other types of sensory alteration such as gustatory, olfactory, or tactile are uncommon in schizophrenia; however, if these are present then there may be a preexisting neurologic or medical illness that the PMH nurse must document or notify the physician about for further investigation. Some patients may experience a "kinesthetic hallucination" that is a sensation of an altered state of bodily organs. The patient may experience burning sensations in the brain, a feeling of rushing in the blood vessels, or a cutting sensation in the bone marrow. A distortion of body image may also occur (Sadock & Sadock, 2008, p. 168). Most clients with schizophrenia may not share openly their hallucinatory experiences with the nurse, so the nurse must indirectly observe the client; for example, the client may look preoccupied during the interview, may respond to internal voices, laugh, or become agitated by the voices. The PMH nurse needs to validate their observation with the patient. The nurse also must assess for a possible substance abuse-related cause for the hallucinations.

Thoughts

There is an alteration in thoughts in terms of content, forms, and processes in schizophrenia. Assessment of thoughts is vital since they are hallmark symptoms in schizophrenia; they are also considered positive symptoms.

Delusions are the most common form of alteration in thought content. Delusion reflects the patient's ideas, beliefs, and interpretations of stimuli (Sadock & Sadock, 2008, p. 168). The most common forms of delusion are persecutory, grandiose, religious, or somatic. During the nursing assessment, the PMH nurse must distinguish bizarre delusions from nonbizarre ones.

Nonbizarre delusion usually have themes of jealousy and persecution and are derived from a person's life experiences. For example, a client believes that their significant other—who is separated from them—is now trying to kill them, or they believe that the police are trying to catch them because they tried drugs when they were 14 years old. Bizarre delusions are not derived from ordinary life situations and are usually exhibited in the form of delusions of control. Examples of some of the common thought control delusions include: (1) the client believes that some outside forces are controlling their thoughts and behavior; (2) the client may state that the other can read their mind or actions (i.e., thought broadcasting), that the other person has placed thoughts into the client's mind (i.e., thought insertion), that the other person is removing thoughts from the client's mind (i.e., thought withdrawal); or (3) the client may believe that they can control outside events with some extraordinary power they have within themselves (APA, 2000).

The PMH nurse also needs to assess the client's forms of thought; a form of thought is objectively observable in the client's spoken and written language. Examples of disorders of thought include looseness of association, derailment, incoherence, tangentiality, circumstantialities, neologism, echolalia, verbigeration, world salad, and mutism (Sadock & Sadock, 2008, p. 168).

In assessing thought processes, the PMH nurse must pay attention to both what the client communicates and how they communicate—in speech, writing, or drawing during activity sessions. Some examples of disorders of thought process include flights of ideas, thought blocking, preservation, clang association (words are repeated based on similar sound) and circumstantialities, poverty of thought content, and poor abstraction ability.

Impulsiveness, Violence, and Suicide

The PMH nurse needs to understand that the client with schizophrenia generally has poor impulse control as well as poor tolerance when they are acutely ill; some clients may even exhibit impulsive behavior such as a suicide or homicide attempt due to hallucinatory experiences as well other stresses affecting their life. During the assessment, the nurse must pay attention to current suicidal ideation or a suicide attempt in the past. Usually suicides occur in clients who have a persecutory delusion, which may exalt violent behavior. The PMH nurse needs to remember that if the patient exhibits violent behavior, the assessment must be discontinued until the client calms down. Suicide attempts can occur without prior warning since a patient who also has severe depressive symptoms may not verbalize about having suicidal ideation or a plan (Sadock & Sadock, 2008, p. 169).

Cognition

Orientation

The PMH nurse first needs to assess the client's orientation to place, person, situation, and time. Usually clients with schizophrenia are oriented to person, place, and time. The nurse should be alert to a lack of such orientation in the client they are assessing since it will require further investigation for the possibility of a neurologic or other medical problem (Sadock & Sadock, 2008, p. 178).

It is important for the nurse to understand that the clinical assessment is not adequate to recognize cognition impairment in schizophrenia. The patient must also be screened using a standardized instrument that is available in the agency. Two examples of the available instruments are the Mini-Mental Status Examination (MMSE) and Cognitive Assessment Screening Instrument (CASI). If there is cognitive impairment detected, then further testing will be done by a psychologist.

Memory

The PMH nurse may find memory intact using standardized instruments such as the MMSE; however, some impairment may be detected such as problems with recall of newly learned information within seconds and the client's ability to focus on abstract thinking.

Judgment and Insight

Insight is an individual's ability to know their own thoughts, the reality of external objects, and their relation to each other (Boyd, 2000, p. 301). Judgment is the ability to make a decision according to a given situation. Insight and judgment are associated with each other, and are dependent on cognitive functions. The nurse should assess various aspects of insight during the cognitive assessment, such as the client's awareness of their own symptoms, ability to cope with others, and their understanding of the reason for seeking care.

Behavior

Bizarre behavior is usually seen in schizophrenia during an acute psychotic episode. The nurse needs to understand that the client may be experiencing disturbed thoughts and/or auditory or visual hallucinations due to external or internal stimuli. It is important to analyze behavior in the context of the client's altered thinking process. A client may not participate in daily living activities due to negative symptoms such as lack of motivation or experiencing avolition or no motivation/apathy. Other negative behaviors seen in schizophrenia are purposeless moving, pacing, echopraxia (i.e., mimicking the interviewer's posture), having an odd or fixed posture for an extended time (i.e., waxy flexibility). During the behavioral assessment the nurse must also be aware that the client's exhibition of abnormal behavior and movement could be related to a side-effect of psychotropic medication, so all clients need to be screened with the Abnormal Involuntary Movement Scale (AIMS) to collect baseline data or to rule this out as the cause of such behavior. Clients may also exhibit low or poor self-concept due to their illness, from hearing comments from others that they are crazy and bearing the overall societal stigma about mental illness.

NURSING INTERVENTIONS AND RATIONALES

Nursing interventions need to focus on developing a trusting relationship with the client, as well as on the specifics of positive and negative symptoms, depression, suicidal ideation and behavior, substance abuse problems, comorbid medical disorders, posttraumatic stress disorder (PTSD), and a range of potential community adjustment problems or situations, such as homelessness, social isolation, unemployment, legal problems, age, education level, cultural background, and religious preference (APA, 2004). Because of all the factors involved, interventions need to be customized to the individual client's needs. For specific nursing diagnoses, outcomes, and evaluation criteria, refer to a general psychiatric-mental health nursing textbook such as *Psychiatric-Mental Health Nursing: Introduction to General Theory and Practice*, O'Brien, Kennedy, & Ballard (2008); *Mental Health Nursing*, Fontaine (2009); *Psychiatric Nursing: Contemporary Practice*, Boyd (2008); *Psychiatric Mental Health Case Studies and Care Plans*, Jakopac & Patel (2009); and psychiatric care plan books such as *Psychiatric Nursing Care Plans*, Fortinash & Holoday-Worret (2007) or *Manual of Psychiatric Nursing Care Plans*, Varcarolis (2006). Goals for nursing care in schizophrenia are to prevent harm; control disturbed behavior; reduce severity of psychosis and related symptoms such as aggression, negative symptoms, and affective symptoms; identify triggers that lead to an acute episode; and develop partnerships with the client and family for the long- and short-term plan of care for aftercare. The nursing interventions described in **Table 11-1** apply to adult clients.

Table 11-1   Nursing Interventions and Rationales for Schizophrenia

Problems	Interventions	Rationales
Establishing trust and therapeutic relationships for planning care	1. Use appropriate therapeutic communication techniques for developing rapport and trust with the client (see also Chapters 4 and 5).	1. Clients with schizophrenia are usually guarded and hesitant to communicate or engage in developing trusting relationships due to previous rejections they may have experienced. Also, their symptoms such as feelings of paranoia or suspiciousness toward others may play an important role in hindering development of trust in others (Boyd, 2008).
	2. Involve the client and family (with client permission) in planning and goal setting for care.	2. A supportive therapeutic alliance allows the nurse to gain essential information about the client and allows the client to develop trust in the nurse so that they are willing to cooperate with the care plan. Involving the client as well as significant others in identification of goals relating to treatment or care outcomes fosters and strengthens the therapeutic relationship as well as treatment adherence.
Suicidal or homicidal ideation and presence of command hallucinations	1. Assess for suicidal and homicidal ideations, plan, lethality of plan, access to the means to carry out plan, prior attempts, and chemical dependency and take precautions as per agency protocol for client's and others' safety. Obtain an order from the psychiatrist to place the client on 1:1 observation for safety.	1. Suicidal and/or homicidal ideations are common in clients in the acute phase of psychosis due to command hallucinations in which the client may act on the commands given to them by the heard voices. Clients with chemical abuse/dependency problems are also at higher risk to act on impulse to harm self or others due to poor impulse control.

(continues)

Table 11-1   Nursing Interventions and Rationales for Schizophrenia *(continued)*

Problems	Interventions	Rationales
	a. If the client reports homicidal thoughts toward a specific person, follow the agency protocol. The nurse needs to obtain as much information as possible and report this to the psychiatrist and immediate nursing supervisor, and document this information including who the information was reported to.	a. Suicidal/homicidal thoughts and urges are not always constant. They can be triggered by something that another client says, a phone call, visitor or something viewed on TV; therefore, documenting and reporting of observations as well as actions taken to the health team as well as to the next shift is vital for the client's as well as others' safety (see also Chapter 9).
	b. If the client is having command hallucinations, such as voices telling them to harm themselves or others, then the client needs to be placed on 1:1 supervision for safety and this information must be reported to the treatment team.	b. When client has command hallucinations, with threatening voice, client safety is prime concern for nurse, so protecting the client from the self-harm due to internal or external stimuli is vital.
	c. Offer antipsychotic medications if they are ordered.	c. The client needs to feel safe, and antipsychotic medications can be very helpful in reducing psychotic symptoms.
	d. Obtain at least a verbal no-self-harm or harm to others contract at admission and every shift change.	d. 1. There is a need for additional assessment and obtaining at least a verbal no-self-harm or harm to others contract. Follow agency protocol for obtaining a verbal or written contract from the client. This measure helps decrease the possibility of the client hurting themselves or others.

	e. Provide hope and a safe therapeutic milieu free from contraband/items that could be potential weapons (see Chapter 3).	d. 2. Assisting the client with verbalization of feelings, thoughts, concerns, or fears helps decrease the possibility of physical acting upon them. This also shows the client that the nurse is listening, is genuinely concerned, helps build rapport, trust, and the therapeutic nurse relationship.
	f. For delusional thinking, provide reassurance to the client and family members for measures taken for the safety of the client and/or others. See Chapter 9 for more information related to working with suicidal clients.	e. This approach shows the client that the nurse provides hope that the client can be helped, and that the client is a valuable human being worthy of help. Nurses also maintain the safe therapeutic milieu for the client's safety.
		f. Contents of delusion reflect the client's underlying fear and anxiety related to the perceived threat of lived experiences of distrust and unsafe feelings. Delusion is the client's defense mechanism to protect the self from painful feelings.
Delusions	1. Do not argue with the client about their delusions nor reinforce the delusions. Acknowledge the client's delusion and provide a reality-based explanation to client. Redirect or distract the client in matter-of-fact way to reality, and focus on real people and real situations.	1. Challenging the client's delusion or getting into an argument about the client's delusions or belief system can make the client angry. Provide reality-based explanation about the client's delusion when client is receptive later in therapy.
Hallucination/ hearing voices	1. Stress reduction activities may help the client to reduce anxiety and therefore hallucinations. Use behavioral and cognitive interventions to assist the client to refocus thoughts and feelings; teach thought stopping techniques.	1. The nurse needs to help the client develop strategies to cope with the alteration in sensory perception as medications may relieve positive symptoms, they may not eliminate the hallucinations and delusion (Boyd, 2008).

(continues)

Table 11-1   Nursing Interventions and Rationales for Schizophrenia *(continued)*

Problems	Interventions	Rationales
	2. Monitor client for any sign that may indicate hallucination (hearing voices or seeing visual images). Examples include noticing client talking, laughing, or arguing with self and, during socialization time, noticing the client looking preoccupied and/or unfocused on a given task. a. Encourage the client to verbalize feelings about the hallucinatory experience and anxiety; however, do not move within close proximity of the client or touch the client. Approach the client in a nonthreatening way. b. Use a nonjudgmental, respectful, and accepting approach with the client through therapeutic use of self (see Chapters 2, 4, and 5). c. Monitor the TV programs the client is watching to reduce perceptual problems.	2. Close observation provides the nurse with clues as to whether or not the client is having hallucinatory experiences and any alteration in their emotional or behavioral system. This observation prompts the nurse to provide timely therapeutic interventions to reduce the client's fear and anxiety and to prevent violent outbursts toward self or others due to heard voices. a. A client who has paranoid ideation or has suspiciousness feelings is very sensitive to close proximity, perceives it as a threat, and may become aggressive. b. Approaching the client in a nonjudgmental way and providing respect and acceptance of them helps the client trust the nurse and opens up the opportunity to discuss their hallucinatory experiences and associated feelings of fear or anxiety. c. Some scenarios such as horror or violent acts in the TV programs, may cause perceptual disturbances in some clients, particularly those who exhibit psychotic symptoms; such programs may increase their anxiety and fear level.
Impaired communication	1. Use an empathetic approach with validation techniques while communicating with the client with schizophrenia to seek clarity from the client.	1. In schizophrenia, the client has communication problems as well as having disorganized or disruptive behavior among other symptoms that may be frightening to the client and others. Some

clients may use symbolic, idiosyncratic, or metaphorical language during communication.

   a. Use of validation techniques is beneficial for the nurse for clarity and in receiving accurate feedback or inferences from the client about his use of symbolic language or behavior.

   b. Validation techniques also help the client to feel their input is important to help the nurse understand what meaning they have for a particular word or behavior.

a. Be patient and do not force or pressure the client to talk.

b. Provide group activities that can motivate the client and help in increasing self-esteem and enjoyment of the sessions.

| Adherence to medications/treatment plan | 1. Provide psychoeducation for psychotropic and other medications involving the client, family and/or significant others. | 1. Psychoeducation sessions are beneficial to the client and family as these sessions can help them learn about the importance of adherence to medication to prevent relapses and sustain recovery from the symptoms of illness. The client and family need to know that psychoeducation sessions are vital for adherence to medications as well as the overall treatment plan. |
| | a. Teach clients who are on psychotropic medications the importance of adherence to medications for their efficacy, effectiveness, and side-effects. Explore the client's reason for nonadherence to medications. Use motivational enhancement, behavioral training approaches, and tailoring medications according to individual client's needs along with social skills training to facilitate adherence to medication management. | a. Gaining knowledge about medications will help the client and family to feel empowered in self-care and instill hope for recovering from symptoms of schizophrenia. |

(continues)

Table 11-1   Nursing Interventions and Rationales for Schizophrenia *(continued)*

Problems	Interventions	Rationales
Self-care deficit	1. Encourage the client to take care of ADLs including personal hygiene when psychotic symptoms are at a manageable level. a. Encourage the client to attend scheduled group sessions, such as psychotherapy, psychoeducation groups, activities therapy, medication education, etc. b. Provide the client a copy of the daily therapeutic activities plan that includes rest periods, so client can rest during rest period and be able to attend the plan sessions.	1. The client may avoid getting dressed or bathing due to decreased energy levels or psychotic symptoms. The client does need to know that the nurse or other staff members can provide assistance if needed. a. The client will be taught about the disease process of schizophrenia, related brain chemicals or neurotransmitters, and medications individually and in psychoeducation groups. b. This helps prevent the client from becoming overwhelmed. Elderly clients may need scheduled rest periods between groups/activities.
Changes in appetite/weight	1. Obtain a baseline weight on admission, assess skin turgor, and take vital signs (temp, pulse, respiration, & blood pressure). Assess laboratory values such as glucose, total protein, albumin, RBCs, WBCs, Hgb, Hct, MCV, MCH, CMP, thyroid level, if ordered. Weigh at least once a week before breakfast on the same scale.	1. Obtaining a baseline weight and assessing skin turgor and vital signs provide information to compare to normal height/weight charts and a general idea of fluid intake. Increased glucose level may be due to an antipsychotic medication such as ziprasidone (Geodone) or aripiprazole (Abilify) as these medications can cause metabolic syndrome and mimic symptoms of diabetes. Total protein and albumin levels may indicate poor nutrition. Decreased RBCs, Hgb, and Hct may indicate nutrition-related anemia. Elevated MCV and MCH values may also indicate nutrition-related anemia. This information will be used to compare to future assessment data to see if the client is improving.

2. Ask the client to complete a food/fluid intake diary for at least the past 3 days.

2. This helps provide a more accurate account of what the patient is eating, drinking, and eliminating. For severely malnourished or elderly clients, the nurse may need to continue monitoring intake and output each shift.

a. Refer the client to a dietician for dietary consult if there is a need for further evaluation.

a. The nurse will need to obtain an order from the psychiatrist for a dietary consult. Consultation by a dietician will assist the client to make necessary changes in dietary intake and help with the weight gain side-effect of many psychiatric medications.

b. Obtain information regarding the client's food preferences, food restrictions due to allergies or religious/cultural practices.

b. Frequently diabetic or elderly clients need temporary supplements until their appetite returns.

Sleep pattern disturbances

1. Assess the client's specific sleep pattern disturbance, number of total hours slept per night, whether or not the client feels rested, and whether or not the client naps during the day. For detail interventions, see Chapter 8.

1. This establishes baseline information.

Helplessness/ hopelessness/ powerlessness

1. Provide emotional support and reassure the client that help is available.

1. This intervention shows the client that they are not alone, there is hope, and that the nurse cares about them.

a. Assist the client to identify factors that they can control and focus on these when the client has hallucinatory experiences.

a. The client can be empowered by identifying and focusing on what they can control when hallucinating or having paranoid ideation.

b. Discuss the importance of trying to be flexible with situations not within the client's control.

b. Focus on teaching the client what can be done to feel safe and in control.

(continues)

Table 11-1   Nursing Interventions and Rationales for Schizophrenia *(continued)*

Problems	Interventions	Rationales
	c. Explore with the client their support system or resources they have to work with such as family members, friends, an employer, church, religious/spiritual leader, and others who can help the client in recovery and preventing relapses.	c. Clients may not be able to perceive how many resources or what support they actually have due to illness. The client may have a tendency to focus on negative problems instead of positive factors. Exploring resources increases their awareness. This helps clients gain a sense of hope, increased control, and empowerment over their situation and assists them to adhere to the treatment plan after discharge from the hospital.
Social isolation/ withdrawn behavior	1. Provide nonthreatening activities to engage the client to do some things such as walking in a designated place, painting, drawing, writing, etc.	1. Initially the client may want to isolate in their room rather than attend scheduled activities. The therapeutic milieu is designed to encourage social interaction. Clients who experience symptoms of schizophrenia will socially isolate themselves and need an environment that discourages social isolation.
	a. Organize the meeting place in a semi-circle or a round table so clients can sit side by side or facing each other.	a. This type of situation will facilitate client interactions with each other in a nonthreatening manner.
	2. Inform the client that the therapeutic milieu includes eating meals with other clients in a common dining room. Discourage the client from eating alone in their room.	2. This intervention demonstrates that the nurse cares about the client and helps decrease isolation.

3. Initially provide frequent interaction one-on-one with the client, then introduce the client to other peers in the presence of a staff member.

4. Provide positive reinforcement for any attempts made by the client to come out of isolative behavior; however, do not force the client to interact in group.

5. Implement behavioral modification if ordered.

3. A smaller group is less overwhelming than being with all the clients on the unit at the same time. This type of setting encourages socialization even if initially the client is just sitting with others and not interacting.

   Having a nurse or other staff member present provides emotional support and conveys caring and interest in the client as a person.

4. Positive reinforcement helps increase the likelihood that the behavior will be repeated.

5. Behavior modification is used to reinforce positive behavior. There are many types of behavior modification systems, such as token economy systems, behavioral contracts, etc. Behavior modification is a useful intervention strategy for encouraging clients to attend groups, perform ADLs, or practice more self-control.

REFERENCES

American Psychiatric Association. (2000). *Diagnostic and statistical manual of mental disorders* (4th ed., Text Revision). Washington, DC: American Psychiatric Association.

American Psychiatric Association. (2000). *Handbook of psychiatric measures* (2nd ed.). Washington, DC: American Psychiatric Association.

American Psychological Association. (2004). *Practice guide line for the treatment of patient with schizophrenia* (2nd ed.). Washington DC: American Psychological Association.

American Psychological Association. (2007). *Practice guide line*. Washington, DC: Author.

Boyd, M. A. (2008). *Psychiatric nursing: Contemporary practice* (4th ed.). Philadelphia, PA: Wolters-Kluwer Health/Lippincott, Williams, & Wilkins.

Fortinash, K. M., & Holoday-Worret, P. A. (2007). *Psychiatric nursing care plans*. St. Louis, MO: Mosby, Elsevier.

Jakopac, K. A., & Patel, S. C. (2009). *Psychiatric mental health case studies and care plans*. Sudbury, MA: Jones and Bartlett Publishers.

O'Brien, P. G., Kennedy, W. Z., & Ballard, K. A. (2008). *Psychiatric mental health nursing: An introduction to theory and practice*. Sudbury, MA: Jones and Bartlett Publishers.

Sadock, B. J., & Sadock, V. A. (2008). *Concise textbook of clinical psychiatry* (3rd ed.). Philadelphia, PA: Lippincott, Williams, & Wilkins.

Varcarolis, E. M. (2006). *Manual of psychiatric nursing care plans*. St. Louis, MO: Saunders, Elsevier.

SUGGESTED READINGS

Antai-Otong, D. (2003). *The client with schizophrenia and other psychotic disorders*. Clifton Park, NY: Thomson Delmar Learning.

Fontaine, K. (2009). *Mental health nursing* (6th ed.). Upper Saddle River, NJ: Pearson Education, Inc.

Fontaine, K. L., & Fletcher, J. S. (2003). *Mental health nursing* (5th ed.). Upper Saddle River, NJ: Pearson Education, Inc.

Frisch, N. C., & Frisch, L. E. (2011). *Psychiatric mental health nursing* (4th ed.). Clifton Park, NY: Delmar.

Mohr, W. K. (2009). *Psychiatric-mental health nursing: Evidence based concepts, skills, and practices* (7th ed.). Philadelphia, PA: Wolters Kluwer/Lippincott, Williams, & Wilkins.

Mosby's medical, nursing & allied health dictionary (6th ed.). (2002). St. Louis, MO: Author.

Sadock, B. J., & Sadock, V. A. (2005). *Kaplan & Sadock's comprehensive textbook of psychiatry* (8th ed.). Philadelphia, PA: Lippincott, Williams, & Wilkins.

Townsend, M. C. (2009). *Psychiatric mental health nursing: Concepts of care in evidence-based practice* (6th ed.). Philadelphia, PA: F. A. Davis.

CHAPTER 12

Restriction to Locked Seclusion and Physical/Mechanical Restraints

Kim A. Jakopac

OBJECTIVES

The nursing student will be able to:

1. Recognize legal–ethical concepts and principles related to the use of locked seclusion and physical/mechanical restraints
2. Discuss patient/civil rights regarding the use of behavioral control measures such as seclusion and physical/mechanical restraints
3. Identify situations where it is necessary to use more restrictive measures when providing patient safety, behavioral control, or helping patients deal with psychotic symptoms
4. Provide nursing care for patients in seclusion and physical/mechanical restraints according to protocols
5. Recognize documentation requirements for clients who require behavioral control in the form of seclusion and physical/mechanical restraints according to protocols
6. Discuss special considerations regarding children/adolescents and elderly clients

KEY TERMS

Assault	False imprisonment
Autonomy	Fidelity
Battery	Justice
Beneficence	Least restrictive alternative doctrine
Bioethics	Nonmaleficence
Civil rights	Psychiatric code
Confidentiality	Restraint
Debriefing	Seclusion
Deescalation	Show of force/crisis team
Ethical dilemma	Veracity
Ethics	

The Joint Commission defines *seclusion* as "the involuntary confinement of a patient alone in a room or area from which the patient is physically prevented from leaving." *Restraint* is defined as "any manual method, physical or mechanical device, material, or equipment that immobilizes or reduces the ability of a patient to move his or her arms, legs, body, or head freely." The definition of restraint also includes medication: "A drug or medication when it is used as a restriction to manage the patient's behavior or restrict the patient's freedom of movement and is *not a standard treatment or dosage* for the patient's condition." (The Joint Commission Accreditation Program, 2009). The focus of this chapter will be on the use of locked physical seclusion and physical/mechanical restraints (otherwise referred to as "behavioral" restraints); hereafter referred to as seclusion and restraints. Medication will be addressed in Chapters 13 and 15.

Complex decisions must be made every day when providing health care and making decisions that affect the health and well-being of patients. Actions of the psychiatric-mental health (PMH) nurse must be consistent with the Nurse Practice Act of the state in which they are practicing in addition to the American Psychiatric Nurses Association (APNA) scope and standards and the American Nurses Association (ANA) code of ethics (Frisch & Frisch, 2011, p. 147). The PMH nurse must recognize and understand basic legal–ethical principles to practice within these parameters. Safety is always the highest priority. The authors of this book do not wish to encourage a stereotype of all people diagnosed with psychiatric illness or mental health problems as violent, but wish to assist all nurses to practice with compassion and safety within legal–ethical guidelines when situations requiring the use of seclusion and restraints occur. Unfortunately the use of seclusion and restraints has been necessary in emergency rooms/departments and other areas of inpatient care rather than being exclusively utilized in specific psychiatric-mental health areas.

LEGAL–ETHICAL CONSIDERATIONS

Legal–ethical considerations include bioethics, bioethical principles, and emphasis on least restrictive alternative doctrine. The major bioethical principles include:

- Autonomy
- Beneficence
- Fidelity
- Justice
- Nonmaleficence
- Veracity
- Least restrictive alternative doctrine

Failure to understand and appropriately apply legal principles as well as a patient's civil rights can lead to improper use of seclusion and restraints. Cultural variations in expression should be taken into account when making clinical judgments for nursing interventions. The PMH nurse and other staff members may be legally liable for charges of assault, battery, and false imprisonment if seclusion and restraints are used without legal justification or with excessive force (Keltner, Schwecke, & Bostrom, 2007, p. 57). The nurse will also be guilty of practicing outside of their scope of nursing practice and not providing the required standard of patient care.

Least restrictive alternative doctrine means using other treatment methods that do not isolate or restrict a patient to the full degree that seclusion or both seclusion and restraints do to handle potentially and actually violent or destructive situations. These methods include the use of therapeutic communication, limit setting, deescalation techniques, relaxation techniques, and other methods of stress management including deep breathing, soft music, guided imagery if patient is not psychotic; distraction, exercise, managing the therapeutic environment including taking the person to a quieter area; assigning an experienced staff member to be with the patient for 1:1 or constant observation (COs); judicious or cautious offering of prn medication (offering oral route first); or using a "show of force" stopping short of a full psychiatric code.

However, there are certain situations when less restrictive alternative methods fail. Some examples would include persons with hostile behavior, physical aggression, or violence related to or not related to psychosis (see appropriate topics in Chapters 9, 10, and 11). In these circumstances people are in crisis and vulnerable, but are too ill to understand and accept any help offered. In these *special circumstances*, The Joint Commission addresses the use of seclusion and restraint. Seclusion and/or seclusion and restraints may be used *only* for the management of violent or self-destructive behavior. Also, according to Varcarolis and Halter (2010), seclusion or seclusion and restraints is authorized when evidence exists and is documented by "nursing and medical staff" showing "substantial risk of harm to others or self is clear," inability to control one's own actions, sustained "problematic behavior" that continues or escalates in spite of other measures, and failure of other measures including "chemical restraints" (pp. 297–298). This is true for both voluntary and involuntary status patients. Contraindications to the use of seclusion and physical/mechanical restraints include "extremely unstable medical conditions" (e.g., unstable cardiac conditions) including delirium, dementia, and punishment or convenience (Varcarolis & Halter, 2010, p. 125).

Ethical dilemmas exist when situations arise that may require the use of only locked seclusion or both seclusion and physical/mechanical restraints. Patients do have the right to refuse treatment and exercise autonomy, but in situations where the patient's behavior is harmful to themselves or others, PMH nurses must balance these rights with the safety needs and legal–ethical principles of least restrictive alternative doctrine, beneficence, nonmalficence, and the safety of others. Such situations and circumstances are very difficult for both patients and nurses. Informing patients of the reasons for taking these measures, providing safety, and debriefing are critical for everyone involved. Providing safety and reassurance for all other patients in the area is extremely important as well.

In 2007, the American Psychiatric Nurses Association (APNA) position paper included the problem of ethical dilemmas in the use of seclusion and restraints, past histories of patient deaths when proper care was not rendered, patient rights, and the possibility of behavior being caused by organic or other medical problems needing attention. Also mentioned are studies on the impact of assault on nurses as well as studies showing that violence on inpatient units does occur and is unpredictable. The APNA paper states that skilled assessments must be performed for individuals in seclusion or seclusion and restraints to ensure both safety and discontinuation as soon as it is safe to release them. Individuals deserve humane, safe treatment that protects their dignity. Needless trauma must be avoided by using preventative measures, intervening early with less restrictive measures, and never using seclusion or seclusion and restraints for convenience, coercion, or punishment. These safety measures should only be used when less restrictive measures are ineffective and for the minimum amount of time needed to provide safety for individuals themselves and others. "The least number of restraint points must be utilized and the individual must be continuously observed" (APNA, 2007, p. 3).

Therefore, seclusion alone or with restraints is used *only when less restrictive methods have failed*, for the *shortest* amount of *time* possible and *only in special circumstances of violent or self-destructive behavior.* Orders for the use of locked seclusion or both locked seclusion and restraints are *always* time limited for specific behavior and are *never* "prn" orders. Typically 4 hours is the maximum amount of time an adult patient may be in seclusion or seclusion and restraints (refer to state statutes for specific rules in your state). If another episode occurs after a patient has been completely taken out of seclusion and restraints, it is treated as a separate, different episode, and a separate order must be obtained (Keltner, Schwecke, & Bostrom, 2007, p. 63).

The Substance Abuse and Mental Health Services Administration's (SAMHSA) Center for Mental Health Services 2009 Practice Guidelines for responding to mental health crisis include avoiding harm and preventing future emergencies in their core elements competencies. Regarding avoiding harm: "An appropriate response to mental health crises considers the risks and benefits attendant to interventions and whenever possible employs alternative approaches, such as controlling danger sufficiently to allow a period of 'watchful waiting.' In circumstances where there is an urgent need to establish physical safety and few viable alternatives to address an immediate risk of significant harm to the individual or others, an appropriate crisis response incorporates measures to minimize the duration and negative impact of interventions used." SAMHSA also addressed taking measures to reduce the likelihood of future emergencies: "Although addressing certain unmet needs may be beyond the purview of one facility or program, capturing and transmitting information about unmet needs to entities that have responsibility and authority (e.g., state mental health programs, housing authorities, foster care, and school systems) is an essential component of crisis services" (HHS Publication No. SMA-09-4427, pp. 5, 12; SAMHSA, 2009).

SECLUSION ROOMS

Seclusion rooms are special safe rooms. Common names for these special rooms include seclusion rooms, behavioral control rooms (BCRs) or "quiet" rooms. Seclusion rooms typically are similar to a regular patient room, but contain only a bed that is a standard twin size seclusion room bed containing a mattress in a wooden box style frame fitted with areas where restraints may be applied. In many facilities the bed is bolted to the floor to provide safety. Alternately, in some facilities a more traditional medical–surgical style bed is used to facilitate raising the head of the bed if necessary in a medical emergency situation. The wheels of these beds are usually kept in locked position, again to provide safety. Standard bed linens are used except in cases where the patient is at high risk for attempting suicide and then only a heavy blanket is used making it more difficult to form a knot and attempt strangulation. Windows typically contain unbreakable glass or have covers allowing light to enter, but preventing access to the actual window to prevent patient injury. Some seclusion rooms may also have special padding on the interior to prevent patients from injuring themselves. A bathroom is available in the seclusion room, but is kept locked unless the patient is actually using it with staff assistance and supervision. At other times a bedpan or urinal are offered. The Joint Commission conducts inspection of these rooms as well as documentation related to the use of these rooms on a regular basis. Example photos of a typical seclusion room and psychiatric-mental health bed are provided in **Figure 12-1** and **Figure 12-2**.

Use of Seclusion

Locked seclusion or removing a patient from a violent or destructive situation involves using temporary isolation therapeutically for the shortest amount of time

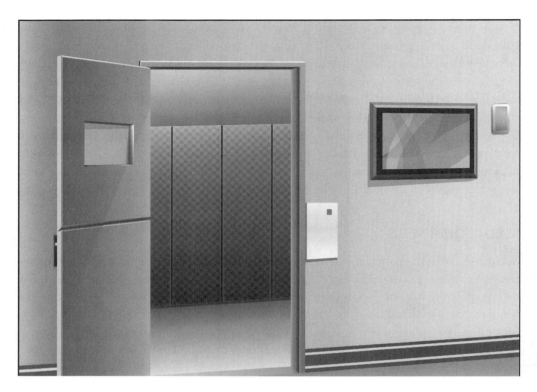

FIGURE 12-1   Seclusion room.

Source: Adapted from Gold Medal Safety Padding. Available at http://www.goldmedalsafetypadding.com.au/product_details.php. Accessed December 30, 2010.

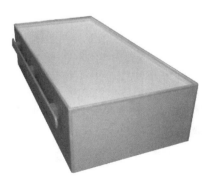

FIGURE 12-2   Restraint bed.

Source: Courtesy of Encore Medical Technologies, Inc.

possible in a safe, secure special room in accordance with facility, state, and federal guidelines. The patient is educated or told the reason for using locked seclusion, reassured that this measure is for safety and not punishment, that basic care needs will be met, and what the release criteria are. The patient also must be observed continuously as part of providing safety. An experienced staff member (e.g., mental health technician [MHT], certified nursing assistant [CNA], licensed practical–vocational nurse [LPN–LVN], or registered nurse [RN]) is assigned to perform 1:1 observation or constant observation (COs) as well as being observed via camera. A small shatterproof window in the door and a camera allow for continuous observation while the staff member is stationed directly outside of the door to the locked seclusion room. In most situations having a staff member in the seclusion room continuously is too stimulating for the patient, who needs a calm, quiet environment. However, the staff member is available if the patient wishes to talk.

Patient dignity must be preserved in various ways such as keeping the immediate area free from other patients, visitors, and individuals who are not part of the crisis team; manner of speaking to the patient; therapeutic use of self; allowing choices when possible (e.g., offering oral medication before IM medication; assisting the patient to walk into the seclusion room vs being carried); keeping the patient physically covered or shielded from the view of others while searching clothing for contraband and in facilities where policy requires placing the patient in a hospital gown with snap-only closures (see Chapter 3). Unfortunately, patients may find ways to harm themselves even in this secure setting if contraband is available and continuous observation is not maintained. Assigning experienced psychiatric-mental health staff members greatly decreases the potential for patient harm. Many patients become calmer in a quiet, less stimulating physical environment where they are able to move about freely, and likely will not require the additional step of applying restraints.

A seclusion order must be obtained from a licensed independent practitioner (LIP) such as a physician, APRN or physician assistant (PA) for specific use, patient behavior, and amount of time. Time frames are limited by the age of the patient. For examples, up to 4 hours from the time the order is obtained for adults 18 years or older, up to 2 hours for children and adolescents 9 to 17 years, and up to 1 hour for children younger than 9 years of age (Joint Commission Standard PC.03.05.05, EP4; also refer to additional guidelines in your state). Time frames begin *from the time the order was received*. Orders may be renewed according to the time limits for a maximum of 24 consecutive hours (Joint Commission FAQs, 2010).

If a physician is not in the immediate area, in most states an RN is permitted to place a patient in locked seclusion, provided the patient's behavior meets criteria for this safety measure and an LIP order is obtained "within 1 hour" (Keltner, Schwecke

& Bostrom, 2007, p. 63). An order should include the reason for seclusion (e.g., behavior), time frame, and criteria for release. The patient must be evaluated "face-to-face . . . within 1 hour" of placing a patient in locked seclusion. This also applies to the use of physical/mechanical restraints (Joint Commission FAQs, 2010; University of Texas Health Science Center at Houston, 2010). Example of an LIP order for an adult patient: "Place patient in locked seclusion and 4-point restraints not to exceed 4 hours for punching another patient and attempting to punch staff."

Additional provision is made by The Joint Commission for alternative ways to meet the face-to-face evaluation. "A registered nurse or a physician assistant may conduct the in-person evaluation within one hour of the initiation of restraint or seclusion if this person is trained in accordance with requirements in Standard PC.03.05.17, EP3. If the one hour face-to-face evaluation is completed by a trained nurse or trained physician assistant, he or she would consult with the attending physician or other licensed independent practitioner responsible for the care of the patient after the evaluation, as determined by hospital policy (PC.03.05.11 EP2). Some states may have statue or regulation requirements that are more restrictive than the requirements in this standard" (Joint Commission FAQs, 2010). According to The Joint Commission, a "telemedicine link" used for patient evaluations by an LIP may not be used to "fulfill the in-person requirement for the evaluation by an LIP of the individual in restraint or seclusion" (Joint Commission FAQs, 2010).

USE OF LOCKED SECLUSION AND RESTRAINTS

When locked seclusion alone is not effective to provide safety, restraints are applied using the same guidelines as previously mentioned for locked seclusion. When a patient is in restraints they are extremely vulnerable, and the door to the seclusion room should be locked with continuous observation via staff and a camera as previously mentioned for use of a seclusion room. "The least number of restraint points must be utilized and the individual must be continuously observed" (APNA, 2007, p. 3). The numbers of limbs or body areas restrained are referred to as "points." For example, a 4-point restraint means that all four of a patient's limbs are individually restrained. Restraints are applied at both wrists and ankles and may be made of leather or nylon. Restraints have padding for comfort and help prevent nerve injury, undue pressure, or impeding of circulation. Restraints additionally have quick release locks or are secured with quick release knots. Example photo of nylon and leather restraints and a simulated patient in restraints can be found in **Figure 12-3**.

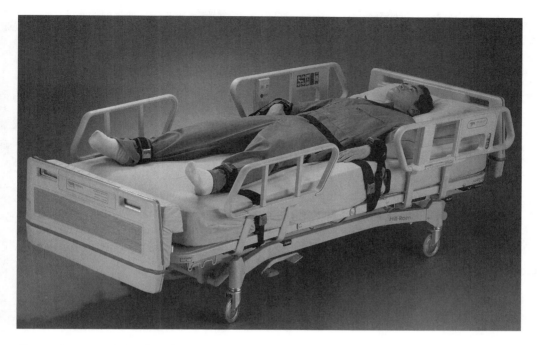

FIGURE 12-3   A simulated patient in restraints.
Source: Images provided courtesy Posey Company, Arcadia, California.

Applying Restraints

Enough staff members should be present to control all of the patient's limbs and head. The patient is placed in a supine position, avoiding a "spread-eagle" position, which would be uncomfortable and potentially cause injury. The nurse or other staff member applying the restraints should be able to put one finger (or the space of one finger) between the restraint and the patient's skin to allow for assessing circulation, sensation, and movement (CSM) and to help prevent nerve injury, undue pressure, or impeding of circulation. Care should be taken when applying restraints to both wrists and ankles to provide support for limb joints, including elbows and knees, which will help provide control of the patient's limbs and help prevent injury. Staff members should be supporting and controlling the patient's unrestrained limbs and head while restraints are applied to a specific location beginning with the wrists to provide safety. The patient should be told what is being done and reassured that these are safety measures, not a punishment, and will be removed as soon as the patient can regain self-control.

NURSING CARE

Care and consideration must be given for the patient's physical as well as psychological/emotional, cognitive, and spiritual needs during this time; this care and consideration should be offered on a regular basis *and prn*. The nurse should have another staff member accompany them into the seclusion room for safety reasons, and in case additional assistance is needed when providing nursing care. For patients in locked seclusion only, many of the same interventions and documentation are necessary and legally required. The PMH nurse should follow The Joint Commission, individual state, and facility protocols for nursing care and frequency. Also, as soon as the patient is safely placed in seclusion and restraints, the nurse assesses and determines if other patients and staff members require treatment for possible injuries incurred during the psychiatric code. **Table 12-1** provides more detailed information on nursing interventions and rationales for working with clients in seclusion and/or restraints.

DOCUMENTATION

Documentation in the patient's legal record is very important to provide an account of the entire situation for current and future treatment decisions, as well as providing a reference for future legal, health insurance, and facility certification questions. In addition to the initial narrative nurse's note, most facilities have forms and flow sheets for patient care as well as every-15-minute observation/safety checks and monitoring of patient behavior. The following information should be included in the patient's record (the PMH nurse should also refer to specific facility and state regulations):

- Specific patient behavior
- Less restrictive alternative interventions attempted
- Ineffectiveness of less restrictive alternatives
- Offer and administration of medication (first oral, then IM/IVP)
- Notification of psychiatrist/LIP
- Order for "locked seclusion" or "seclusion and 4-point restraints" including specific behavior, time frame, date, and time of order being written/receiving telephone order (e.g., "not to exceed 4 hours" for an adult)
- Show of force and psychiatric code
- Placement of patient in locked seclusion only or seclusion and application of restraints

- Informing/teaching patient of reason for safety measure and emphasis that patient is not being punished as well as patient responses to information or teaching provided
- Assessing restraints, CSMs, comfort level, and performance of ROM
- Assessing vital signs and pain level
- Assessing therapeutic effects and side/adverse effects of medication administered
- Offer of fluids, food, hygiene, and addressing elimination needs
- Patient mental status and behavior including self-control
- Additional medication administered
- Debriefing
- Reducing the number of restraints and complete removal
- Discontinuing locked seclusion
- Return to the therapeutic community

REMOVING RESTRAINTS

As soon as it is safely possible or no later than 2 hours after being placed in restraints, whichever occurs first, the nurse should begin to reduce the number of restraints moving toward complete removal. For example, if the patient can maintain control of their behavior for approximately 20 minutes (also refer to specific facility and state regulations) begin with the upper extremities:

1. Remove one wrist restraint and document.
2. Observe patient's ability to maintain self-control for approximately 20 minutes.
3. Remove the alternating ankle restraint and document.
4. Observe patient's ability to maintain self-control for approximately 20 minutes.
5. Remove both remaining restraints simultaneously (i.e., last wrist restraint and last ankle restraint) and document.

Note: If during the process the patient shows an inability to control their behavior, the restraints are reapplied under the same orders. If the patient requires seclusion and restraints for longer than 4 hours, the order must be renewed. If the patient is completely out of restraints and becomes violent or physically aggressive, it is a new episode and a new physician order must be obtained.

Table 12-1   Nursing Care of Patients in Seclusion and Restraints

Needs	Nursing interventions	Rationales
Basic physical care	1. Search clothing and shoes for contraband and remove.	1. Care must be taken to prevent the patient from accidentally or intentionally injuring themselves. Unfortunately, items considered to be contraband may be passed from other patients in the area or from visitors to patients.
	2. Remove any objects from the patient's clothing/body that have not already been removed and can cause injury including eye glasses, earrings and rings in other pierced body areas, belts, and bra for female patients.	2. Again, care must be taken to prevent the patient from accidentally or intentionally injuring themselves. Clothing such as a bra may move up as the patient moves about on the bed potentially impinging on the patient's diaphragm, or higher, decreasing the ability to breathe and lead to accidental strangulation.
	3. Depending on facility policy, place patient in a hospital gown with snap closures only.	3. Refer to #2 previously. Hospital gowns with ties can pose a physical risk when dealing with patients who are suicidal or psychotic. Also, some patients have hidden contraband in the seams and hems of their clothing, making it more difficult for staff members to find. Placing patients in hospital gowns increases the staff's ability to keep patients safe. There are situations where patients have hidden contraband in their body cavities, but a body cavity search is not routinely done due to legal–ethical considerations. If evidence suggests this type of situation is occurring, the nurse will discuss it with the psychiatrist/LIP, who will make the decision on whether or not to order and initiate a body cavity search.

4. Maintain 1:1 or COs.

   a. Document every 15 minutes. See Emotional needs #4 in this table.

5. Assess restraints, CSMs, skin, body alignment, and provide range of motion (ROM) at least every 15 minutes.

6. Assess, evaluate, and document behavior and mental status every 1–2 hours.

7. Assess vital signs, pain level, and any actual or potential medical problems at least every 1–2 hrs.

4. This must be done to maintain patient safety at all times.

   a. See the rationale in Emotional needs #4 in this table regarding every-15-minute safety checks/observation.

5. Care must be taken to provide not only safety, but prevent injury and physical complications of being placed in restraints, including nerve damage and decreased circulation.

6. Although the nurse may delegate every-15-minute safety checks/observation to other experienced staff members (as mentioned previously in this chapter) the RN legally is required to assess, evaluate, and document the patient's condition. Assessing and evaluating behavior will assist the nurse to provide care and make decisions regarding the patient's safety and readiness to begin reducing the restraints and debriefing.

7. Actual medical problems may be exacerbated or potential medical problems may be avoided by careful assessment and early intervention. A situation may occur indicating anything from a need for repositioning to possible early removal of restraints and release from the seclusion room if needed related to changes in condition (refer to contraindications previously mentioned).

(continues)

Table 12-1 Nursing Care of Patients in Seclusion and Restraints *(continued)*

Needs	Nursing interventions	Rationales
		Medications are frequently given before and/or during seclusion and restraint. The nurse must assess for side/adverse effects as well as therapeutic effects, including hypotension, cardiac arrhythmias, extrapyramidal side-effects (EPS), anticholinergic effects, or neuroleptic malignant syndrome (NMS).
		Unfortunately, patients may experience pain after physical resistance during a psychiatric code or due to improper restraint application or body positioning. Pain may also occur due to an unexpected medical event. Any of these situations must be assessed, reported, addressed, and documented.
	8. Offer food, fluids, use of bathroom/bedpan/urinal, provide for hygiene and skin care at least every 1–2 hrs.	8. While in seclusion and restraints the patient is totally dependent on staff members for basic physical needs as well as safety.
	9. Document (see the Documentation section later in this chapter).	9. All assessments and intervention implemented must be entered into the patient's legal record as well as evaluation of their effectiveness or ineffectiveness.
Psychological/emotional care	1. Reassure the patient that they are in a safe area and these measures are being taken to provide safety.	1. At this time the patient is emotionally vulnerable, fearful, anxious, or angry and needs to be reassured of their safety. The patient at some point in the process will derive some feeling of safety from external control being used since they have lost their ability to internally control themselves. This loss of internal control creates emotional distress that may be demonstrated in agitation and physical aggression.

2. Reinforce that these measures are not a punishment and the patient will be released as soon as they demonstrate the ability to control their own behavior.

3. Acknowledge, accept, and assist the patient to verbalize feelings and anxiety.

4. Assess and document the patient's behavior every 15 minutes (may be delegated to an experienced CNA, MHT, LPN/LVN or RN).

5. Assess the patient's ability to participate in the debriefing process and begin if able to do so.

2. The patient may feel that they are being punished and need to hear more than once that these measures are for their safety and possibly the safety of others. The patient also needs to know that they will not be kept in seclusion and restraints indefinitely and that they do have some control in the situation.

3. This is an emotionally intense and distressing time. The nurse needs to maintain and convey a nonjudgmental attitude and acceptance of the patient. The patient will need to feel the nurse's acceptance and be able to express their own feelings to help decrease the psychological and emotional negative effects of the experience.

4. Behavior is an indicator of the patient's emotional and psychological status and is analyzed when determining if a patient is able to cooperate and meet criteria for self-control.

5. The patient may or may not be able to participate in debriefing at this time. If they are, then the nurse will begin to do this. If not, the nurse will wait and attempt to do so when the patient is calmer. Some patients do not remember some of or even the entire situation that precipitated their loss of control or the process of and application of seclusion and restraints due to the intense emotional impact of the situation.

(continues)

Table 12-1   Nursing Care of Patients in Seclusion and Restraints (continued)

Needs	Nursing interventions	Rationales
		6. All interventions and interactions must be documented in the patient's legal record.
Cognitive	1. Teach the patient the reason for the safety measure being used.	1. Patients have legal rights, including being informed of any treatment and safety measures being implemented on their behalf whether or not they agree with emergency safety measures. Patients may not understand or agree with the safety measure being implemented. The nurse has a legal–ethical obligation to inform patients.
	2. Reinforce that these measures are not a punishment, but are used for the safety of the patient and others.	2. Again, patients may not agree with the emergency safety measure being taken and may mistakenly perceive they are being punished.
	3. Document (see the Documentation section later in this chapter).	3. All patient teaching and patient responses must be documented in the patient's legal record.
Spiritual	1. Acknowledge the patient's spiritual distress prior to entering and being in seclusion and restraints.	1. Patients in crisis, seriously mentally ill, or psychotic experience spiritual crisis that can lead to aggressive behavior. Even though patients cannot control their behavior, they may still feel they are "bad" people or that the nurse does not like them, which lowers self-esteem and can cause disturbances in self-concept. They need help dealing with these feelings to reduce the negative effects. Also, the experience of being in seclusion and restraints, although necessary in an emergency situation for safety, can be spiritually distressing and patients need help coping with the situation.
		6. Document (see the Documentation section later in this chapter).

2. Offer to stay with the patient and actively listen.

3. Use additional therapeutic communication techniques to convey that the patient is not alone, is still a human being worthy of care, and will have help during this difficult time.

4. Assess if the patient is calm enough to begin debriefing.

5. Offer to contact the patient's family or support person.

6. Offer to contact the patient's spiritual advisor or facility chaplain after the patient is released from seclusion and restraints.

2. These interventions reinforce that the nurse is available and cares about the patient.

3. Refer to item #2 previously. Even though the patient has demonstrated inappropriate behavior, they are still a human being worthy of care who is experiencing spiritual distress.

4. During the debriefing process, possible reasons for the development of spiritual distress and crisis development can be explored, inaccurate perceptions can begin to be corrected, and possible alternatives to inappropriate behavior can be discussed. This process is helpful in decreasing spiritual distress.

5. Although this may not be done very often, the patient has the legal right to request notification of family or support persons (Keltner, Schwecke, & Bostrom, 2007, p. 63). However, family members are not permitted to visit the patient in the seclusion room for safety reasons.

6. This offer can help the patient utilize their spiritual system and respects their rights. However, no one other than staff members and healthcare professionals are permitted in the seclusion room for safety reasons.

DEBRIEFING

The entire situation is discussed or processed with the patient during debriefing. The debriefing process includes:

- Exploring precipitating event(s) and reasons for crisis development
- Providing factual information to help correct inaccurate perceptions
- Possible alternatives to inappropriate behavior that has occurred
- Future ways to deal with situations and circumstances in early stages and attempting to avoid experiencing a full crisis

The patient may not remember everything that has occurred due to the intense nature of the experience, but this process helps to increase understanding, provides opportunities to learn new coping skills, and reestablishes trust between the patient and the nurse as well as other staff members. The patient will need much emotional support to return to the therapeutic community, and during the debriefing process, the nurse and other staff members convey their empathy and support for the patient, thus helping to make a smoother transition back into the therapeutic community.

Debriefing is also done with other patients and staff members. The nurse provides emotional support, facilitates expression of feelings, and educates other patients as to the need for safety measures when someone temporarily loses the ability to use self-control during periods of acute mental illness or crisis. Ways in which other patients and staff members may possibly have contributed to the patient's inability to maintain self-control are explored. Alternatives are also discussed.

SPECIAL CONSIDERATIONS

When working with children/adolescents and the elderly there are special considerations due to age, developmental issues, and medical conditions.

Children/Adolescents

As previously mentioned, time frames for seclusion and restraint are up to 2 hours for children and adolescents 9 to 17 years, and up to 1 hour for children younger than 9 years of age (also refer to additional guidelines in your specific state). The seclusion room is referred to as the "quiet room." Restraints are used that fit a child/adolescent vs adult-size restraints. Great care must be taken to avoid injury or compromising the child/adolescent's respiratory, circulatory, or nervous system. Informed consent is obtained from the parent or guardian upon admission for general care and potential safety measures if needed. Separate, specific consent for medication to be administered to children/adolescents must be obtained from the parent or guardian http://www.natsap.org/behavior_support_management.asp.

Children and adolescents may quickly become angry and physically act upon their intense emotions. They also may quickly de-escalate especially if they trust the nurse and believe she/he truly will listen. Early assessment and intervention can help prevent escalation of intense emotion and the need for more restrictive interventions. There are several less restrictive alternatives to using seclusion and restraints including time-outs, facilitating verbal expression of feelings, relaxation and stress management techniques including deep breathing, medication, yoga mats; behavioral modification programs using points and level systems (rewards vs. consequences), limit setting, engaging in problem-solving, physical exercise/use of gymnasium, use of soft objects that can be punched or thrown (i.e., pillows, Nerf footballs or basketballs), art supplies or play therapy (Varcarolis and Halter, 2010, pp. 635–637).

When using time outs, the general rule of thumb is to use time frames of 1 minute per year of age (ex. 5 minutes for a 5 yr. old child). However, for children/adolescents who are diagnosed with problems such as Attention Deficit Hyperactivity Disorder (ADHD) or for other reasons do not cope well with frustration, the time frame is adjusted to ½ or even ¼ of the usual amount, otherwise the experience is not therapeutic and can increase frustration, agitation, and aggression (ex. 2 and ½ minutes vs. 5 minutes for a 5 yr. old child). The time out area or chair is strategically placed away from other children/adolescents to decrease the amount of attention received from others, is free from toys, computers or televisions, and is within view of the nurse or other staff member giving the time out. Locked rooms are never used for time outs. No talking is allowed until the time out session is completed and the child/adolescent is encouraged to think about their behavior. If the child/adolescent becomes disruptive during the time out session, the original time frame begins again until it is completed. After the time out is completed, the person who gave the child/adolescent the time out debriefs or processes with them the reason for the time out being given, precipitating event(s), child/adolescent's behavioral response, and engages in problem-solving future potential responses (Boyd, 2008, p. 656; http://www.natsap.org/ and http://www.natsap.org/behavior_support_management.asp).

Therapeutic holding is defined as the physical restraint of a child by one or more people to assist the child who has lost control of behavior to regain control of strong emotions (Committee on Pediatric Emergency Medicine, 1997, p. 497). These techniques are considered an alternative to traditional seclusion and restraint safety measures. A common technique includes standing behind the child, crossing the child's arms across their chest with their hands under opposite elbows while the nurse holds the child's hands and leans the child slowly backwards against the nurse. Criteria for using therapeutic holding includes danger to self or others or destruction of property and is typically used for a period of no longer than 30 minutes (also refer to specific facility and state regulations). If other less restrictive alternatives attempted and therapeutic holding for 30 minutes are not effective, then locked seclusion or seclusion and restraints may be the last resort depending on facility policy and procedure and state regulations (Behavioral Support Management, 2010).

Elderly

When working with elderly patients, the PMH nurse and other nursing staff will attempt to avoid using seclusion and restraints to avoid physical injury and emotional distress. Many elderly patients have serious medical problems causing mental confusion and misinterpretation of the environment as well as the actions of others. Many elderly clients experience delirium and dementia, making it difficult to reason with them. They also experience decreased visual and auditory acuity secondary to the aging process, making environmental stimuli more difficult to interpret. It is important that these patients have access to their eye glasses and hearing devices and that they are in proper working order.

When dealing with elderly patients, less restrictive alternative methods include those previously mentioned when working with adults. Additional methods include decreasing environmental stimuli (e.g., decreasing noise, using softer lights, eliminating offensive odors, regulating room temperature, having fewer people in the general area); providing increased space to wander; assigning an experienced staff member for 1:1 observation or COs; providing toileting every 2 hours and prn; and assessing for pain. When communicating, keep sentences short and use simple language to decrease misunderstanding and avoid frustrating patients. Refrain from joking, using sarcasm, or whispering to other staff members, which can be misinterpreted by confused, elderly patients and could increase agitation. Approach patients slowly and from the front so that they can see you and explain what you are going to do before touching them, otherwise they may become fearful and aggressive to protect themselves. Medication may be offered (oral first), but the nurse may need to be even more cautious due to Axis III diagnoses. If the patient is experiencing delirium, additional medication can worsen the condition. Additionally, there are FDA warnings for all antipsychotic medications used for psychosis related to dementia due to an increase in cardiovascular-related deaths (Evans, 2008, p. 9).

REFERENCES

American Psychiatric Nurses Association. (2007). 2007 position statement on the use of seclusion and restraint. Washington, DC: Author.

Boyd, M. A. (2008). *Psychiatric nursing: Contemporary practice* (4th ed.). Philadelphia, PA: Wolters-Kluwer Health/Lippincott, Williams, & Wilkins.

Committee on Pediatric Emergency Medicine. (1997). The use of physical restraint interventions for children and adolescents in the acute care setting. *Pediatrics, 99*, 497–498.

Evans, J. (Jul., 2008). All antipsychotics to get warnings about elderly. *Clinical Psychiatry News, 36*(7), 9.

Frisch, N. C., & Frisch, L. E. (2011). *Psychiatric mental health nursing* (4th ed.). Clifton Park, NY: Delmar.

Joint Commission on Accreditation of Healthcare Organizations (JCAHO) Accreditation. (2009). Retrieved from http://www.jointcommission.org/AccreditationPrograms/Hospitals/Standards/09_FAQs/PC/Restraint+_Seclusion+For+Hospitals+That+Use+The+Joint+Commission+For+Deemed+Status+Purposes.htm

Joint Commission on Accreditation of Healthcare Organizations (JCAHO) *Standards and frequently asked questions* (2010). Retrieved from http://www.jointcommission.org/Standards/FAQs

Keltner, N. L., Schwecke, L. H., & Bostrom, C. E. (2007). *Psychiatric nursing* (5th ed.). St. Louis, MO: Mosby, Elsevier.

National Association of Therapeutic Schools and Programs (NATSAP). (2004). Behavioral support management in therapeutic schools, therapeutic programs, and outdoor behavioral health programs. Principles of good practice. Retrieved from http://www.natsap.org/ and http://www.natsap.org/behavior_support_management.asp

Substance Abuse and Mental Health Services Administration Center for Mental Health Services (SAMHSA). (2009). *Practice guidelines: Core elements for responding to mental health crises.* HHS Publication No. SMA-09-4427. Retrieved from http://www.samhsa.gov

University of Texas Health Science Center at Houston. (2010). Mechanical restraints. Retrieved from http://www.uth.tmc.edu/uth_orgs/hcpc/procedures/volume2/chapter3/treatment_services-40.htm

University of Texas Heath Sciences Center at Houston. (2010). *Seclusion/Restraint Process.* Retrieved from http://www.uth.tmc.edu/uth_orgs/hcpc/procedures/volume2/chapter3/treatment_services-39.htm

Varcarolis, E. M., & Halter, M. J. (2010). *Foundations of psychiatric mental health nursing: A clinical approach* (6th ed.). St. Louis, MO: Saunders, Elsevier.

SUGGESTED READINGS

American Psychological Association. (2007). *APA dictionary of psychology.* Washington, DC: Author.

Bazelon Center for Mental Health. (2010). Retrieved from http://bazelon.org.gravitatehosting.com/Where-We-Stand/Self-Determination/Forced-Treatment/Restraint-and-Seclusion.aspx

Beech B. F., & Leather, P. (2003). Evaluating a management of aggression unit for student nurses. *Journal of Advanced Nursing, 44*(6), 603–612.

Centers for Medicare and Medicaid Services (CMS) Certification. (2010). *Psychiatric hospitals*. Retrieved from http://www.cms.gov/CertificationandComplianc/ and http://www.cms.gov/CertificationandComplianc/14_PsychHospitals.asp#TopOfPage

Fontaine, K. (2009). *Mental health nursing* (6th ed.). Upper Saddle River, NJ: Pearson Education, Inc.

Guido, G. W. (2007). *Legal & ethical issues in nursing* (4th ed.). Upper Saddle River, NJ: Pearson/Prentice Hall.

How to provide crisis intervention and de-escalate an angry person (2010). Retrieved from http://www.ehow.com/how_5702408_provide-intervention-de_escalate-angry-person.html

Joint Commission and CSM Rules for Restraint and Seclusion (2010). Retrieved from http://www.crisisprevention.com/Resources/Knowledge-Base/CMS-and-Joint-Commission

Krakowski, M. (2007). Violent behavior: Choosing antipsychotics and other agents. *Current Psychiatry*, 6(4), 63–70.

Miller, D., Walker, M. C., & Friedman, D. (May, 1989). Use of a holding technique to control the violent behavior of seriously disturbed adolescents. *Hospital Community Psychiatry*, 40, 520–524. Retrieved from http:www.psychservices.psychiatryonline.org/cgi/content/abstract/40/5/520

Mohr, W. K. (2009). *Psychiatric-mental health nursing: Evidence based concepts, skills, and practices* (7th ed.). Philadelphia, PA: Wolters Kluwer/Lippincott, Williams, & Wilkins.

Physical intervention training (2010). Retrieved from http://www.crisisprevention.com/Resources/Knowledge-Base/Physical-Intervention-Training

Seclusion room. (2010). Retrieved from www.goldmedalsafetypadding.com.au/advantages.php

Sourander, A., Ellila, H., Valimaki, M., & Piha, J. (Aug., 2002). Use of hold, restraints, seclusion, and time-out in child and adolescent in psychiatric in-patient treatment. *European Child & Adolescent Psychiatry*, 11(4), 162–167.

Stuart, G. W., & Laraia, M. T. (2005). *Principles and practice of psychiatric nursing* (8th ed.). St. Louis, MO: Mosby, Elsevier.

Townsend, M. C. (2009). *Psychiatric mental health nursing: Concepts of care in evidence-based practice* (6th ed.). Philadelphia, PA: F. A. Davis.

Unruh, L., Joseph, L., & Strickland, M. (Dec., 2007). Nurse absenteeism and workload: Negative effect on restraint use, incident reports, and mortality. *Journal of Advanced Nursing*, 60(6), 673–681.

Whitman, G. R., Davidson, L. J., Rudy, E. B., & Sereika, S. M. (Jul.–Sept., 2001). Practice patterns related to mechanical restraint use across a multi-institutional healthcare system. *Outcomes Management in Nursing Practice*, 5(3), 102–111.

Whitman, G. R., Davidson, L. J., Sereika, S. M., & Rudy, E. B. (Nov.–Dec., 2001). Staffing and pattern of mechanical restraint use across a multiple hospital system. *Nursing Research*, 50(6), 356–362.

Wilder, S. S., & Sorenson, C. (2001). *Essentials of aggression management in health care*. Upper Saddle River, NJ: Prentice-Hall, Inc.

CHAPTER 13

Administration and Monitoring of Psychotropic Medications: Antipsychotics

Kim A. Jakopac

OBJECTIVES

The nursing student will be able to:

1. Explain the basic neurobiologic basis for patient treatment with psychotropic medication specific to antipsychotics
2. Describe variations in therapeutic effects among different ethnic groups
3. Identify nursing responsibilities related to the administration of psychotropic medications including patient education
4. Recognize potential serious adverse effects of antipsychotic medications
5. Discuss patient civil rights regarding the use of chemical restraint in emergency situations
6. Discuss special considerations regarding children/adolescents and elderly clients

KEY TERMS

Agonist
Agranulocytosis
Akathisia
Akinesia
Antagonist
Anticholinergic
Antipsychotic(s)
Autonomic nervous system
Blood–brain barrier
Central nervous system
Cytochrome P450
Depot injection
Dystonia

Ethnopharmacology
Extrapyramidal symptoms
Gynecomastia
Hyperkalemia
Hyponatremia
Metabolic syndrome
Neuroleptic
Neuroleptic malignant
  syndrome
Neurons
Neurotransmitters
Orthostatic hypotension
Parasympathetic

Peripheral nervous system
Pharmacodynamics
Pharmacogenomics
Pharmacokinetics
Pseudoparkinsonism
Psychoactive
Psychopharmacology
Psychotropic
Rhabdomyolysis
Sympathetic
Synaptic junction/gap
Tardive dyskinesia

*P*sychotropic or *psychoactive medications* are a broad category or classification of medications that significantly affect psychological processes such as thinking, perception, and emotion, thus causing alteration in a person's state of consciousness (APA, 2007, pp. 749, 757).

When administering psychotropic medications, the psychiatric-mental health (PMH) nurse must have an understanding of basic concepts and principles of pharmacology and psychopharmacology as well as the purpose for specific medications being prescribed. Therapeutic and adverse effects of psychotropic medications are due to a complex balance of pharmacodynamics, pharmacokinetics, P450 cytochrome system function, levels of neurotransmitters, cell receptors, nutrition, and the blood–brain barrier. Ethnopharmacology must also be considered, and there are indications that metabolism of medications or substances may differ in some racial/ethnic populations, resulting in faster or slower metabolism. For example, people who are considered to be "fast metabolizers" may experience a decreased response to medication at standard dose ranges because it takes longer to establish and maintain a steady serum level. They may require larger doses of medication. For people who are considered to be "slow metabolizers," there is an increased risk for developing side-effects or toxicity because medication is not excreted in the normal amount of time from the body. Some African Americans and some Asians are either slow or fast metabolizers. Some Hispanics may respond more quickly to antipsychotics at low dose ranges, but may also experience side- or adverse effects at low dose ranges (Keltner, Schwecke, & Bostrom, 2007, pp. 169–170; Fontaine, 2009, p. 215).

Antipsychotic medications traditionally have been used to control symptoms of psychosis (e.g., delusions, hallucinations) or agitation associated with psychiatric illnesses secondary to neurotransmitter imbalances in the brain, including schizophrenia, schizoaffective disorder, and psychosis occurring at times with mania, depression, temporal lobe epilepsy, adverse effects of steroid therapy, and delirium (see also the Delirium section in this chapter). More recently newer antipsychotics have been approved by the Food and Drug Administration (FDA) for use in mood disorders without psychosis. Antipsychotics have been found to be more effective in the treatment of schizophrenia than placebo (Sadock & Sadock, 2005, p. 1468). These medications have also been used to treat symptoms of psychosis occurring in survivors of torture and to help decrease psychosis, nightmares, and flashbacks in posttraumatic stress disorder (PTSD). However, use of antipsychotic medications in the treatment of impulse-control disorders is controversial (Sadock & Sadock, 2005, p. 2828).

Agitation can result from disturbing or frightening psychotic symptoms including delusions and hallucinations. "The term agitation refers to a broad range of inappropriate verbal or motor behaviors, and pharmacological interaction is reserved for situations in which distress is prominent or safety or basic care is compromised" (Sadock & Sadock, 2005, p. 3732). In emergency situations when the patient is exhibiting dangerous behavior towards self or others or their condition is deteriorating, chemical restraint or forced medications (see Chapter 12) consisting of antipsychotics, certain benzodiazepine type anxiolytics (See Chapter 15/Anxiolytics), or both may be administered. This is true for both voluntary and involuntary status patients. The same legal–ethical concepts and principles—including least restrictive alternative doctrine—apply to the use of chemical restraint or forced medication. Threatening with or actually forcing a calm, cooperative, voluntary patient to take medication may be legally viewed as assault and battery. Even a patient admitted involuntarily has the right to refuse medication unless an emergency situation exists (Keltner, Schwecke, & Bostrom, 2007, p. 57). The PMH nurse should also refer to individual state mental health regulations regarding court ordered treatment. Medication "used as a restriction to manage the patient's behavior or restrict the patient's freedom of movement and is *not a standard treatment or dosage* for the patient's condition" is considered to be "chemical restraint" (Joint Commission Accreditation Program, 2009) (see Chapter 12).

Patients receiving antipsychotic medication for psychosis-related illnesses have less severe relapse of symptoms, less self-destructive behavior or violence toward others, and less antisocial behavior than patients who stopped taking medication or were not being treated with antipsychotics. Other less common uses for traditional antipsychotics include intractable hiccups and severe nausea and/or vomiting in patients receiving chemotherapy (Sadock & Sadock, 2005, pp. 1474, 2826, 2829). A large, nationwide controlled research study, Clinical Antipsychotic Trials of Intervention Effectiveness (CATIE), showed that traditional antipsychotics were as effective as atypical antipsychotics in the treatment of schizophrenia (NIMH, 2005/2006). The research included perphenazine (Trilafon), clozapine (Clozaril), and olanzapine (Zyprexa). However, there was concern that since traditional antipsychotics cost less that there would be pressure for licensed independent practitioners (LIPs) to use them even though there is a greater risk of adverse effects.

Prior to starting antipsychotic medication therapy, patients should receive the following:

- Complete physical examination
- Neurologic examination
- Mental status examination
- Laboratory/diagnostic tests

Laboratory/diagnostic tests should include:

- EKG/ECG
- CBC
- Electrolytes
- Fasting glucose
- Liver function tests
- Renal function tests
- Thyroid function tests
- Lipid profile
- Pregnancy test for females of childbearing age
- Syphilis test if indicated by history and/or symptoms
- HIV test if indicated by history and/or symptoms
- Hepatitis testing if indicated by history and/or symptoms

Note: In emergency situations, antipsychotic medications may be administered before completion of the medical evaluation or if patients refuse to complete the evaluation (Sadock & Sadock, 2005, pp. 1468, 2835) unless contraindications are known (e.g., history of cardiac disease, syncope, electrolyte imbalances, family history of sudden death) (Sadock & Sadock, 2005, p. 3730) and other medications could be considered (e.g., antianxiety medications).

PREGNANCY

Regarding pregnancy, all psychotropic medications cross the placenta, and there have not been adequate, well-controlled human medication studies (Einarson & Boskovic, 2009). Yet according to Sadock and Sadock (2005), there is "very little evidence to suggest that there is an association between prenatal exposure to antipsychotics and an increased incidence of congenital malformation" (p. 2833). Also, Bezchlibnyk-Butler and Jeffries (2005), state that "antipsychotics have not been clearly demonstrated to have teratogenic effects" (p. 98). These authors may mean that there is not *enough* human research to be conclusive, and these texts predate the 2009 article. However, Sadock and Sadock and Bezchlibnyk-Butler and Jeffries do not advise breast feeding while taking antipsychotics because these medications are secreted in low levels in breast milk.

ANTIPSYCHOTIC MEDICATIONS

Antipsychotic medications are classified or categorized as "traditional, conventional, typical, or first generation" and "atypical, second generation antipsychotics (SGAs) or novel" (Keltner, Schwecke, & Bostrom, 2007, p. 213; Varcarolis & Halter, 2010, pp. 68–70). Traditional antipsychotics are also classified by degree of potency (i.e., low, moderate, high) or chemical composition (e.g., phenothiazines, butyrophenones, thioxanthenes). Another term used for antipsychotics is *neuroleptics*. These medications accumulate in fat tissue, the brain, and lungs. Brain levels are higher than serum levels. Antipsychotics are protein-bound, and malnutrition can affect the amount of medication available to control symptoms (Sadock & Sadock, 2005, p. 2823). Antipsychotic medications are available in various forms including oral delivery, liquid concentrates, IM injections, and IV/IVP (e.g., haloperidol [Haldol]) forms. A few traditional and atypical antipsychotics are able to be given as depot injections, and most recently atypical antipsychotics in the form of oral dissolving tablets that provide an alternative to injections in emergency situations when available.

According to neurobiologic theory, psychiatric illnesses or mental health problems occur due to genetic variations, neurotransmitter imbalances, problems with cell membrane receptors, brain structure abnormalities, endocrine disorders, and malnutrition or exposure to toxins during the prenatal period. A large enough biologic or psychological stressor can trigger a genetic response manifesting the symptoms of psychiatric illness. Antipsychotic medications are used to help restore the balance of neurotransmitters at the synaptic junction/gap, which in turn alleviates symptoms. Many substances act as neurotransmitters in the body including monoamines (e.g., dopamine, serotonin, norepinephrine), cholinergics (acetylcholine), amino acids (gamma-aminobutyric acid, glutamate), hormones, neuropeptides (endorphins, enkephalins, substance P) and histamine (Keltner, Schwecke, & Bostrom, 2007, p. 80). In addition, research is being done on new medications that act on these various substances.

Traditional Antipsychotics

As previously stated, traditional antipsychotic medications are also referred to as conventional, typical, or first generation as well as of low, moderate, or high potency. These medications were developed prior to atypical antipsychotics and are very effective for treating the psychotic symptoms also known as the "positive" symptoms of schizophrenia (see Chapter 11) and agitation. The main mechanism of action is the blockade of the dopamine (DA)—usually at the D2 neuron receptor site—resulting in a DA antagonist effect. For various reasons including effectiveness in controlling symptoms and lower cost, these medications are still frequently prescribed, although in some cases such as chlorpromazine (Thorazine) in much lower doses than in the past. Patient collaboration, risks vs benefits, and patient and family medical history are all taken into consideration when any medications are prescribed.

Unfortunately, the traditional antipsychotics are more likely to cause serious adverse effects including cardiac effects (e.g., potentially fatal cardiac arrhythmias, orthostatic/postural hypotension); anticholinergic effects; extrapyramidal symptoms (EPS) including akathesia, dystonia, tardive dyskinesia (TD), pseudoparkinsonism, akinesia; and neuroleptic malignant syndrome (NMS) (see **Table 13-1** and **Box 13-1** as well as other related areas of this chapter). For further information also refer to pharmacology texts such as *Mosby's Pharmacology in Nursing*, McKenry, Tessier, and Hogan (2006); *Clinical Handbook of Psychotropic Drugs*, Bezchlibnyk-Butler and Jeffries (2005); *Essential Psychopharmacology: Neuroscientific Basis and Practical Applications*, Stahl (2005); and websites including those of the National Institutes of Mental Health (NIMH) and the FDA.

Atypical Antipsychotics

As previously stated, atypical antipsychotic medications are also referred to as second generation antipsychotics (SGAs) or novel (Bezchlibnyk-Butler & Jeffries, [2005], classify aripiprazole [Abilify] as a "third generation" atypical antipsychotic). Not only are these medications very effective for treating psychotic symptoms, including positive symptoms of schizophrenia and agitation, but also have a beneficial effect on what are termed the "negative" symptoms as well as being "somewhat" more helpful for "cognitive" symptoms of schizophrenia (see Chapter 11) (Sadock & Sadock, 2005, pp. 1445–1446, 1473, 2826, 3729). Clozapine (Clozaril) has been shown to be effective for treating resistant symptoms. Atypical antipsychotic medications are beneficial for treating mood disorder symptoms, decreasing excitement in the manic phase of Bipolar I disorder and psychotic symptoms in mood disorders. According to Sadock and Sadock (2005), antipsychotic medications have a faster onset than mood stabilizing/antimanic (anticonvulsant) medications, but as soon as mood stabilizing/antimanic (anticonvulsant) medication is effective, the dose of antipsychotic medication should be decreased and discontinued. There is some evidence that patients diagnosed with mood disorders may be more "vulnerable to developing tardive dyskinesia" than patients diagnosed with schizophrenia, and antipsychotics should be used "only when clearly indicated" for as short a time as possible (p. 2827).

The main mechanism of action includes at least two major neurotransmitters: (1) blockade of serotonin (5-HT2) antagonist, which causes an inhibition of DA release; and (2) blockade of DA at more than one neuron receptor site, including more specific affinity for the D1, D3, and D4 neuron receptor sites, and lower affinity for the D2 neuron receptor site, all of which resulting in a DA antagonist effect. The degree

Table 13-1   Common Antipsychotic Medications

Traditional medications	Daily dose ranges	Side/adverse effects
	(For adults 18 years old or older; see Special Considerations section for consideration of children/adolescents and elderly; doses are adjusted for patients with hepatic or renal problems and the elderly typically by at least half of the adult dose)	Potential interactions occur with other CNS depressants, antihypertensives, anti-arrhythmia medications, and any other medications that cause sedation or lower BP and pulse).
High potency		
Haloperidol (Haldol) Available in oral tablets, oral liquid concentrate, and injectable forms (haloperidol lactate for IM or IVP; haloperidol decanoate for depot IM). *Note: Do not use decanoate form for IV administration; dose ranges in Table 13-3.*	Adults/children older than 12 years: 1–50 mg po; may be given in divided doses; may be given hourly until control is achieved (max dose = 80–100 mg in 24 hours)

Children ages 3–12 years weighing 15–40 kg (33–88 lbs): 0.05–0.15 mg/kg po in divided doses (max dose = 6 mg in 24 hours for *nonpsychotic behavior*)

Elderly: 0.25–0.5 mg IVP every 4 hours.

Delirium: Adults/elderly 1–2 mg IVP every 2 to 4 hours; may require higher doses for severe agitation

Can increase risk of lithium toxicity | General and specific side/adverse effects of all traditional antipsychotics:

Weight gain
Dry mouth
Blurred vision
Constipation
Urinary retention
CNS sedation
Hypotension or orthostatic hypotension
Reflex tachycardia

QRS changes on EKG including QTc interval prolongation (increased risk for fatal cardiac arrhythmias including Torsades de point)

EPS

NMS

Seizures
Shaking tremor
Muscle spasms
Agranulocytosis
Aplastic anemia (bone marrow suppression) |

(continues)

Table 13-1 Common Antipsychotic Medications (continued)

Traditional medications	Daily dose ranges	Side/adverse effects
Fluphenazine (Prolixin) Available in oral tablets, oral liquid concentrate, oral elixir, and injectable forms (prolixin hydrochloride for IM injection; prolixin decanoate for depot IM) injection; prolixin decanoate for depot IM) *Note: Prolixin is not administered IV/IVP; dose ranges for decanoate in Table 13-3.*	Adults: 0.5–40 mg po in divided doses. Usual IM dose = 1.25 mg (IM doses are one-third to one-half of oral doses) Elderly: 1–1.5 mg po	Thrombocytopenia Sexual side-effects (decreased libido, erectile dysfunction, decreased orgasm) Increased sensitivity to sun (photosensitivity increasing risk of sunburn and skin rashes) Endocrine—increased prolactin levels = lactation, amenorrhea in females & gynecomastia in males; increased glucose levels Jaundice Elevated liver enzymes SGPT/ALT and SGOT/AST, liver function tests (LFTs) Hypersalivation May increase glucose and cholesterol levels Problems with thermoregulation
Thiothixene (Navane) Available in oral tablets, oral solution, and IM injection.	Adults: 10–60 mg po	See previous list of side/adverse effects for haloperidol.

Pimozide (Orap) Available in oral tablets	Adults/children 12 years and older: 2–20 mg po (maximum dose = 20 mg in 24 hours; see max dose below for children) Children younger than 12 years: 0.05 mg/kg (maximum dose = 0.2 mg/kg or 10 mg in 24 hours)	See previous list of side/adverse effects for haloperidol.
Moderate potency Perphenazine (Trilafon) Available in oral tablets, oral liquid concentrate, and IM injection	Adults/children older than 12 years: typically 12–24 mg po in divided doses, up to 64 mg po for adults in divided doses	See previous list of side/adverse effects for haloperidol.
Loxipine (Loxitane) Available in oral tablets or capsules, oral solution, and IM injection	Adults: 20–60 mg po in divided doses; higher dose ranges up to 100 mg Elderly: Initially 10 mg po in divided doses	See previous list of side/adverse effects for haloperidol.
Molindone (Moban) Available in oral capsules and oral liquid	Adults and adolescents 18 years and older: 50–200 mg po	See previous list of side/adverse effects for haloperidol.
Low potency Chlorpromazine (Thorazine) Available in oral tablets, oral concentrate, rectal suppositories, and IM injection	Adults oral dose: 75–1000 mg po; IM dose 30–150 mg Epinephrine and other phenothiazines may cause severe hypotension (Frisch & Frisch, 2011, p. 774).	See previous list of side/adverse effects for haloperidol. Vision—granular deposits on anterior lens and posterior cornea seldom affect vision and resolve when medication is discontinued or changed to another antipsychotic (Sadock & Sadock, 2005, p. 2833).

(continues)

Table 13-1   Common Antipsychotic Medications (continued)

Traditional medications	Daily dose ranges	Side/adverse effects
Thioridazine (Mellaril) Available in oral tablets and oral concentrate	Adults oral dose: 200–800 mg po Children ages 2–12 years: 0.5 mg/kg (maximum dose = 3.0 mg/kg in 24 hours) Only generic form FDA approved for children Elderly: typical dose = 25 mg po tid	See previous list of side/adverse effects for haloperidol. Vision–high doses (≥ 1000 mg) can result in pigmentation of the retina leading to visual impairment or blindness (Sadock & Sadock, 2005, p. 2833).

Atypical medications	Daily dose ranges	Side/adverse effects
Clozapine (Clozaril) Available in oral tablets or oral dissolving tablets	Adults: 300–900 mg po Give oral dissolving tablets without water (place in buccal pouch)	See previous list of side/adverse effects for haloperidol. *Note: Agranulocytosis is a major concern with the medication. Medication protocol includes weekly laboratory testing of WBC for the first 6 months; if WBC values continue to be normal then the frequency is reduced to every 2 weeks thereafter (Sadock & Sadock, 2005, pp. 1470, 1472).* Myositis, cardiomyopathy Hypersalivation
Risperidone (Risperdal) Available in oral tablets, oral solution, oral dissolving tablets (M-tab), and long acting depot IM injection *Note: Dose ranges for long acting depot injection (Consta) in Table 13-3.*	Adults: 4–6 mg po Children 13 years and older for *schizophrenia* **or** 10 years and older for *bipolar mania and mixed episodes*: 0.5–1 mg po (max dose = 6 mg in 24 hours)	See previous list of side/adverse effects for haloperidol. Arthralgia, myalgia, back, or leg pain

Medication	Dosage	Side/Adverse Effects
	Children ages 5 to 16 years for *irritability associated with autism*: 0.25 mg if < 20 kg; 0.5 if ≥ 20 kg (maximum 3 mg in 24 hours)	
	Give oral dissolving M-tabs without water (place in buccal pouch)	
	May be given with lithium or divalproex	
Olanzapine (Zyprexa) Available in oral tablets, oral dissolving tablets, and IM injection	Adults: 5–20 mg po (max dose = 20 mg in 24 hours) Place oral dissolving tablets directly onto patient tongue	See previous list of side/adverse effects for haloperidol.
	For agitation: 2.5–10 mg IM; a second dose may be given in 2 hours if necessary; a 3rd dose may be given 4 hours after the 1st injection if necessary	
	Elderly or debilitated patients: 2.5–10 mg	
Quetiapine (Seroquel) Available in oral tablets and extended release capsules	Adults: 200–800 mg po	See previous list of side/adverse effects for haloperidol.
	May be given with lithium or divalproex	May increase risk of developing cataracts and seizures.
Ziprasidone (Geodon) Available in oral tablets, IM	Adults: 40–160 mg po	See previous list of side/adverse effects for haloperidol. QRS changes on EKG including QTc interval prolongation (increased risk for fatal cardiac arrhythmias including Torsades de point) seen more often.

(continues)

Table 13-1   Common Antipsychotic Medications *(continued)*

Atypical medications	Daily dose ranges	Side/adverse effects
Paliperidone (Invega) Available in oral extended release tablets and long acting depot IM *Note: Dose ranges for long acting depot injection (Sustenna) in Table 13-3*	Adults: 6–12 mg po	See previous list of side/adverse effects for haloperidol. EKG changes including AV block, bundle branch block, and QTc interval prolongation.
Asenapine (Saphris) Available in oral *sublingual* tablets.	Adults: 5–20 mg po	See previous list of side/adverse effects for haloperidol.
Aripiprazole (Abilify) (also classified as "novel" or third generation) Available in oral tablets, oral dissolving tablets, and IM injection	Adults: 10–30 mg po Children 13–17 yrs: 2–10 mg (max dose = 30 mg in 24 hours; irritability in autistic disorder: maximum dose = 15 mg in 24 hours)	See previous list of side/adverse effects for haloperidol.

Notes: **Low potency** *traditional antipsychotic medications are more likely to cause orthostatic hypotension,* **but all** *antipsychotic medications* **can** *cause orthostatic hypotension, and patients should be assessed and evaluated to avoid complications including risk for falls.*

High potency *traditional antipsychotic medications are more likely to cause EPS,* **but all** *antipsychotic medications* **may** *cause EPS, and patients should be assessed and evaluated to avoid complications and potentially permanent problems.*

Any medications in liquid form should be stored in dark containers.

Sources: Bezchlibnyk-Butler & Jeffries, 2005, pp. 73–117, 299–300; McKenny, Tessier, & Hogan, 2006, pp. 378–413; *Nursing 2010*, pp. 648–681; Varcarolis, & Halter, 2010, pp. 327–329; Internet Mental Health—Thioridizine, 2008; NIMH, 2010, schizophrenia medications; and NIMH, 2010, alphabetical medications list FDA–main website, 2010.

of control depends on the neural pathway affected (Sadock & Sadock, 2005, pp. 2824–2825; Stahl, 2005, p. 414).

Although atypical antipsychotics are less likely to cause the same adverse effects of traditional antipsychotics, they still can, and the PMH nurse must continue to assess for adverse effects as well as provide patient education regarding them. Serious adverse effects including agranulocytosis and myositis occur with individual atypical antipsychotics such as clozapine (Clozaril) and QTc interval prolongation with ziprasidone (Geodon) (Sadock & Sadock, 2005, p. 2155) (see Table 13-1). For further information also refer to pharmacology texts previously listed.

NURSING RESPONSIBILITIES AND IMPLICATIONS

Psychotropic medications are a major treatment modality for psychiatric-mental health problems. There is a collaborative legal–ethical responsibility with LIPs, pharmacists, and patients when using these medications. Common nursing responsibilities and implications include:

- Communicating clearly with LIPs and pharmacists
- Maintaining the "five rights" of medication administration and national safety goals, including using two forms of patient identification
- Being aware of and questioning contraindications (refer to pharmacology texts such as *Mosby's Pharmacology in Nursing*, *Clinical Handbook of Psychotropic Drugs* by Bezchlibnyk-Butler and Jeffries, and *Physicians' Desk Reference*)
- Continuing professional and self-education
- Assessing therapeutic medication effects and side/adverse effects
- Preventing when possible and intervening early when side/adverse effects are identified
- Educating patients and families with patient permission
- Advocating for patients
- Maintaining documentation of all medication administration and related patient care

According to Sadock and Sadock (2005), emphasis should be placed on patient collaboration, and risks vs benefits should be explained to the patient (and family with patient permission). Initially, information may have to be focused on benefits of medication as well as reinforcing the most common side-effects depending on the patient's ability to cognitively process information. More detailed information is given as the patient's thoughts become more organized and their ability to understand improves (p. 1469). Patients and families need much emotional support when dealing with psychiatric illnesses and the need to take medications. It may take several medication trials and some time to find a medication that treats symptoms and is well tolerated (see **Table 13-2**).

Table 13-2 Nursing Implications of Antipsychotic Medication and Medication Used to Treat EPS	
(See also previous bulleted list in this chapter)	(See also Tables 13-1, 13-3, and 13-4; Box 13-1)
Assessing therapeutic and side/adverse effects	• Assess vital signs every 8 hours, prior to medication administration, and prn • Perform cardiovascular and neurologic assessments as well as a mental status examination on admission and prn • Perform Autonomic Involuntary Movement Scale (AIMS) prior to beginning antipsychotics (or on admission if patient has been taking antipsychotic medications prior to admission) (See **Figure 13-1**) • Assess elimination patterns and provide adequate fluid intake to prevent urinary retention and paralytic ileus • Monitor laboratory/diagnostic test results; report abnormal results to LIP who ordered them and assess body system corresponding to abnormal test results • Document all therapeutic and side/adverse effects • Notify LIP prescribing medication of side/adverse effects
Patient/family education (Permission must be obtained from the patient for family or friends to have information; if the patient has a guardian, permission must be obtained from the guardian for anyone else to have information.)	(See also Tables 13-1, 13-3 and 13-4; Box 13-1) • Benefits of medications ordered and emphasis on increased potential to function as well as relief of symptoms • Common side-effects and ways to relieve dry mouth (e.g., increase fluid intake if not contraindicated, use ice chips, more frequent oral care, sugarless gum/candy) • Initial sedation feeling and blurred vision will decrease as the body adjusts to the medication

(continues)

Table 13-2 Nursing Implications of Antipsychotic Medication and Medication Used to Treat EPS *(continued)*

- Change positions slowly and ask for help ambulating
- Reporting immediately of cardiac symptoms (e.g., dizziness, syncope, palpitation, funny feeling, heaviness or pain in chest, difficulty breathing)
- Antipsychotics: Signs of EPS and NMS to watch for and report
- Antipsychotics: Signs of agranulocytosis, aplastic anemia or other hematologic problems to watch for an report
- Antipsychotics: Signs of cardiovascular, neurologic (both antipsychotics and anticholinergic/antiparkinsonian), endocrine, and hepatic problems to watch for and report
- Take medication exactly as prescribed in order to have the most possible benefit; inform that while these medications do not cause tolerance or dependence (nonaddicting), stopping them suddenly can lead to increased anticholinergic rebound symptoms including nausea, vomiting or diarrhea, additional symptoms of headache, restlessness, insomnia or diaphoresis. Withdrawal symptoms can last from 2 days to 2 weeks.
- Do not drive or operate machinery until patient knows how medication will affect them (e.g., sedation, drowsiness, blurred vision, decreased reaction time).
- Acknowledge embarrassment of potential sexual side-effects and importance of reporting these rather than just stop taking medication.
- Importance of nutrition to mental health and how to eat a balanced diet to help balance weight gain and risk of metabolic syndrome
- Importance of physical exercise to help balance weight gain; advise to obtain physician's approval for specific types of exercise to avoid injury

(continues)

Table 13-2   Nursing Implications of Antipsychotic Medication and Medication Used to Treat EPS *(continued)*

- Inform all healthcare providers of all the medication taken (e.g., any physicians, nurse practitioners, dentist, chiropractor, massage therapist, naturopathic/homeopathic practitioner).
- Report all side-effects rather than just stop taking medications so can work together with the psychiatrist or APRN to obtain best approach and result.
- Take medications even though you may feel well enough to not need them anymore to maintain the highest level of symptom relief and functioning.
- Avoid use of alcohol, drugs, narcotics, OTC medications, herbs, or other supplements because these will interfere with how well the medication works, increase or decrease medication serum levels, and in some cases can lead to life-threatening side-effects.
- Cigarette smoking can reduce serum/blood levels of antipsychotic medications; if patients decrease the amount they smoke or stop smoking, they should tell the psychiatrist so that the dose of antipsychotics can be adjusted downward to avoid overmedicating and risk of increased side/adverse effects.
- Antipsychotics: Periodic, and in some cases weekly, blood tests will need to be done so medications effects can be monitored and adverse effects prevented/early intervention.
- Eye exam prior to starting medications that may affect vision longer term (e.g., quetiapine [Seroquel], thioridazine [Mellaril]) and at least every 6 months.
- Keep a list of medications in their wallet; wear a medic alert identification bracelet or chain.
- Decide on a way to remember to take medications—calendar, pill box, putting the bottles near the coffee pot, etc.

(continues)

Table 13-2	Nursing Implications of Antipsychotic Medication and Medication Used to Treat EPS *(continued)*
	• Do not store medications in the bathroom, near the stove, in the refrigerator (unless specifically instructed to do so), or any other area where they may be exposed to excessive heat, moisture, or light; this will decrease the strength of the medication and it will not work as well.
	• Throw away any medications that are no longer prescribed to avoid medication interactions or accidental overdose (can take them to own pharmacy/hospital pharmacy to dispose of).
	• After discharge, if serious side-effects are experienced, and psychiatrist or other physician is not available (e.g., at night, weekends, holidays) call whoever they were told to call or their local emergency room.
	• Caution women regarding potential effects of antidepressant medications on fetal development and plans to breast feed. Women of child-bearing age should discuss birth control methods and plans to become pregnant with their physician.

DEPOT INJECTIONS

Depot injections are long acting forms of antipsychotic medications. Not all antipsychotic medications are available in depot or long acting forms. Most of these medications are oil suspensions that result in storage of the medication in body fats/tissues with a gradual release of the medication into the circulation over several days. They are beneficial for patients who have problems with medication adherence, problems with medication absorption from the GI tract, or first-pass hepatic effects. Initially, oral doses of antipsychotics will continue to be ordered and administered until a steady state of depot medication is reached, and then the oral doses will be discontinued. In some cases it may take up to 3 months to reach steady state (Sadock & Sadock, 2005, pp. 2823, 2838) (see **Table 13-3)**.

Table 13-3   Depot Injections

Traditional	Typical dose range and schedule	Nursing implications
		(Note: Patients receiving oral doses should be instructed when to stop taking them)
Haloperidol decanoate (Haldol [D])	Adults: 25–50 mg every 2 wks OR 50–100 mg every 4 weeks (maximum dose = 250 mg in 4 weeks)	See "Side/adverse effects" in Tables 13-1, 13-2, 13-4; also Boxes 13-1 and 13-2 Administer **deep IM/gluteal** sites, Z-track technique using a 1.5 to 2 inch, 20 G needle. Change needle after drawing up and before administering injection. Rotate injection sites. Do not massage injection sites.
Fluphenazine decanoate (Prolixin [D])	Adults: 12.5 mg every 1–2 weeks OR 25–50 mg every 4 weeks (maximum dose = 75 mg in 4 weeks)	See previous nursing implications for haloperidol.

Atypical	Typical dose range and schedule	Nursing implications
Risperidone (Risperdal) Consta	Adults: 25, 37.5, or 50 mg every 2 weeks	See "Side/adverse effects" in Tables 13-1, 13-2, 13-4; also Boxes 13-1 and 13-2. Package provided includes needle and is a powder requiring reconstituting. Administer **deep IM/gluteal** sites. Rotate injection sites. Do not massage injection sites.
Invega/paliperidone (Sustenna)	Adults: 234 mg 1st dose on day 1; 156 mg 2nd dose 1 week later; then 117 mg monthly dose (monthly maintenance dose individualized ranges 39–234 mg)	See "Side/adverse effects" in Tables 13-1, 13-2, 13-4; also Boxes 13-1 and 13-2. 1st two injections **must be** given in the **deltoid muscle** 1.5 inch 22G for ≥ 90 kg (200 lb) or 1-inch 23G needle for < 90 kg (< 200 lb) May use either deltoid or gluteal sites for **monthly** doses For gluteal injection (monthly) use a 1.5-inch 22G needle **regardless of weight.** Rotate injection sites. Do not massage injection sites.

Sources: Bezchlibnyk-Butler & Jeffries, 2005, pp. 78–79,111–112; DailyMed, 2010, website.

EXTRAPYRAMIDAL SYMPTOMS (EPS)

The term extrapyramidal symptoms (EPS) refers to various types of abnormal, involuntary movements that are a result of adverse effects of antipsychotic medication related to blocking the neurotransmitter DA or unmasking of abnormal movements already present at low levels when antipsychotic medication is administered. General categories of EPS include dystonic reactions or dystonia, akathesia, akinesia, tardive dyskinesia (TD), and pseudoparkinsonism. Risk factors for developing EPS include advanced age, duration of medication use, female sex, genotype, mood disorders, anticholinergic medications, medical illnesses, and the presence of subtle movement symptoms before the start of antipsychotic medication treatment (Sadock & Sadock, 2005, p. 3731).

Dystonic reactions or dystonia are muscle spasms or uncoordinated spastic muscle movements that can involve the face, tongue, extraocular muscles (i.e., oculogyric crisis), trachea/larynx (i.e., laryngospasm), esophagus, neck (i.e., torticollis), thorax/respiratory muscles (i.e., respiratory problems), trunk (i.e., opisthotonus or arching of the back), or pelvis (i.e., swaying or difficulty walking). These reactions can be very frightening for patients, but are easily treated.

Akathesia is described as motor restlessness. The patient has difficulty sitting still or staying in one position for any length of time. The patient may pace, fidget, shift their weight frequently from one foot to another or tap their foot, or they are unable to sit still in a chair. The patient may also make statements of feeling as if they are going to "jump out of" their "skin." These reactions can cause extreme distress for the patient to the point of them preferring to be ill rather than experience this side-effect or even contemplating suicide. Early identification of akathesia, as well as any EPS, is extremely important for the patient's well-being and increased adherence to prescribed treatment. Also, since akathesia may be difficult to assess, care must be taken to avoid misinterpreting it as agitation (Sadock & Sadock, 2005, p. 1471).

Akinesia refers to a decrease in motor movement or muscle weakness. The patient may complain of fatigue or tiring easily with physical activity and is at risk for falls.

Tardive dyskinesia (TD) refers to abnormal or purposeless muscle movements, including the extremities, trunk, face, jaw, and oral-buccal muscles causing rocking or twisting motions, pelvic thrusting or gyrations, tremors, tongue darting or writhing, spastic facial movements, frowning, blinking, blowing, teeth grinding, lip smacking, or chewing movements as if the patient has food or gum in their mouth. This type of EPS may be irreversible and can also be extremely distressing for the patient. The dose of the prescribed antipsychotic may be decreased or totally discontinued. In the past, anticholinergic or antiparkinsonian medications were used to treat these adverse effects, but more recently it is thought that these medications may worsen TD. Unfortunately, regardless of these efforts, the TD symptoms may be permanent.

Pseudoparkinsonism refers to signs and symptoms similar to those seen in Parkinson's disease including slow motor movements, tremors, muscle rigidity, cogwheel rigidity, stooped posture, shuffling gait, facial masking or flattened affect, and pill rolling finger movements. Medication may be given to counteract the adverse effects, and the dose of the prescribed antipsychotic may be decreased or totally discontinued.

Anticholinergic Medications

Certain anticholinergic or antiparkinsonian medications may be prescribed for EPS, including akathesia, pseudoparkinsonism, or dystonic reactions. Additionally the antihistamine diphenhydramine (Benadryl) may be prescribed for dystonic reactions (see **Table 13-4**).

Table 13-4   Medications to Treat EPS

Medication	Typical daily dose	Side/adverse effects
Anticholinergic/ antiparkinsonian Benztropine (Cogentin)	Adults: 1–4 mg in divided doses po, IM or IVP (maximum dose = 6 mg in 24 hours)	Blurred vision, mental confusion, delirium, psychosis including hallucinations, urinary retention, and constipation
Trihexyphenidyl (Artane)	Adults: 1–2 mg daily po or tid in divided doses Children: Up to 80 mg (Bezchlibnyk-Butler & Jeffries, 2005, p. 122; Mckenry, Tessier, & Hogan, 2006, p. 471; Medline Plus, 2010, pediatric disorders)	See previous side/adverse effects for benztropine.
Biperiden (Akineton)	Adults: 1 mg po; increase to usual dose range of 5–15 mg po in divided doses	See previous side/adverse effects for benztropine.

(continues)

Table 13-4   Medications to Treat EPS *(continued)*

Medication	Typical daily dose	Side/adverse effects
Procyclidine hydrochloride (Kemadrin)	Adults: 2.5–5 mg po tid in divided doses	See previous side/adverse effects for benztropine.
Amantadine hydrochloride (Symmetrel)	Adults: 100–300 mg po bid in divided doses	Dizziness, insomnia, orthostatic hypotension, heart failure, mental confusion, hallucinations, nausea, and constipation
Antihistamine Diphenhydramine (Benadryl)	Adults: 25–50 mg tid or qid po, IM or IVP Children ages 6–11 years: 12.5–25 mg po	Sedation, dry mouth, hypotention, urinary retention and constipation

Sources: Bezchlibnyk-Butler & Jeffries, 2005, pp. 120–127; Sadock & Sadock, 2005, pp. 2829–2830; Fontaine, 2009, p. 203; *Nursing 2010*, pp. 628–634, 827–828; Medline Plus, 2010, trihexiphenidyl.

NEUROLEPTIC MALIGNANT SYNDROME (NMS)

Neuroleptic malignant syndrome (NMS) is a potentially fatal adverse effect of antipsychotic medications. Traditional antipsychotics are more likely to cause NMS, but there have been cases of NMS related to atypical antipsychotics (Sadock & Sadock, 2005, p. 2830; Zarrouf & Bhanot, 2007). Cases of NMS in patients receiving atypical antipsychotic medications have been missed in early stages because of reliance on the fact that NMS occurs less often in patients prescribed atypical antipsychotics versus traditional ones. It is still important for the PMH nurse to be aware of this possibility and assess these patients for signs and symptoms of NMS:

- Elevated temperature (i.e., 101–108°F)
- Respiratory difficulty
- Muscle rigidity (i.e., "lead pipe" rigidity)
- Tachycardia; labile pulse
- Hypertension; labile blood pressure
- Diaphoresis
- Mental confusion, delirium, altered LOC
- Hyperreflexia
- Elevated WBCs
- Hyperkalemia

- Hyponatremia
- Elevated CPK
- Rhabdomyolysis (see **Box 13-1**)

(Sadock & Sadock, 2005, pp. 997, 2714; Keltner, Schwecke, & Bostrom, 2007, pp. 219, 221, 223; Antai-Otong, 2009, pp. 70–71; Fontaine, 2009, p. 201). For treatment modalities, see Table 13-2.

BOX 13-1   Rhabdomyolysis/Acute Tubular Necrosis/Renal Failure

- Abnormal urine color (dark, red, or cola colored)
- Muscle pain, tenderness, weakness, stiffness
- Fatigue
- Joint pain
- Seizures
- Increased serum CPK
- Increased serum K+ (hyperkalemia)
- + Serum and/or urine myoglobin
- Urine contains casts, hemoglobin without RBCs

Source: Medline Plus: http://www.nlm.nih.gov/medlineplus/ency/article/000473.htm

---

BOX 13-2   Treatment of NMS

- Stop all antipsychotic medication
- IV fluids
- Antipyretics (acetaminophen [Tylenol])
- Cooling blanket
- Dantrium (Dantrolene) 1 mg/kg IVP; may repeat up to 10 mg/kg
- Change to po dosing 4–8 mg/day in 4 divided doses x 3 days

OR

- Dantrium (Dantrolene) 0.8–3 mg/kg/day IVP in 4 divided doses; max 10 mg/kg/day; then po maintenance dose ranges 50–200 mg/day
- Bromocriptine (Parlodel) 2.5–10 mg tid po initially; if no improvement in 24 hours, increase to max dose of 20 mg po qid
- Bromocriptine (Parlodel) 1.25–2.5 mg/day po for *milder* cases
- Mechanical ventilation may be needed

Sources: Keltner & Folks, 2005, p. 498; Sadock & Sadock, 2005, p. 2830; Keltner, Schwecke, & Bostrom, 2007, pp. 219, 221, 223; Antai-Otong, 2009, pp. 70–71, Fontaine, 2009, p. 201.

METABOLIC SYNDROME

Metabolic syndrome, previously referred to as "central obesity" or "Syndrome X," is a collection of signs and symptoms including elevated glucose levels ($\geq$ 110); elevated cholesterol levels (triglycerides $\geq$ 150; HDL < 40 in men & < 50 in women); increased insulin levels (insulin resistance); obesity (BMI $\geq$ 25; waist circumference > 40 inches in men & > 35 inches in women); and hypertension ($\geq$ 135/85). The presence of at least three of these signs or symptoms may lead to increased risk for diabetes mellitus type 2 or cardiovascular disease. All antipsychotic medications can increase a patient's risk for developing metabolic syndrome, but there are some patients who have increased glucose and cholesterol levels prior to starting antipsychotic therapy (Fontaine, 2009, p. 202). Because atypical antipsychotics have been approved by the FDA for other uses (e.g., mood disorders) there is concern that metabolic syndrome may effect more people.

DELIRIUM

Haloperidol (Haldol), a traditional, high-potency antipsychotic medication, has been used in low doses for the longest amount of time to treat delirium. chlorpromazine (Thorazine) and thioridazine (Mellaril) are *not* recommended for use in treating delirium. Atypical antipsychotics have had the most research for use in delirium. Patients should be monitored for cardiac arrhythmias, including prolonged QTc intervals, when antipsychotic medications are administered IV/IVP (Sadock & Sadock, 2005, pp. 1065, 2155). Antipsychotics should be tapered off as soon as the delirium improves. Pseudoparkinsonism has occurred several weeks to months after administration of risperidone (Riperdal). For patients with contraindications to antipsychotic medications, benzodiazepines are used short term (Sadock & Sadock, 2005, p. 1066).

It is also common for all medications that may be causing or contributing to the symptoms of delirium to be discontinued or held. The PMH nurse should manage the environment, including low level lighting, decreasing environmental stimuli (e.g., noise, overcrowding), and assigning an experienced staff member to stay with patients experiencing delirium before administering medication to avoid potentially exacerbating symptoms.

DEMENTIA

Although according to Sadock and Sadock (2005, p. 2828) and Frisch and Frisch (2011, p. 775), antipsychotics have been shown in double-blind studies to reduce agitation and psychosis in patients diagnosed with dementia, the FDA has issued black box warnings for all antipsychotics in the treatment of psychosis related to dementia due to an increase in cardiovascular-related deaths.

SPECIAL CONSIDERATIONS

Due to age and side/adverse effects, antipsychotic medications are used more cautiously in the treatment of children/adolescents and the elderly.

Children/Adolescents

"Research shows that half of all lifetime mental illness begins by age 14" and neurologic changes begin before symptoms become apparent (NIMH, 2009). A complete history and physical examination should include questions about psychological trauma including natural disasters and deaths in the family. Diagnoses and treatment need frequent review due to changes related to normal growth and development and the resulting influence on child/adolescent symptoms. Not all antipsychotics should be used in this patient population and more research is needed regarding the use of psychotropic medications in children/adolescents. The risks vs benefits of their use and potential future developmental consequences make it more difficult to conduct research. Doses are usually calculated by weight. For further information, see Tables 13-1, 13-2, 13-4 and Boxes 13-1 and 13-2 as well as previous sections of this chapter regarding EPS and NMS. You may also refer to pharmacology texts such as *Mosby's Pharmacology in Nursing* and *Clinical Handbook of Psychotropic Drugs* by Bezchlibnyk-Butler and Jeffries.

Although rare, childhood schizophrenia has been diagnosed, and there are a few controlled studies of antipsychotics use in children. According to Sadock & Sadock (2005), high potency antipsychotics may help with symptoms of agitation such as combativeness, screaming or hyperactivity in children/adolescents diagnosed with pervasive developmental disorders, but antipsychotics may also impair learning, so the lowest possible dose should be prescribed when it is necessary to use antipsychotics in child/adolescent populations (p. 2828). Use of antipsychotic medications is controversial in impulse control disorders, but can help reduce the severity of neurologic motor or vocal tics in Tourette's syndrome (Sadock & Sadock, 2005, p. 2828). There is also increasing concern regarding the risk of developing metabolic syndrome.

According to a National Institutes of Mental Health (NIMH) 2008 press release regarding a 6-year, multisite research study of traditional and atypical typical antipsychotic medications, atypical antipsychotics "were no better" in treating child and adolescent schizophrenia. The medications used in this research study included molindone

ABNORMAL INVOLUNTARY MOVEMENT SCALE (AIMS)

Name: _____   Date: _____

Instructions: Complete the examination procedure before making ratings. Rate the highest severity of movement for each movement observed. Circle the number corresponding to the severity of movement observed. Ask the patient being assessed to remove any gum or candy from their mouth before beginning.

Rating scale: 0 = none/normal, 1 = minimal, may be extreme normal; 2 = mild, 3 = moderate, 4 = severe

FACIAL AND ORAL MOVEMENTS

1. Muscles of facial expression (i.e., movements of eyebrows, forehead, periorbital area, checks; include blinking, smiling, frowning, grimacing).   0   1   2   3   4

2. Lips and perioral area (i.e., smacking, pouting, puckering).   0   1   2   3   4

3. Jaw (i.e., chewing, clenching, biting, mouth opening, lateral movements).   0   1   2   3   4

4. Tongue—Rate only an increase in movements both in and out of the mouth, not an inability to sustain movement.   0   1   2   3   4

EXTREMITY MOVEMENTS

5. Upper (arms, wrists, hands, fingers). Include choreic movements (i.e., rapid, purposeless, irregular, spontaneous) and athetoid movements (i.e., slow, irregular, serpentine, complex). Do not include tremor (i.e., regular, repetitive, rhythmic).   0   1   2   3   4

6. Lower (legs, knees, ankles, toes). (i.e., foot tapping, lateral knee movement, heel dropping, foot squirming, inversion and eversion of foot).   0   1   2   3   4

TRUNK MOVEMENTS

7. Neck, shoulders, hip (i.e., twisting, rocking, squirming, pelvic gyrations).   0   1   2   3   4

GLOBAL JUDGEMENTS

8. Severity of abnormal movements.   0   1   2   3   4

9. Incapacitation due to abnormal movements.   0   1   2   3   4

10. Patient's awareness of abnormal movements.   0   1   2   3   4

DENTAL STATUS

Any current problems with teeth? With dentures?   Yes   No

Does the patient usually wear dentures?   Yes   No

FIGURE 13-1 AIMS Form

Sources: Jakopac, K. A., & Patel, S. C. (2009). *Psychiatric-mental health case studies and care plans.* Sudbury, MA: Jones and Bartlett; Mullen, J., Endicott, J., Hirschfeld, R. M., Yonkers, K., Tarcum, S., & Bullinger, A. L. (Eds.). (2004). *Manual of rating scales: For the assessment of mood disorders.* Wilmington, DE: Astrazeneca Pharmaceuticals LP.

(Moban), olanzapine (Zyprexa), and risperidone (Risperdal). There still is concern about side/adverse effects, and researchers are asking for the development of safer medications for the child/adolescent population. According to the NIMH, eskalith (Lithium) (mood stabilizer, antimanic), aripiprazole (Abilify) and risperidone (Risperdal) "are the only medications approved by the U.S. Food and Drug Administration (FDA) to treat bipolar disorder in young people" (2010). However, included in the same document was the (off-label) use of atypical antipsychotics including quetiapine (Seroquel), olanzapine (Zyprexa), and ziprasidone (Geodon) as well as mood stabilizers (antimanic, anticonvulsants) valproic acid or divalproex sodium (Depakote), lamotrigine (Lamictal) and selective serotonin reuptake inhibitors (SSRIs). Refer to Chapters 9, 14, and 15 for more information as well as the previously mentioned pharmacology texts.

Elderly

Due to the aging process, elderly patients have decreased cardiac output, renal clearance, liver size, and P450 cytochrome enzyme system function. This patient population is also more sensitive to pseudoparkinsonism, dystonic, and akathesia types of adverse effects. For these reasons most medication doses prescribed are half of typical adult doses unless otherwise indicated. For further information, see Tables 13-1, 13-2, 13-4 and Boxes 13-1 and 13-2. Clozapine (Clozaril) is generally avoided due to anticholinergic, cardiac, and sedative effects. Also, chlorpromazine (Thorazine) and thioridazine (Mellaril) are not recommended for use in the elderly due to susceptibility to anticholinergic toxicity. This susceptibility makes it difficult to treat EPS. Also, "advanced age is one of the strongest risk factors" for developing TD (Sadock & Sadock, 2005, pp. 2823, 3728–3731). The FDA has issued black box warnings for all antipsychotics in the treatment of psychosis related to dementia due to an increase in cardiovascular-related deaths.

Regarding delirium, refer to the previous sections in this chapter. According to Sadock & Sadock (2005), elderly patients may demonstrate delirium due to medical problems including infections, dehydration, electrolyte imbalances, urinary retention, pain, or adverse medication effects. Medical intervention and behavioral intervention should be attempted before administering antipsychotic medications (p. 3732).

REFERENCES

American Psychological Association (APA). (2007). *APA dictionary of psychology*. Washington, DC: Author.

Antai-Otong, D. (2009). *Psychiatric emergencies: How to accurately assess and manage the patient in crisis* (2nd ed.). Eau Claire, WI: PESI HealthCare, LLC.

Bezchlibnyk-Butler, K. Z., & Jeffries, J. J. (2005). *Clinical handbook of psychotropic drugs* (15th ed.). Ashland, OH: Hogrefe & Huber.

Daily Med, 2010. *Invega/Sutenna; Saphris/Ascenapine.* Retrieved from http://dailymed.nlm.nih. gov/dailymed/drugInfo.cfm?id=10704

Einarson, A., & Boskovic, R. (2009). Use and safety of antipsychotic drugs during pregnancy. *Journal of Psychiatric Practice*, *15*(3), 183–192. Retrieved from http://journals.lww.com/practical psychiatry/Abstract/2009/05000/Use_and_Safety_of_Antipsychotic_Drugs_During.4.aspx.

Fontaine, K. (2009). *Mental health nursing* (6th ed.). Upper Saddle River, NJ: Pearson Education, Inc.

Frisch, N. C., & Frisch, L. E. (2011). *Psychiatric mental health nursing* (4th ed.). Clifton Park, NY: Delmar.

Internet Mental Health. (2009). Retrieved from http://www.mentalhealth.com/drug/p30-m01. html#Head_7

Jakopac, K. A., & Patel, S. C. (2009). *Psychiatric-mental health case studies and care plans.* Sudbury, MA: Jones and Bartlett.

Joint Commission. (2009). Accreditation programs. Retrieved from http://www.jointcommission. org/standards_information/standards.aspx

Keltner, N. L., & Folks, D. G. (2005). *Psychiatric drugs* (4th ed.). St. Louis, MO: Elsevier/Mosby.

Keltner, N. L., Schwecke, L. H., & Bostrom, C. E. (2007). *Psychiatric nursing* (5th ed.). St. Louis, MO: Mosby, Elsevier.

McKenry, L., Tessier, E., & Hogan, M. (2006). *Mosby's pharmacology in nursing* (22nd ed.). St. Louis, MO: Mosby, Inc.

Medline Plus. (2010). *Rhabdomyolysis.* Retrieved from http://www.nlm.nih.gov/medlineplus/ency/ article/000473.htm

Medlineplus (2010). *Treatment of pediatric movement disorders.* Retrieved from http://www. wemove.org/pediatric_treatment

Medlineplus (2010). *Trihexiphenidyl.* Retrieved from http://www.nlm.nih.gov/medlineplus/ druginfo/meds/a682160.html

Mullen, J., Endicott, J., Hirschfeld, R. M. Yonkers, K., Tarcum, S., & Bullinger, A. L. (Eds.). (2004). *Manual of rating scales: For the assessment of mood disorders.* Wilmington, DE: Astrazeneca Pharmaceuticals LP.

National Institutes of Mental Health (NIMH) 2005 and 2006. *Clinical antipsychotic trials of effectiveness.* Retrieved from http://www.nimh.nih.gov/trials/practical/catie/index.shtml

National Institutes of Mental Health (NIMH) 2009. Document Fact Sheet: *Children with mental illness: Frequently asked questions about the treatment of mental disorders in children.* Retrieved from http://www.nimh.nih.gov/health/publications/treatment-of-children-with-mental-illness-fact-sheet/index.shtml

National Institutes of Mental Health (NIMH) 2010. *Mental health medications.* Retrieved from http://www.nimh.nih.gov/health/publications/mental-health-medications/alphabetical-list-of-medications.shtml

National Institutes of Mental Health (NIMH). Press Release September 15, 2008: *Newer antipsychotics no better than older drug in treating child and adolescent schizophrenia.* Retrieved from http://www.nimh.nih.gov/science-news/2008/newer-antipsychotics-no-better-than-older-drug-in-treating-child-and-adolescent-schizophrenia.shtml

National Institutes of Mental Health (NIMH) 2010. *What medications are used to treat schizophrenia?* Retrieved from http://www.nimh.nih.gov/health/publications/mental-health-medications/what-medications-are-used-to-treat-schizophrenia.shtml

National Institutes of Mental Health (NIMH) 2010. *What treatments are available for children and teens with bipolar disorder?* Retrieved from http://www.nimh.nih.gov/health/publications/bipolar-disorder-in-children-and-teens-a-parents-guide/what-treatments-are-available-for-children-and-teens-with-bipolar-disorder.shtml

Nursing 2010 drug handbook, 30th anniversary edition. Philadelphia, PA: Wolters Kluwer/Lippincott, Williams, & Wilkins.

Sadock, B. J., & Sadock, V. A. (2005) *Kaplan & Sadock's comprehensive textbook of psychiatry* (8th ed.). Philadelphia, PA: Lippincott, Williams, & Wilkins.

Stahl, S. M. (2005). *Essential psychopharmacology: Neuroscientific basis and practical applications* (2nd ed.). New York, NY: Cambridge University Press.

United States Food and Drug Administration. (2009). *Abilify.* Retrieved from www.accessdata.fda.gov/drugsatfda_docs/label/2009/021436s027lbl.pdf

United States Food and Drug Administration. (2010). *FDA approved drug products* (2010). Retrieved from http://www.accessdata.fda.gov/scripts/cder/drugsatfda/index.cfm?fuseaction=Search.Overview&DrugName=RISPERDAL and http://www.accessdata.fda.gov/scripts/cder/drugsatfda/index.cfm?fuseaction=Search.Label_ApprovalHistory and http://www.accessdata.fda.gov/drugsatfda_docs/label/2010/021444S-030S-033S-036S-037lbl.pdf

United States Food and Drug Administration (2010). Retrieved from http://www.fda.gov

Varcarolis, E. M., & Halter, M. J. (2010). *Foundations of psychiatric mental health nursing: A clinical approach* (6th ed.). St. Louis, MO: Saunders, Elsevier.

Zarrouf, F. A., & Bhanot, V. (Aug., 2007). Neuroleptic malignant syndrome: Don't let your guard down yet. *Current Psychiatry*, *6*(8), 89–95.

SUGGESTED READINGS

Appel, S. J., Jones, E. D., & Kennedy-Malone, L. (Aug., 2004). Central obesity and metabolic syndrome: Implications for primary care providers. *Journal of the American Academy of Nurse Practitioners*, *16*(8), 335–342.

Beebe, L. H. (2003). Health promotion in persons with schizophrenia: Atypical medications. *Journal of the American Psychiatric Nurses Association*, *9*(4),115–121.

Boyd, M. A. (2008). *Psychiatric nursing: Contemporary practice* (4th ed.). Philadelphia, PA: Wolters-Kluwer Health/Lippincott, Williams, & Wilkins.

Bradshaw, T., Lovell, K., & Harris, N. (2005). Healthy living interventions and schizophrenia: A systematic review. *Journal of Advanced Nursing*, *49*(6), 634–654.

Courey, T. J. (July/Aug., 2007). Detection, prevention, and management of extrapyramidal symptoms. *JNP: The Journal for Nurse Practitioners*, 464–469.

Eli Lilly. (2006). *Zyprexa, Zyprexa Zydis, Zyprexa Intramuscular.* Retrieved from http://www.accessdata.fda.gov/drugsatfda_docs/label/2007/020592s042s043,021086s022s023,021253s026lbl.pdf

Evans, J. (Jul., 2008). All antipsychotics to get warnings about elderly. *Clinical Psychiatry News*, *36*(7), 9.

Fontaine, K. L., & Fletcher, J. S. (2003). *Mental health nursing* (5th ed.). Upper Saddle River, NJ: Pearson Education, Inc.

Gene alterations could mean new treatments for schizophrenia. (June, 2007). *NeuroPsychiatry Reviews, 8*(6), 10.

Josiassen, R. C. (2007). IM aripiprazole for acute agitation. *Current Psychiatry, 6*(7), 103–106.

Keltner, N. (2005). Genomic influences on schizophrenia-related neurotransmitter systems. *Journal of Nursing Scholarship,* Fourth Quarter, *37*(4), 322–328.

Kirn, T. F. (Aug., 2007). Ethnic differences seen in drug metabolism. *Clinical Psychiatry News, 35*(8), 17.

Krakowski, M. (2007). Violent behavior: Choosing antipsychotics and other agents. *Current Psychiatry, 6*(4), 63–70.

Lauriello, J., & Keith, S. J. (April, 2005). Using IM antipsychotics: Lessons from clinical practice. *Current Psychiatry, 4*(4), 44–53.

Marcus, P. (2007). Understanding the use of genetics in psychiatry. Psychiatric Nursing Conference, New Orleans, LA.

Marder, S. R., Essock, S. M., Miller, A. I. et al. (2004). Physical health monitoring of patients with schizophrenia. *American Journal of Psychiatry, 161,* 1334.

Meyer, J. (2004). Managing metabolic risks of antipsychotic therapy. *A Supplement to Clinical Psychiatry News, Clinical Update Continuing Education,* 3.

Mohr, W. K. (2009). *Psychiatric-mental health nursing: Evidence based concepts, skills, and practices* (7th ed.). Philadelphia, PA: Wolters Kluwer/Lippincott, Williams, & Wilkins.

Mosby. (2002). *Mosby's medical, nursing & allied health dictionary* (6th ed.). St. Louis, MO: Author.

Nihart, M. (2007). Psychopharmacology update. Psychiatric Nursing Conference, New Orleans, LA.

Otsuka American Pharmaceutical, Inc. (2004). *Abilify.* Retrieved from www.accessdata.fda.gov/drugsatfda_docs/label/2004/21436slr006_abilify_lbl.pdf - 2009-03-31.

Pinto, S., & Pravikoff, D. (Nov., 2007). Agitation, acute: Treatment with benzodiazepines and antipsychotics. *Evidence based care sheet: CINAHL nursing guide.* Dupre Library On-line Nursing Data Base.

Prussian, K. H., Barksdale-Brown, D. J., & Diekmann, J. (April, 2007). Racial and ethnic differences in presentation of metabolic syndrome. *JNP: The Journal for Nurse Practioners, 3*(4), 229–240.

Psychiatry.com (2010). Retrieved from http://www.psychiatry.com

Sherman, C. (Aug., 2005). Factor ethnicity into drug treatment-Part 2. *Clinical Psychiatry News, 33*(8), 42.

Townsend, M. C. (2009). *Psychiatric mental health nursing: Concepts of care in evidence-based practice* (6th ed.). Philadelphia, PA: F. A. Davis.

Wynd, C. (2005). Guided health imagery for smoking cessation and long-term abstinence. *Journal of Nursing Scholarship,* Third Quarter, *37*(3), 245–250.

CHAPTER 14

Administration and Monitoring of Psychotropic Medications: Antidepressants

Kim A. Jakopac

OBJECTIVES

The nursing student will be able to:

1. Explain the basic neurobiologic basis for patient treatment with psychotropic medication specific to antidepressants
2. Describe variations in therapeutic effects among different ethnic groups
3. Identify nursing responsibilities related to the administration of psychotropic medications including patient education
4. Recognize potential serious adverse effects of antidepressant medication
5. Discuss special considerations regarding children/adolescents and elderly clients

KEY TERMS

Antidepressants	Priapism
Asthenia	Serotonin discontinuation syndrome
Enuresis	Serotonin syndrome
Hypertensive crisis	Tyramine

See also key terms Chapter 13.

---

*A*ntidepressants are a broad category of psychotropic medications used to treat mood disorders, mood symptoms occurring in other medical disorders, anxiety disorders, and various other mental health problems (APA, 2007, p. 61).

Antidepressant medications are used to treat symptoms of depressed mood, sleep disturbances, cognitive disturbances, decreased energy, suicidal thoughts, and anxiety (see also Chapters 7, 8, and 9). There has been "cautious" use of antidepressants in the treatment of the depressed phase of bipolar disorders as augmentation to prescribed mood stabilizing (antimanic) medications. According to Sadock and Sadock (2005), "some studies have reported an increased incidence of switches into hypomania or mania observed during Tricylic (TCAs) or Monoamine oxidase inhibitors (MAOIs) antidepressant augmentation therapy that is higher than expected for the patient's natural course of illness" and "there is evidence that these compounds (antidepressants) can speed up the rate of cycling in rapid cycling patients" (p. 1695). Selective serotonin reuptake inhibitors (SSRIs) may be less likely to cause these phenomena, but more research is needed because "commencement of rapid or continuous rapid cycling has been observed anecdotally" (Sadock & Sadock, 2005, pp. 1695–1701). Antidepressants are also prescribed for patients with other medical disorders to treat mood symptoms, including cognitive disturbances, occurring in traumatic brain injury (TBI), human immunodeficiency virus (HIV), premenstrual dysphoria and depressed mood occurring in patients diagnosed with dementia (Sadock & Sadock, 2005, pp. 401, 435–436, 485–486, 1075, 2320–2321).

Antidepressant medications are very effective for treating anxiety that can occur as a symptom of major depression or if the client meets DSM IV-TR criteria for anxiety disorders including panic disorder, social anxiety disorder, generalized anxiety disorder, pain disorder, neuropathy pain, fibromyalgia, pathological gambling, and symptoms of PTSD, including survivors of torture (Sadock & Sadock, 2005, pp. 1783–1785, 1822, 2041, 2403). Some antidepressants have been approved for use in obsessive-compulsive disorder (OCD) as an alternative to benzodiazepines including SSRIs (e.g., fluvoxamine [Luvox], fluoxetine [Prozac]), and the TCA clomipramine [Anafranil]). See also Chapters 7 and 8. Antidepressants have also been prescribed for bulimia nervosa and anorexia nervosa. Prophylactic treatment of migraine headaches is another potential reason for antidepressant treatment. For further information refer to pharmacology texts such as *Mosby's Pharmacology in Nursing* by McKenry, Tessier, and Hogan; *Clinical Handbook of Psychotropic Drugs* by Bezchlibnyk-Butler and Jeffries, *Essential Psychopharmacology: Neuroscientic Basis and Practical Applications* by Stahl, and websites including the National Institutes of Mental Health (NIMH) and the FDA.

As previously mentioned in the chapter on antipsychotics, patients should have complete physical, neurologic, and mental status examinations as well as laboratory/diagnostic tests. Factors regarding ethnic populations are becoming more a focus of attention regarding the pharmacodynamics, pharmacokinetics, and effect of P450 cytochrome enzyme systems on all medications including antidepressants (see also Chapter 13).

Medications, including many psychotropic medications, may be prescribed for "off-label" use. Usually this involves the use of the medication for other purposes than the FDA-approved use, but may also include doses or time frames/durations and dose schedules outside of the FDA-approved guidelines. According to Mossman (2009), "off-label prescribing is legal," and he quotes material from the *Physician's Desk Reference* (PDR) explaining that once medications or products are FDA-approved for marketing, they may be prescribed for patients or treatments "that are not included in approved labeling" and that federal statutes "do not limit or interfere with the authority of a health care practitioner to prescribe" approved medications or products "for any condition or disease." While this is true, it is acknowledged that healthcare providers can be found legally negligent "if their decision to use an off-label (medication, product) is sufficiently careless, imprudent (unwise), or unprofessional." The courts have also determined that off-label use does not require special informed consent different from standard informed consent (pp. 19–21). The psychiatric-mental health (PMH) nurse needs to be aware of typical use and doses of common psychotropic medications and keep current with literature, news, and scientific evidence related to psychotropic medications in order to maintain safe nursing practice and fulfill legal–ethical responsibilities.

CLASSIFICATIONS/CATEGORIES

Antidepressants are classified or categorized into various groups by pharmacologic action. Some antidepressants affect the serum levels, neuron receptors, and actions of mainly one neurotransmitter while others affect more than one. For some antidepressants, the classification or category includes the name of the neurotransmitter affected:

- Selective serotonin reuptake inhibitors (SSRIs)
- Selective serotonin-norepinephrine reuptake inhibitors (SNRIs)
- Norepinephrine-dopamine reuptake inhibitors (NDRIs)
- Tricyclics (TCAs)
- Noradrenergic-specific antagonists (NaSSAs)
- Serotonin-2 antagonist/reuptake inhibitors (SARIs)
- Monoamine oxidase inhibitors (MAOIs)

TCAs were the first antidepressants developed, and MAOIs have been available for some time. Both TCAs and MAOIs are very effective for treating symptoms, but their side/adverse effects and medication interactions can limit their use (see also the

MAOIs section in this chapter and the pharmacology reference texts mentioned in Chapter 13).

SSRIs have fewer side/adverse effects and usually do not have the potential cardiac effects, with the exception of serotonin syndrome (see the Serotonin Syndrome section in this chapter). SNRIs, NDRIs, Noradrenergic-specific antagonists, and Serotonin-2 antagonist/reuptake inhibitors allow medication therapy to be tailored even more for individual patient needs.

Caution: Some patients, especially those younger than 18 years of age, have reported increased aggression, suicidal ideation, or thoughts of harming others, which has led to mandatory "black box" warnings for SSRIs. These symptoms should be reported immediately. Precautions to be taken include informing patients and their families as well as more frequent assessment by the psychiatrist after discharge from the hospital (e.g., every week for the first 4 weeks). "In 2007, the FDA proposed that makers of all antidepressant medications extend the warning to include young adults up through age 24" (for weekly follow-up for generally the first 1 to 2 months) (NIMH, 2010, treatment of children with mental illness; FDA, 2010, pediatric use of antidepressants; FDA, 2007, young adults and antidepressants). Warnings regarding suicidal ideation and increased aggression more recently have been issued for all antidepressant medications and anticonvulsants used as mood stabilizers for all age ranges (see Chapter 15 and refer to individual medication pharmaceutical company information on package inserts). The benefits of improving functioning and preventing suicide due to depression or anxiety must be weighed against the risks when antidepressants are prescribed.

SSRIs

SSRIs act mainly by selectively blocking the reuptake of serotonin in the synaptic junction/gap affecting more than one receptor site (e.g., 5-HT1A, 5-HT2, 5-HT3, etc.). This classification or category includes many antidepressants. They are routinely ordered for symptoms of major depression, depressive symptoms occuring as a result of other medical conditions, anxiety related to depression, and anxiety disorders (refer to previously mentioned conditions on page 348 in this chapter). These medications have fewer side/adverse effects (see **Table 14-1**) than other types of antidepressants and usually do not have the potential cardiac effects, with the exception of serotonin syndrome, or anticholinergic effects. SSRIs cause fewer problems related to overdose. Sexual dysfunction is one of the most common reasons for medication nonadherence (noncompliance) or discontinuation. The LIP may decrease the dose, change to another SSRI, SNRI, or NDRI; or augment the original SSRI with bupropion (Wellbutrin) (an NDRI), mirtazapine (Remeron) (an NaSSA), sildenafil (Viagra) or the herbal supplement yohimbe (Sadock & Sadock, 2005, p. 1784).

Abruptly stopping SSRIs, and possibly SNRIs, can cause symptoms referred to as serotonin discontinuation syndrome. Due to the long half-life of fluoxetine (Prozac), serotonin discontinuation syndrome (withdrawal) may be less likely to occur with this antidepressant. Symptoms of serotonin discontinuation syndrome include:

- Anxiety
- Agitation
- Palpitations
- Tremor
- Lethargy
- GI distress
- Flu-like symptoms minus fever
- Myalgias
- Electric-shock sensations in extremities
- Irritability
- Slowed thinking
- Confusion
- Dizziness

(Keltner, Schwecke, & Bostrom, 2007, p. 238; McKenry, Tessier, & Hogan, 2006, p. 403; Sadock & Sadock, 2005, p. 2890)

Serotonin Syndrome

Serotonin syndrome is a potentially fatal collection of symptoms that can occur as a result of excessively high serum levels of the neurotransmitter serotonin. This syndrome can occur from the combination of more than one medication affecting serotonin levels (e.g., SSRIs, SNRIs, MAOIs, TCAs, desyrel [Trazodone]) and the combination of antidepressant medications and herbal supplements (e.g., St. John's Wort). Combinations of other medications including the opioid analgesic meperidine (Demerol) with antidepressants, antidepressants with eskalith (Lithium) or the cough syrup ingredient dextromethorphan (DM) and antidepressants may also cause serotonin syndrome (McKenry, Tessier, & Hogan, 2006, p. 406; Fontaine, 2009, p. 205). "The FDA has warned that combining the newer SSRI or SNRI antidepressants with one of the commonly-used 'triptan' medications used to treat migraine headaches" could cause serotonin syndrome (NIMH, 2010). Symptoms of serotonin syndrome can begin 2–72 hrs *or* several weeks after beginning medication and include:

- Restlessness
- Excitement
- Agitation
- Mental confusion
- Delirium
- High fever (i.e., 101 to 107°F)
- Elevated blood pressure
- Muscle twitching
- Muscle spasms
- Seizures
- Hyperreflexia
- Chills/shivering or shaking chills
- Nausea
- Diarrhea
- Coma
- Death

(McKenry, Tessier, & Hogan, 2006, p. 406; Keltner, Schwecke, & Bostrom, 2007, p. 239; Fontaine, 2009, p. 205; Varcarolis & Halter, 2010, p. 262).

SNRIs

SNRIs, also known as "dual Serotonin and Norepinephrine reuptake inhibitors," affect the serum levels of more than one neurotransmitter, mainly two, and their influence is "dose dependent." For example, at lower doses these medications mainly inhibit the reuptake of serotonin. At moderate-to-high doses, SNRIs also have more of an inhibitory effect on norepinephrine (NE), and at high doses they also have a small amount of dopamine (DA) inhibitory effect (Stahl, 2005, pp. 246–247; Keltner, Schwecke, & Bostrom, 2007, pp. 234–235). Venlafaxine (Effexor) has been shown to be as effective as SSRIs in random, controlled medication trials (Sadock & Sadock, 2005, p. 1784), although it has been reported to be related to increased aggression and suicidal thinking in children/adolescents (FDA, 2010, pediatric medication labeling).

Regarding duloxetine (Cymbalta), short-term studies did not show an increase in the risk of suicidality with antidepressants compared to placebo in adults older than age 24; there was a reduction in risk with antidepressants compared to placebo in adults aged 65 and older. Depression and certain other psychiatric disorders are themselves associated with increases in the risk of suicide. Patients of all ages who are started on antidepressant therapy should be monitored appropriately and observed closely for clinical worsening, suicidality, or unusual changes in behavior. Families and caregivers should be advised of the need for close observation and communication with the prescriber. Duloxetine is not approved for use in pediatric patients (RxList, 2010) (see Table 14-1).

NDRIs

There is only one NDRI, bupropion (Wellbutrin), and this is a unique category because this is "the only antidepressant medication that primarily inhibits DA reuptake and does not affect serotonin systems" and "also inhibits norepinephrine uptake" (Stahl, 2005, p. 241; Keltner, Schwecke, & Bostrom, 2007, p. 235). This medication is also used as a smoking cessation treatment (i.e., bupropion [Zyban]). Bupropion (Wellbutrin) is less likely to cause sexual side-effects. It is, however, contraindicated in patients who have a history of seizure disorders especially if "any single dose exceeds 150 mg," including sustained release forms, in total daily doses of greater than 400 mg or if the dosage is increased too quickly. Also, caution is advised when using this medication for patients with hepatic or renal impairment (Bezchlibnyk-Butler & Jeffries, 2005, pp. 16–17; Sadock & Sadock, 2005, p. 3368) (see Table 14-1).

TCAs

TCAs are generally considered to be "nonselective" in their inhibitory reuptake action (Bezchlibnyk-Butler & Jeffries, 2005, p. 33). However, some TCAs (i.e., secondary amines) are more potent NE reuptake inhibitors than others. Some exert more of an effect on serotonin (i.e., tertiary amines) than NE (Sadock & Sadock, 2005, p. 3366; Keltner, Schwecke, & Bostrom, 2007, p. 235). Other actions included antagonist effects at histamine (H1) and alpha 1 adrenergic receptors (Bezchlibnyk-Butler & Jeffries, 2005, p. 35). Some TCAs may also have a small effect on DA (Stahl, 2005, pp. 219–220). Although very effective, they have significant cardiac and anticholinergic side/adverse effects. These antidepressants are particularly dangerous for patients at risk to overdose. Withdrawal symptoms can occur when TCAs are abruptly stopped (i.e., discontinuation syndrome) (see Table 14-1).

NaSSAs

There is only one NaSSA, mirtazapine (Remeron), which acts by "increasing the availability of both serotonin and norepinephrine by antagonizing alpha-2 autoreceptors." Mirtazapine (Remeron) is unique in that it blocks serotonin 5-HT2, 5-HT2A, and 5-HT3 receptors and seems to not cause GI symptoms or sexual side-effects (Keltner, Schwecke, & Bostrom, 2007, p. 235). At lower dose ranges this antidepressant also is very effective for improving sleep pattern disturbances, thought to be due to blocking 5-HT2A, 5-HT2C, and histamine (H1) receptors (Bezchlibnyk-Butler & Jeffries, 2005, p. 30; Stahl, 2005, p. 255). This effect is decreased at higher recommended doses (see Table 14-1). Mirtazapine (Remeron) is not FDA-approved for use in children (FDA—Mirtazapine information, 2007).

SARIs

Currently there are two SARIs: desyrel (Trazodone) and nefazadone (Serzone). (Nefazadone [Serzone] was withdrawn from the North American market due to hepatotoxicity, [Bezchlibnyk-Butler & Jeffries, 2005, p. 25] but was reintroduced with a "black box" warning for hepatotoxicity [Frisch & Frisch, 2011, p. 785]). Both antidepressants in this category exert a strong blockade (antagonist action) of serotonin 5-HT2A in one area and less strong reuptake inhibition of serotonin in another area.

Desyrel (Trazodone) is frequently used for sleep pattern disturbances as well as in the treatment of major depression; it has alpha-1 antagonist plus antihistamine effects. Although therapeutically effective and cost effective, desyrel (Trazodone) can cause significant cardiovascular side/adverse effects and may cause priapism in males (Mohr, 2009, p. 296). Nefazadone (Serzone) also has weak alpha-1 antagonist and NE reuptake inhibition (Stahl, 2005, pp. 258–259) (see Table 14-1).

MAOIs

MAOIs are effective medications, but are not prescribed as often due to adherence issues with dietary restrictions. Failure to adhere to dietary restrictions concerning foods containing high amounts of the amino acid tyramine can lead to a potentially life-threatening adverse reaction known as hypertensive crisis (Bezchlibnyk-Butler & Jeffries, 2005, p. 47; McKenry, Tessier, & Hogan, 2006, pp. 77, 404; Keltner, Schwecke, & Bostrom, 2007, p. 249). According to Fontaine (2009), the only exception to the dietary restrictions is when a patient is prescribed selegiline (Eldepryl), a transdermal patch. Although selegiline (Eldepryl) is an MAOI, its "unique properties" prevent food interactions (p. 205). However, Bezchlibnyk-Butler and Jeffries (2005) still suggest dietary restrictions be applied because selegiline (Eldepryl) inhibits "both A + B MAO enzymes" (p. 49), and Townsend (2009) recommends dietary restrictions with doses of 9–12 mg/24 hrs (p. 313).

There are also adverse medication interactions between MAOIs and several other medications (McKenry, Tessier, & Hogan, 2006, p. 404; Keltner, Schwecke, & Bostrom, 2007, p. 248; Frisch & Frisch, 2011, p. 784–785; also refer to the previously mentioned psychopharmacologic texts on page 348 in this chapter), making it extremely important to notify all healthcare providers when a patient is prescribed MAOIs. In general it is recommended that there be at least 2 weeks between the discontinuation of an MAOI medication and the start of other antidepressants or medications known to interact with MAOIs. This time period is also recommended prior to surgery or ECT. However, when patients have been receiving fluoxetine (Prozac), there should be a much longer period of time, up to 5 weeks, due to the long half-life of fluoxetine (Bezchlibnyk-Butler & Jeffries, 2005, p. 52; Sadock & Sadock, 2005, p. 3366).

MAOIs inhibit the action of the enzyme monoamine oxidase, which is responsible for the breakdown of neurotransmitters in the synaptic junction/gap (Stahl, 2005, p. 155; Keltner, Schwecke, & Bostrom, 2007, p. 235). This results in neurotransmitters remaining in the synaptic junction/gap for longer periods of time and continuing to exert their effects, including CNS stimulation. MAOIs may be further categorized

Table 14-1 Common Antidepressant Medications

Medications	Daily dose ranges	Side/adverse effects
	(Adults = 18 years or older; see also Special Considerations section in this chapter; doses are adjusted for patients with hepatic, renal problems; for the elderly typically reduce to at least half of the adult dose)	(Potential interactions occur with other medications or supplements that increase serotonin levels, norepinephine levels, and triptans; alcohol and other CNS depressants; caffeine; see also previous information in this chapter and specific antidepressant information in this table)
SSRIs		
Fluoxetine (Prozac)/serafem Available in oral tablets, oral capsules for daily or delayed release for weekly dosing, and oral solution	Adults: 10–80 mg po Weekly medication form dosing: 90 mg weekly to begin 7 days after the last daily dose form Children ages 8–17 years for OCD: 10–20 mg po (maximum dose = 60 mg/24 hours) Children ages 8–18 years for depression: 10–20 mg po	General and specific side/adverse effects of all SSRI antidepressants: GI symptoms including nausea, diarrhea Lightheadedness Headache Insomnia Vivid dreams Nervousness or "jittery" feeling Drowsiness Fine tremor Sexual dysfunction (i.e., men—erectile dysfunction, delayed or painful ejaculation; women—decreased libido or orgasm) Diaphoresis Weight loss or gain Dry mouth Flu-like symptoms minus fever (exception see Serotonin Syndrome section of this chapter) Occasional bleeding Painful menstruation Increase in suicidal thinking or agitation (refer to "black box" warnings)

Interaction effects with:
SNRIs, MAOIs, TCAs—serotonin syndrome

Valproic acid (Depakene)—may experience increased serum levels of fluoxetine (Prozac) (Bezchlibnyk-Butler & Jeffries, 2005, p. 10).

St. John's Wort—may increase serotonergic effects, levels (Bezchlibnyk-Butler & Jeffries, 2005, p. 14).

Protease inhibitor ritonavir (Norvir)—"Cardiac and neurological side effects . . . due to elevated ritonavir level"; "moderate increase" in fluoxetine (Prozac) and paroxetine (Paxil) levels; "increased" sertraline (Zoloft) serum levels (Bezchlibnyk-Butler & Jeffries, 2005, p. 14).

Anticoagulants—"data contradictory" for increased bleeding (Bezchlibnyk-Butler & Jeffries, 2005, p. 10).

Children—may be more prone to experience restlessness, irritability, agitation, insomnia, hypomania activation, or social disinhibition (Bezchlibnyk-Butler & Jeffries, 2005, p. 8).

(continues)

Table 14-1   Common Antidepressant Medications (*continued*)

Medications	Daily dose ranges	Side/adverse effects
		Elderly—higher doses associated with delirium, falls, and impaired balance; hyponatremia; may take longer to excrete medication and also may take longer for symptoms to respond to medication (Bezchlibnyk-Butler & Jeffries, 2005, pp. 8–9).
		Note: Fluoxetine (Prozac) has the longest half-life of SSRIs, "2 to 9 days" (Mohr, 2009, p. 294) and may be less likely to cause serotonin discontinuation syndrome; it is recommended that fluoxetine be discontinued for up to 5 weeks before beginning MAOI antidepressant therapy rather than the standard 2 weeks because of the long half-life (Sadock & Sadock, 2005, p. 3366).
Olanzapine and Fluoxetine (Symbyax) Available in oral capsules; combination antipsychotic and antidepressant product	Adults: 1 capsule po in the evening	See information on Olanzapine (Zyprexa) in Chapter 13, Table 13-1, and fluoxetine (Prozac) in this table.
Sertraline (Zoloft) Available in oral tablets, capsules, and oral concentrate	Adults: 25–200 mg po	See General and specific side/adverse effects of all SSRI antidepressants previously in this table. *Interaction Effects:* Anticoagulants—increased INR or PT (Bezchlibnyk-Butler & Jeffries, 2005, p. 10).

Drug	Dosage	Side/Adverse Effects
Paroxetine/pexeva (Paxil) Available in oral tablets, oral controlled release (CR) tablets, and oral suspension	Adults: 10–50 or 60 mg po; for CR tablets 12.5–75 mg po Elderly: 10–40 mg po (maximum dose = 40 mg/24 hours; CR tablets maximum dose = 50 mg 24 hours)	See General and specific side/adverse effects of all SSRI antidepressants previously in this table. Elderly—some reports of increased agitation *Interaction Effects:* Anticoagulants—increased INR or PT (Bezchlibnyk-Butler & Jeffries, 2005, p. 10).
Fluvoxamine (Luvox) Available in oral tablets and continuous release (CR) capsules	Adults: 50–300 mg po Children ages 11–17 years, 25–300 mg (maximum dose = 300 mg) and 8–10 years: 25–200 mg (maximum dose = 200 mg/24 hours) Administer daily amounts greater than 50 mg in two divided doses FDA Pediatric Medication Labeling of SSRIs (2010)–determined that a dose adjustment (increased dose) may be necessary in adolescents, and girls 8–11 years of age may require lower doses.	See General and specific side/adverse effects of all SSRI antidepressants previously in this table.
Citalopram (Celexa) Available in oral tablets, oral disintegrating tablets, and oral solution	Adults: 10–60 mg po Elderly: 10–40 mg po	See General and specific side/adverse effects of all SSRI antidepressants previously in this table. May cause myalgia, arthralgia, muscle cramping
Escitalopram (Lexapro) Available in oral tablets and oral solution	Adults: 10–20 mg po Elderly: 10 mg po	See General and specific side/adverse effects of all SSRI antidepressants previously in this table.

(continues)

Table 14-1   Common Antidepressant Medications *(continued)*

Medications	Daily dose ranges	Side/adverse effects
SNRIs Venlafaxine (Effexor) Available in oral tablets, oral extended release (ER) tablets, and ER capsules	Adults: 75–375 mg po	General and specific side/adverse effects of all SNRI antidepressants: Increase in suicidal thinking or agitation (refer to "black box" warnings) Asthenia Nervousness Dizziness Hypertension Tachycardia Vasodilation Headache Somnolence Insomnia Abnormal dreams Tremor Agitation Nausea Dry mouth Anorexia Hyponatremia Weight gain/loss Discontinuation syndrome/withdrawal symptoms if medication stopped abruptly (reportedly "self-limited," Weyth.com, 2010) include: Irritability Anxiety Depressed mood

Labile emotions including hypomania
Agitation
Headache
Lethargy
Dizziness
Mental confusion
Seizures
Paresthesias/electric shock sensations)
Insomnia
Tinnitus
(Campagne, 2005; MentalHealth.com, 2010; Weyth.com, 2010)

Interaction effects with:

SNRIs, MAOIs, TCAs, triptans, and tryptophan supplements—serotonin syndrome

NSAIDS, ASA, and warfarin (Coumadin)—increased risk of bleeding (Weyth.com, 2010)

Pregnancy/lactation—breastfeeding is not advised while taking this medication (Weyth.com, 2010)

Desvenlafaxine (Pristiq)

Available in extended release (ER) oral tablets

Adults: 50 mg po

ESRD: 50 mg po every other day

See General and specific side/adverse effects and interaction effects of all SNRI antidepressants previously in this table.
Elderly—greater risk of systolic orthostatic hypotension seen in patients 65 years or older (Pfizer, 2009)

(continues)

Table 14-1   Common Antidepressant Medications (continued)

Medications	Daily dose ranges	Side/adverse effects
Duloxetine (Cymbalta) Available in delayed-release oral capsules	Adults: 20–60 mg po (maximum dose = 60 mg/24 hours)	*Caution*—unstable heart disease, preexisting or uncontrolled hypertension, cerebrovascular disease, lipid metabolism disorders, seizure disorders, or family history of mania/hypomania—has not been evaluated systemically in patients with a recent history of myocardial infarction (Pfizer, 2009) See General and specific side/adverse effects of all SNRI antidepressants previously in this table. FDA alerts for "suicidality risk" in young adults and aggravation of preexisting liver disease; liver toxicity in moderate-to-heavy alcohol users (Campagne, 2005). *Interaction effects with:* Other SNRIs, SSRIs, MAOIs, amphetamines, desyrel (Trazadone) (Campagne, 2005). Avoid in severe renal insufficiency (Bezchlibnyk-Butler & Jeffries, 2005, p. 20).
NDRIs Bupropion (Wellbutrin) Available in oral tablets, oral extended and sustained release tablets	Adults: 150–450 mg po	General and specific side/adverse effects include: Agitation Tremors Increased risk of seizures (refer to previously mentioned information on pages 353–354 in this chapter and information below in this column in Table 14-1 under "Caution").

Cardiac arrhythmias

Insomnia, abnormal dreams

Diaphoresis

Weight changes

Increase in suicidal thinking or agitation

May cause increased liver function test results

Least likely antidepressant to cause sexual dysfunction

Used alone or as adjunct/augmentation when patents experience sexual side-effects of other antidepressants

Additionally used as a smoking cessation treatment

Caution—with patient history of seizure disorder; seizure risk increases especially when "any single dose exceeds 150 mg" including sustained release forms, in total daily doses of greater than 400 mg or if the dosage is increased too quickly. Patients diagnosed with bulimia have experienced seizures. Also caution is advised when using this medication for patients with hepatic or renal impairment (Bezchlibnyk-Butler & Jeffries, 2005, pp. 16–17; Sadock & Sadock, pp. 2005, 3366, 3368).

(continues)

Table 14-1 Common Antidepressant Medications (continued)

Medications	Daily dose ranges	Side/adverse effects
		Children—exacerbation of tics reported in children diagnosed with ADHD and Tourette's (Bezchlibnyk-Butler & Jeffries, 2005, p. 17).
		Elderly—some patients may experience dizziness and orthostatic hypotension (Bezchlibnyk-Butler & Jeffries, 2005, p. 16).
		Interaction effects with: Antiparkinsonian and antihistamine medications (increased anticholiergic effects)
		Increased serum levels of TCAs (Bezchlibnyk-Butler & Jeffries, 2005, p. 18).
TCAs		
Amitriptyline/endep (Elavil) Available in oral tablets, oral suspension, and IM injection	Adults: 75–300 mg po (maximum dose = 300 mg/24 hours) Elderly: 10 mg po tid; 20 mg po at bedtime	General and specific side/adverse effects of all TCAs: Sedation Weakness Fatigue Mental confusion Delirium Disturbed concentration Dry mouth Blurred vision Urinary retention

Constipation

Hypotension/orthostatic hypotension

Tachycardia

Cardiac arrhythmias, heart failure, MI

Diaphoresis

Seizures

Hypomania

Weight gain

Sexual dysfunction

Increase in suicidal thinking or agitation

May cause hypertension in patients diagnosed with bulimia (Bezchlibnyk-Butler & Jeffries, 2005, p. 36).

Caution—Cardiac and cerebral toxicity occur with overdose (Mohr, 2009, p. 290)

Discontinuation syndrome (withdrawal):

Sleep disturbance including nightmares

Irritability

GI symptoms

Malaise

Interaction effects with: Many medications including SSRI, SNRIs, MAOIs, cardiac medications, antihypertensives, CNS depressants or stimulants, antiparkinsonian medications, Disulfiram (Antabuse)

(continues)

Table 14-1   Common Antidepressant Medications (*continued*)

Medications	Daily dose ranges	Side/adverse effects
Clomipramine (Anafranil) Available in oral tablets and oral capsules	Adults: 75–300 mg po	See General and specific side/adverse effects of all TCAs previously in this table. See information regarding overdose, discontinuation syndrome and interaction effects of amitriptyline/endep (Elavil).
Nortriptyline/aventyl (Pamelor) Available in oral capsules and oral syrup	Adults: 25–100 mg po in divided doses; doses higher than 150 mg po daily not recommended (Mohr, 2009, p. 291)	See General and specific side/adverse effects of all TCAs previously in this table. See information regarding overdose, discontinuation syndrome and interaction effects of amitriptyline/endep (Elavil).
Imipramine (Tofranil) Available in oral tablets and oral capsules	Adults: 30–300 mg po in divided doses	See General and specific side/adverse effects of all TCAs previously in this table. See information regarding overdose, discontinuation syndrome and interaction effects of amitriptyline/endep (Elavil).
Desipramine (Norpramin) Available in oral tablets	Adults: 25–300 mg po	See General and specific side/adverse effects of all TCAs previously in this table. See information regarding overdose, discontinuation syndrome and interaction effects of amitriptyline/endep (Elavil).

Protriptyline (Vivactil) Available in oral tablets	Adults: 15–60 mg po	See General and specific side/adverse effects of all TCAs previously in this table. See information regarding overdose, discontinuation syndrome and interaction effects of amitriptyline/endep (Elavil).
Doxepin (Sinequan) Available in oral capsules and oral concentrate	Adults: 25–300 mg po (maximum dose = 300 mg/24 hours)	See General and specific side/adverse effects of all TCAs previously in this table. See information regarding overdose, discontinuation syndrome and interaction effects of amitriptyline/endep (Elavil).
Amoxapine (Asendin) Available in oral tablets	Adults: 50–600 mg po	See General and specific side/adverse effects of all TCAs previously in this table. See information regarding overdose, discontinuation syndrome and interaction effects of amitriptyline/endep (Elavil).
Maprotiline (Ludiomil) Available in oral tablets (*Note:* Amoxapine [Asendin] is technically a dibenzoxapine, and Maprotiline [Ludiomil] is technically a tetracyclic, but their actions and side/adverse effects are similar to TCAs [Bezchlibnyk-Butler & Jeffries, 2005, p. 33])	Adults: 50–225 mg po (maximum dose = 300 mg/24 hours)	See General and specific side/adverse effects of all TCAs previously in this table. See information regarding overdose, discontinuation syndrome and interaction effects of amitriptyline/endep (Elavil).

(continues)

Table 14-1   Common Antidepressant Medications (continued)

Medications	Daily dose ranges	Side/adverse effects
NaSSAs Mirtazapine (Remeron) Available in oral tablets and oral dissolving tablets (Remeron SolTab)	Adults: 15–45 mg po (maximum dose = 60 mg/24 hours)	See general and specific side/adverse effects of all SSRIs previously in this table. Fewer GI symptoms or sexual side-effects than SSRIs Weight gain Drowsiness—at lower recommended doses effective for insomnia, but this effect is lost as the dose approaches the higher recommended levels Increase in suicidal thinking or agitation (see "black box" warnings)
SARIs Desyrel (Trazodone) Available in oral tablets	Adults: 150–400 mg po (maximum dose = 600 mg/24 hours)	General and specific side/adverse effects of all SARIs: Agitation Mental confusion and disorientation Decreased concentration Impaired memory Dizziness Syncope Hypotension, orthostatic hypotension Tachycardia QTc interval prolongation: cardiac Arrhythmia/ventricular arrhythmias Shortness of breath

Sedation
Edema
Lack of muscle coordination
Sexual side-effects, including priapism in males
Nightmares
Hallucinations
Delusions
Hypomania
Dry mouth or bad taste

Increase in suicidal thinking or agitation

Interaction effects with: SNRIs, MAOIs, TCAs, triptans, and tryptophan supplements—serotonin syndrome

Adults: 200–600 mg po

See General and specific side/adverse effects of all SARIs previously in this table.
Diaphoresis
Itching

Increase in suicidal thinking or agitation

"Black box" warnings for hepatotoxicity

Interaction effects with: SNRIs, MAOIs, TCAs, triptans, and tryptophan supplements—serotonin syndrome

Additional drug interactions: With benzodiazepines, steroids, antibiotics, or antifungals (Sadock & Sadock, 2005, p. 3722).

Nefazodone (Serzone)

Available in oral tablets

(continues)

Table 14-1 Common Antidepressant Medications *(continued)*

Medications	Daily dose ranges	Side/adverse effects
MAOIs Irreversible/MAO-B:		General and specific side/adverse effects include: Drowsiness Dizziness Orthostatic hypotension
Isocarboxazid (Marplan)	Adults: 20–60 mg po	Weakness Restlessness Headache Tremors Myoclonic jerking during sleep Edema of lower extremities Urinary retention Weight gain Sexual side-effects (i.e., decreased libido, impotence, decreased orgasm) Constipation Blurred vision Hyponatremia Rare liver toxicity "Black box" warnings for suicidal thinking
Available in oral tablets		Discontinuation syndrome: Headache Chest palpitations Vivid nightmares Muscle weakness Agitation Irritability

Myoclonic jerking

Nausea

Diaphoresis

Interaction effects with:

(See also Hypertensive Crisis section subsequently in chapter)

Dietary:

Foods containing moderate-to-high amounts of tyramine including, but not limited to:

Aged cheeses (e.g., blue, cheddar, brick, Roquefort)

Other cheeses (e.g., parmesan, feta, swiss, mozzarella, muenster)

Dried, salted fish/pickled herring

Aged, smoked meats

Improperly stored or spoiled meats and fruits

Soy sauce/soybean condiments, tofu

Broad bean pods (e.g., Fava beans)

Avocadoes

Bananas

Chianti wine, sherry, champagne

Beer, including alcohol-free

Concentrated yeast

Spinach

Eggplant

(for a more complete list, refer to the previously mentioned psychopharmacology and pharmacology texts on page 348 in this chapter)

Medications:

OTC cold remedies including nasal sprays and any product containing dextromethorphan

(continues)

Table 14-1   Common Antidepressant Medications *(continued)*

Medications	Daily dose ranges	Side/adverse effects
		CNS stimulants including OTCs Narcotics containing codeine Mepheridine (Demerol) Propranolol (Inderol) Fentynl/sublimaze (Duragesic) Carbamazepine (Tegretol) Buspirone (Buspar) Propoxyphene (Darvocet) CNS depressants Antiparkinsonian medications Triptans (for a more complete list refer to the previously mentioned psychopharmacology and pharmacology texts on page 348 in this chapter)
Phenelzine (Nardil) Available in oral tablets	Adults: 45–90 mg po	See General and specific side/adverse effects, discontinuation syndrome, and interaction effects for isocarboxazid (Marplan).
Tranylcypromine (Parnate) Available in oral tablets	Adults: 30–60 mg po	See General and specific side/adverse effects, discontinuation syndrome, and interaction effects for isocarboxazid (Marplan).
Reversible/MAO-A: Moclobemide (Manerix) Available in oral tablets	Adults: 300–600 mg po	See General and specific side/adverse effects, discontinuation syndrome, and interaction effects for isocarboxazid (Marplan). *Interaction effects also with:* Cimetidine (Tagamet)

Other/MAO-A + MAO-B:

Selegiline/emsam (Eldepryl)

Available in transdermal patches (used as adjunct treatment to manage symptoms of Parkinson's disease)

(Selegiline hydrochloride is available in oral capsules and orally disintegrating tablets)

Adults and children ages 12 to adult: 6 mg–12 mg/24 hours for transdermal patch (maximum dose = 12 mg/24 hours)

Elderly: 6 mg po

General and specific side/adverse effects include:

Insomnia

Headache

Hypotension/orthostatic hypotension

Chest pain

Cardiac arrhythmias

Dizziness

Agitation

Confusion

Hallucinations

Delusions

Application site reactions such as itching, redness, rash, edema

See Discontinuation syndrome section of this table for isocarboxazid (Marplan).

See Interaction effects section of this table for isocarboxazid (Marplan).

OTC herbal supplements: Ginseng and St. John's Wort

Sources: Bezchlibnyk-Butler & Jeffries, 2005, pp. 4–45, 47–58, 293–295; Sadock & Sadock, 2005, pp. 402, 924, 1783–1784, 2027, 3366–3368, 3720–3724; McKenry, Tessier, & Hogan, 2006, pp. 397–407; Keltner, Schwecke, & Bostrom, 2007, pp. 235–247; Boyd, 2008, pp. 119–122; Fontaine, 2009, pp. 202–204; Mohr, 2009, pp. 289–296; Townsend, 2009, pp. 305–313; *Nursing 2010*, pp. 583–616, 644, 1422; Varcarolis & Halter, 2010, pp. 262–266; Frisch & Frisch, 2011, pp. 778–786; FDA, (2010), pediatric medication labeling; Internet Mental Health, 2010; Weyth.com, 2010; Psychcentral.com, 2010; Drug Information.com, 2010, Nardil, Parnate.

by subtypes regarding the specific neurotransmitters they affect: A (NE and serotonin; most likely to cause food interactions) vs B (DA; less likely to cause food interactions), or as reversible vs irreversible (destruction of the enzyme) (Stahl, 2005, pp.
213–216; McKenry, Tessier, & Hogan, 2006, p. 405; Varcarolis, 2006, p. 756; Frisch
& Frisch, 2011, p. 783).

NURSING RESPONSIBILITIES AND IMPLICATIONS

See Chapter 13, Tables 14-1 and 14-2 in this chapter and previously mentioned pharmacology texts on page 348 in this chapter.

HYPERTENSIVE CRISIS

Hypertensive crisis is a dangerous elevation in blood pressure secondary to elevation
of NE levels that can be life threatening. It may occur as an adverse medication reaction in patients receiving MAOI antidepressant medications who also eat foods high
in tyramine or as an adverse medication reaction with other medications. Symptoms
of hypertensive crisis can occur suddenly and include:

- Severe increase in blood pressure
- Throbbing headache commonly in the occipital area
- Stiff neck
- Chest pain
- Nausea and/or vomiting
- Diaphoresis
- Cold, clammy skin
- Cardiac arrhythmias
- Intercranial bleeding
- Elevated temperature
- Dilated pupils
- Photophobia
- Sudden nose bleed
- Coma

(Bezchlibnyk-Butler & Jeffries, 2005, p. 51; McKenry, Tessier, & Hogan, 2006, p. 77;
Keltner, Schwecke, & Bostrom, 2007, pp. 247–250; Fontaine, 2009, p. 205; Frisch &
Frisch, 2011, p. 784)

> **BOX 14-2   Treatment of Hypertensive Crisis**
>
> - Stop medication and notify physician
> - Phentolamine (Regitine) 5 mg IV
>   **OR**
>   Hydralazine (Apresoline) 10–40 mg IM or IV
>   **OR**
>   Nifedipine (Procardia) 10 mg sublingual (instruct patient to bite capsule and swallow)
>   **OR**
>   Captopril (Capoten) 25 mg sublingual (instruct patient to bite capsule and swallow)
>
> - Monitor BP and pulse every 5 minutes until stable
> - Monitor temperature and respirations every 5 minutes until stable
> - ECG/EKG
> - Cooling blanket if hyperthermia
> - Supportive care
>
> *Sources:* Bezchlibnyk-Butler & Jeffries, 2005, p. 52; McKenry, Tessier, & Hogan, 2006, pp. 406, 568–569; Keltner, Schwecke, & Bostrom, 2007, pp. 247–250; Lewis, Heitkemper, Dirkson, O'Brien, & Bucher, 2007, p. 775; Townsend, 2009, p. 313; Varcarolis & Halter, 2010, p. 268; Frisch & Frisch, 2011, p. 784.

THYROID SUPPLEMENTATION

Thyroid supplementation may be used to accelerate antidepressant medication therapeutic effects when antidepressant therapy is first initiated in unipolar depression and to treat co-occuring thyroid disorders, but this is to be done cautiously due to the risk of cardiotoxicity (Sadock & Sadock, 2005, pp. 132, 1698). Also, according to Sadock and Sadock (2005), much research has been done with thyroid augmentation of antidepressant therapy in the treatment of resistant depression, but thyroid supplementation proved to be less consistently effective than eskalith (Lithium) supplementation. Medications included in these studies included liothyromine (Cytomel) or T3, TCAs, and SSRIs. Estrogen augmentation has been shown to be both effective and ineffective (pp. 3005–3006).

PREGNANCY

As previously mentioned in Chapter 13, all psychotropic medications cross the placenta, and there have not been enough adequate controlled research studies on humans. TCAs are *not* recommended to be taken during pregnancy (Frisch & Frisch, 2011, p. 779). Although SSRIs have been prescribed more often due to a better side-effect profile, there have been mixed results regarding the use of SSRIs, with some studies showing increased risk of teratogenic effects and miscarriages and others not supporting these findings. There is a lack of long-term studies. Also, infants exposed to SSRIs during the third trimester may experience symptoms of serotonin withdrawal including "breathing problems, jitteriness, irritability, trouble feeding, or hypoglycemia" for up to 2 weeks after birth (Keltner, Schwecke, & Bostrom, 2007, p. 239; Psychiatry.com—medications while pregnant, 2010). These withdrawal symptoms have not been life threatening. There have also been warnings regarding the SSRI paroxetine (Paxil) regarding increased risk of neurologic teratogenic effects during the first trimester of pregnancy (College Urges Pregnant Women to Avoid Paxil, 2007). In 2006 the FDA posted an alert related to SSRIs including the following: "A recently published case-control study has shown that infants born to mothers who took selective serotonin reuptake inhibitors (SSRIs) after the 20th week of pregnancy were 6 times more likely to have persistent pulmonary hypertension (PPHN)." Also, "The study did not find an association between exposure to SSRIs during the first 20 weeks of gestation and PPHN." This information also applies to the combination medication olanzapine (Symbyax) and fluoxetine (Prozac) (FDA Alert, 2006). The risks of the return of symptoms of major depression, suicidal thoughts, and possible suicide attempts must be weighed against teratogenic risks and benefits of antidepressant therapy when these medications are prescribed. According to the results of a longitudinal study of Latina women in New York City, "mental health status affects a pregnant woman's ability to care for herself and her newborn child" (Everest & Nutt, 2007, pp. 61–62). SSRIs and MAOIs do appear in breast milk, and patients are referred to their LIPs for questions related to the safety of any medications while breast feeding (Frisch & Frisch, 2011, pp. 779, 782, 784). According to Bezchlibnyk-Butler and Jeffries (2005), safety data is lacking for MAOI use in pregnancy (p. 48).

Table 14-2 Nursing Implications of Antidepressant Medication	

Assessing therapeutic and side/adverse effects	• Refer to Table 14-1
	• Assess vital signs every 8 hours and prior to medication administration, and prn
	  • Perform orthostatic BP measurements prn (symptoms)
	  • Place on fall risk precautions

(continues)

Table 14-2	**Nursing Implications of Antidepressant Medication** *(continued)*
	• Assess for suicidal thoughts/attempts and increased agitation on admission, every 8 hours and prn (e.g., change in behavior from what nursing staff, family, or friends have previously seen; receiving unwelcome or unexpected news) • Perform cardiovascular and neurologic assessments as well as a mental status examination on admission, every 8 hours, and prn • Assess elimination patterns and provide adequate fluid intake to prevent urinary retention and paralytic ileus • Monitor laboratory/diagnostic test results; report abnormal results to LIP who ordered them and assess body system corresponding to abnormal test results • Assess for signs of liver toxicity • Assess for signs/symptoms of serotonin syndrome • Document all therapeutic and side/adverse effects • Notify LIP prescribing medication of side/adverse effects
Administration	• Prozac—best if taken on empty stomach for better absorption; other SSRIs not affected; administer/take earlier in the day if problems with insomnia (i.e., no later than 5 pm) • Celexa—Do not break or crush oral dissolving tablets, but allow to dissolve on patient's tongue without water/fluids • Remeron SolTab—place oral dissolving on tongue without water/fluids • Wellbutrin—do not crush or split tablets • Eldepryl—do not cut transdermal patches into smaller pieces; apply patches to clean and dry skin surface; rotate application sites (i.e., outer/upper arm, upper torso, upper thigh) • For any orally dissolving tablets—do not give food or liquids at least 5 minutes prior to administering medication

(continues)

Table 14-2   Nursing Implications of Antidepressant Medication *(continued)*

Patient/family education (permission must be obtained from the patient for family or friends to have information; if the patient has a guardian, permission must be obtained from the guardian for anyone else to have information)	• Explain benefits of medications ordered and emphasize increased potential to function as well as relief of symptoms. • Medications typically take an average of 2 weeks (longer with fluoxetine (Prozac)—4–6 weeks) to achieve full therapeutic benefits. • Report immediately any suicidal thoughts/ attempts, agitation, changes in behavior, unusual or strange thoughts, mental confusion or disorientation, hallucinations, delusional thinking (There is an increased risk of suicide when patients are experiencing depression, anxiety, or agitation and have not yet received treatment, and again approximately 1 week after beginning treatment when their energy levels are improving but the other symptoms of depression have not fully been relieved. It is common for only a 2 week supply of psychotropic medication to be prescribed/available to decrease potential for overdosing. Patents/families should be taught this as well as the "black box" warning information). • Report immediately any cardiac symptoms (e.g., dizziness, syncope, palpitation, funny feeling, heaviness or pain in chest, difficulty breathing). • Change positions slowly and ask for help ambulating. • Initial sedation feeling and blurred vision will decrease as the body adjusts to the medication. If these symptoms continue/worsen, report these. • Do not drive or operate machinery until they know how medication will affect them (e.g., sedation, drowsiness, blurred vision, decreased reaction time). • Common side-effects and ways to relieve dry mouth (e.g., increase fluid intake if not contraindicated, ice chips, more frequent oral care, sugarless gum/candy). • Take medication exactly as prescribed in order to have the most possible benefit. Inform that while these medications do not cause tolerance or dependence (nonaddicting), stopping them suddenly can lead to discontinuation syndromes (withdrawal symptoms) (see Table 14-1).

(continues)

Table 14-2   Nursing Implications of Antidepressant Medication *(continued)*

- Avoidance of caffeine (may increase agitation), CNS depressants including alcohol, narcotics, and other drugs (increased sedation and cardiovascular effects), CNS stimulants including drugs and amphetamine-like substances (increased cardiovascular effects, potentially life-threatening), herbal supplements that increase serotonin levels/function (e.g., St. John's Wort).
- Teach signs of serotonin syndrome and to report immediately (see Box 14-1).
- Teach signs of hepatotoxicity and to report immediately (e.g., loss of appetite, abdominal pain, dark urine, jaundice, clay/light colored stools).
- ECG/EKG prior to starting TCAs and periodically while continuing on TCAs.
- Periodic CBC, renal, and liver function laboratory tests will be needed including SSRIs (Varcarolis & Halter, 2010, p. 265).
- Acknowledge embarrassment of potential sexual side-effects and importance of reporting these rather than just stop taking medication.
- Importance of nutrition to mental health and how to eat a balanced diet to help balance weight gain and risk of metabolic syndrome.
- Importance of physical exercise to help balance weight gain; advise to obtain physician's approval for specific types of exercise to avoid injury.
- Inform all healthcare providers of all the medication taken (e.g., any physicians, nurse practitioners, dentist, chiropractor, massage therapist, naturopathic/homeopathic practitioner).
- Report all side-effects rather than just stop taking medications so can work together with the psychiatrist or APRN to obtain the best approach and result.
- Take medications even though may feel well enough to not need them anymore to maintain level of symptom relief and functioning.
- Keep a list of medications in their wallet; wear a medic alert identification bracelet or chain.
- Decide on a way to remember to take medications—calendar, pill box, put the bottles near the coffee pot, etc.

(continues)

Table 14-2 Nursing Implications of Antidepressant Medication *(continued)*	
	• Advise not to store medications in the bathroom, near the stove, in the refrigerator (unless specifically instructed to do so), or any other area where they may be exposed to heat, moisture or light. This will decrease the strength of the medication and it will not work as well. • Advise to throw away any medications that are no longer prescribed to avoid medication interactions or accidental overdose (can take them to own pharmacy/hospital pharmacy to dispose of). • After discharge if experience serious side-effects and psychiatrist or other physician is not available (e.g., at night, weekends, holidays) call whoever they were told to call or their local emergency room. • Caution women regarding the potential effects of antidepressant medications on fetal development and plans to breast feed. Women of childbearing age should discuss birth control methods and plans to become pregnant with their physician. • For MAOIs teach dietary restrictions and medications to avoid as well as signs of hypertensive crisis and to seek immediate medical attention if these signs occur (see Table 14-1).

Sources: Sadock & Sadock, 2005, p. 1784; *Nursing 2010*, pp. 583–616, 1422; Keltner, Schwecke, & Bostrom, 2007, pp. 235–247; Boyd, 2008, pp. 119–122; Fontaine, 2009, pp. 202–204; Mohr, 2009, pp. 289–296; Townsend, 2009, pp. 305–313; Varcarolis & Halter, 2010, pp. 262–266; Frisch & Frisch, 2011, pp. 778–782, 785–786.

SPECIAL CONSIDERATIONS

Children/Adolescents

In 1999 the results of a large scientific study, Methodology for Epidemiology of Mental Disorders in Children and Adolescents (MECA), were published showing that "almost 21 percent" of children 9 to 17 years old in the United States had a diagnosable "mental or addictive disorder that caused at least some impairment" (PsychCentral.com, 2010). As previously stated in the chapter on antipsychotic medications, psychiatric illnesses begin much earlier than the manifestation of symptoms. "Through greater understanding of when and how fast specific areas of children's brains develop, we are learning more about the early stages of a wide range of mental illnesses that appear later in life. Helping young children and their parents manage difficulties early in life may prevent the development of disorders. Once mental illness develops, it becomes a regular part of your child's behavior and more difficult to treat. Even though we know how to treat (though not yet cure) many disorders, many children with mental illnesses are not getting treatment" (NIMH, 2010, treatment of children with mental illness).

According to a 2004 FDA Executive Summary, major depression is a serious illness affecting "up to 2.5 percent of children and about eight percent of adolescents in the United States." Suicide continues to be "the third leading cause of death in the U.S. in the 15–19 year-old age group and accounts for more deaths than all other major physical conditions combined. Older medications are of limited value in the pediatric population because of serious, potentially life–threatening adverse events. Newer medications, such as the selective serotonin reuptake inhibitors (SSRIs), have fewer side-effects than the older drugs, making it easier for people to continue treatment." The Senate Subcommittee on Oversight and Investigations Committee on Energy and Commerce "agreed with FDA's conclusion that the data in aggregate indicate an increased risk of suicidality in pediatric patients and made several recommendations" (Temple, 2004) resulting in changes to medication labeling and "black box" warnings (see previously mentioned information on these warnings in this chapter). However, there was NIMH support for pharmacotherapy treatment in 2007. The NIMH Director, Thomas R. Insel, stated, "Although we cannot ignore the possibility that antidepressants may exacerbate suicidal thoughts and actions in some children, it would be worse to let these children go untreated." Referring to a comprehensive review of pediatric trials conducted between 1988 and 2006 reported in the *Journal of the American Medical Association (JAMA)*, and partially funded by the NIMH regarding the benefits outweighing the risks, he further stated, "This study indicates that more children are ultimately helped by antidepressant treatment than harmed" (NIMH, 2007). "In the FDA review, no completed suicides occurred among nearly 2,200 children treated with SSRI medications (the most commonly prescribed type of antidepressants). However, about 4 percent of those taking SSRI medications experienced suicidal thinking or behavior, including actual suicide attempts—twice the rate of those taking placebo, or sugar pills" (PsychCentral.com, 2010).

Due to the risks previously mentioned, medication therapy is carefully considered and benefits are weighed against risks. Developmental changes as well as differences in pharmacodynamics and pharmacokinetics from adults require close monitoring and frequent adjusting of medications. As previously stated in Chapter 13, medication is usually prescribed by weight. Fluoxetine (Prozac) is the only FDA approved

SSRI antidepressant for treating depression in children and fluoxetine (Prozac), fluvoxamine (Luvox), and sertraline (Zoloft) are approved in children/adolescents 9–18 years of age (Bezchlibnyk-Butler & Jeffries, 2005, p. 8). According to Sadock and Sadock (2005), "several randomized, controlled trials now provide conclusive evidence that SSRIs are useful in the treatment of certain anxiety disorders in children and adolescents" (p. 1784). Regarding children/adolescents diagnosed with pervasive development disorders (PDDs), SSRIs have been beneficial for managing symptoms of anxiety, depression, or OCD, but more research is needed. Small randomized controlled medication trials of TCAs have shown benefit for enuresis (Sadock & Sadock, 2005, pp. 3367–3368).

Regarding citalopram (Celexa) in the treatment of major depression, the "safety and effectiveness in the pediatric population have not been established" and results were pending for escitalopram (Lexapro) (FDA, 2010, pediatric medication labeling). Treatment with medication requires the consent of the parent or guardian (see Chapter 13). Psychotherapy including behavioral interventions is important for the child/adolescent as well as the involvement of parents and teachers. Ethical–legal considerations and future effects of medications in this population have limited research. See Table 14-1 and the previously mentioned pharmacology texts on page 348 in this chapter for more information. An additional clinical psychotropic medications handbook for pediatrics such as *Clinical Handbook of Psychotropic Drugs for Children and Adolescents* by Bezchlibnyk-Butler and Jeffries would be helpful.

Regarding the "off-label" use of antidepressants and other psychiatric medications in the treatment of children/adolescents, "based on clinical experience and medication knowledge, a physician may prescribe to young children a medication that has been approved by the U.S. Food and Drug Administration (FDA) for use in adults or older children. This use of the medication is called 'off-label.' Most medications prescribed for childhood mental disorders, including many of the newer medications that are proving helpful, are prescribed off-label because only a few of them have been systematically studied for safety and efficacy in children. Medications that have not undergone such testing are dispensed with the statement that 'safety and efficacy have not been established in pediatric patients.' The FDA has been urging that products be appropriately studied in children and has offered incentives to drug manufacturers to carry out such testing." (PsychCentral.com, 2010).

Elderly

Depression often is unrecognized and left untreated in elderly patients. For some elderly patients, poor nutrition including folate/folic acid and vitamin B12 deficiencies is the culprit, but others may need medication as well as psychotherapy. As previously stated in Chapter 13, elderly patients have decreased cardiac output, renal clearance, liver size, and P450 cytochrome enzyme system function due to the aging process. These changes make them more sensitive to side/adverse effects, and in most cases elderly patients require typical dose reductions of at least half of the usual adult recommended doses (see Table 14-1).

SSRIs are the first choice for elderly patents because of their better side-effect profile compared to other antidepressant medications. However, according to Sadock and Sadock (2005), fluoxetine (Prozac) and paroxetine (Paxil) interfere with P450 cytochrome enzymes, which can result in higher, even toxic, serum levels of other medications including cardiac anti-arrhythmics, benzodiazepines, steroids, some antibiotics, antifungals, other antidepressants, and neuroleptics (p. 3721). TCAs, nortriptyline (Pamelor), and desipramine (Norpramin), have been effective for relief of symptoms of depression in this population, however, the side/adverse effect profile limits their use (e.g. cardiac, anticholinergic). Therapeutic serum levels for these TCAs are the same as for those of younger patients. Also, although NDRIs (50–300 mg)—and including extended release forms—cause fewer anticholinergic, cognitive, or cardiac side-effects in elderly patients (Sadock & Sadock, 2005, pp. 3721–3722), some elderly patients may experience dizziness and orthostatic hypotension (Bezchlibnyk-Butler & Jeffries, 2005, p. 16). Improvements in cognition have been noted in the elderly with MAOIs, but in that case orthostatic hypotension may present problems (Bezchlibnyk-Butler & Jeffries, 2005, p. 52).

REFERENCES

American Psychological Association (APA). (2007). *APA dictionary of psychology*. Washington, DC: Author.

Bezchlibnyk-Butler, K. Z., & Jeffries, J. J. (2005). *Clinical handbook of psychotropic drugs* (15th ed.). Ashland, OH: Hogrefe & Huber.

Boyd, M. A. (2008). *Psychiatric nursing: Contemporary practice* (4th ed.). Philadelphia, PA: Wolters-Kluwer Health/Lippincott, Williams, & Wilkins.

Campagne, D. M. (2005). Venlafaxine and serious withdrawal symptoms: Warning to drivers. *Medscape General Medicine 2005*, 7(3), 22. Retrieved from http://www.medscape.com/viewarticle/506427

College urges pregnant women to avoid paxil. (April, 2007). *The Journal for Nurse Practitioners—JNP*, 3(4), 218.

Drug Information.com. (2010). *Drugs A-Z: Nardil*. Retrieved from http://www.drugs.com/cdi/nardil.html

Drug Information.com. (2010). *Drugs A-Z: Parnate.* Retrieved from http://www.drugs.com/cdi/parnate.html

Everest, T., & Nutt, B. (July, 2007). Mental health and pregnancy: The link between prenatal and postpartum depression. *Advance for Nurse Practitioners, 15*(7), 61–64.

Fontaine, K. (2009). *Mental health nursing* (6th ed.). Upper Saddle River, NJ: Pearson Education, Inc.

Frisch, N. C., & Frisch, L. E. (2011). *Psychiatric mental health nursing* (4th ed.). Clifton Park, NY: Delmar.

Internet Mental Health—Mentalhealth.com. (2010). *Thioridazine.* Retrieved from http://www.mentalhealth.com/drug/p30-m01.html#Head_7

Keltner, N. L., Schwecke, L. H., & Bostrom, C. E. (2007). *Psychiatric nursing* (5th ed.). St. Louis, MO: Mosby, Elsevier.

Lewis, S. L., Heitkemper, M. M., Dirkson, S. R., O'Brien, P. G., & Bucher, L. (2007). *Medical-Surgical nursing: Assessment and management of clinical problems* (7th ed.). St. Louis, MO: Mosby, Elsevier.

McKenry, L., Tessier, E., & Hogan, M. (2006). *Mosby's pharmacology in nursing* (22nd ed.). St. Louis, MO: Mosby, Inc.

Mohr, W. K. (2009). *Psychiatric-mental health nursing: Evidence based concepts, skills, and practices* (7th ed.). Philadelphia, PA: Wolters Kluwer/Lippincott, Williams, & Wilkins.

Mossman, D. (2009). Why off-label isn't off base. *Current Psychiatry, 8*(2), 19–22.

National Institutes of Mental Health (NIMH). (2007). *Science update: Benefits of antidepressants may outweigh risks for kids.* Retrieved from http://www.nimh.nih.gov/science-news/2007/benefits-of-antidepressants-may-outweigh-risks-for-kids.shtml

National Institutes of Mental Health (NIMH). (2010). *Mental health medications.* Retrieved from http://www.nimh.nih.gov/health/publications/mental-health-medications/what-medications-are-used-to-treat-depression.shtml

National Institutes of Mental Health (NIMH). (2010). *Treatment of children with mental illness fact sheet.* Retrieved from http://www.nimh.nih.gov/health/publications/treatment-of-children-with-mental-illness-fact-sheet/index.shtml

Nursing 2010 drug handbook 30th anniversary edition. Philadelphia, PA: Wolters Kluwer/Lippincott, Williams & Wilkins.

Pfizer Inc. (Dec., 2009). Label information #262294-01. *Current Psychiatry, 9*(6), 1–2.

PsychCentral. (2010). *Medication library.* Retrieved from http://psychcentral.com/drugs/

Psychiatry.com. (2010). *Medications while pregnant.* Retrieved from http://www.psychiatry.com

RxList. (2010). *The internet drug index.* Retrieved from http://www.rxlist.com

Sadock, B. J., & Sadock, V. A. (2005). *Kaplan & Sadock's comprehensive textbook of psychiatry* (8th ed.). Philadelphia, PA: Lippincott, Williams, & Wilkins.

Stahl, S. M. (2005). *Essential psychopharmacology: Neuroscientific basis and practical applications* (2nd ed.). New York, NY: Cambridge University Press.

Temple, R. (Sept., 2004). Anti-depressant drug use in pediatric populations. *Food and Drug Administration News Events—Executive Summary.* Retrieved from http://www.fda.gov/NewsEvents/Testimony/ucm113265.htm

Townsend, M. C. (2009). *Psychiatric mental health nursing: Concepts of care in evidence-based practice* (6th ed.). Philadelphia, PA: F. A. Davis.

U.S. Food and Drug Administration (FDA) Alert. (July, 2006). *Information for healthcare professionals: Fluvoxamine—Selective serotonin reuptake inhibitors (SSRIs) and Olanzapine/fluoxetine (marketed as Symbyax).* Retrieved from http://www.fda.gov/Drugs/DrugSafety/PostmarketDrugSafety InformationforPatientsandProviders/DrugSafetyInformationforHeatcareProfessionals/ ucm085181.htm

U.S. Food and Drug Admisnistration (FDA). (May, 2007). *FDA proposes new warnings about suicidal thinking, behavior in young adults who take antidepressant medications.* News Release PO7-77. Retrieved from http://www.fda.gov/NewsEvents/Newsroom/PressAnnouncements/2007/ ucm108905.htm

U.S. Food and Drug Administration (FDA). (May, 2007). *Mirtazapine (marketed as Remeron).* Retrieved from http://www.fda.gov/Drugs/DrugSafety/PostmarketDrugSafetyInformationfor PatientsandProviders/ucm109344.htm

U.S. Food and Drug Administration (FDA). (2010). *Antidepressant use in children, adolescents, and adults.* Retrieved from http://www.fda.gov/Drugs/DrugSafety/InformationbyDrugClass/ ucm096273.htm

U.S. Food and Drug Administration (FDA). (2010). *Pediatric medication labeling SSRIs.* Retrieved from http://www.fda.gov/ScienceResearch/SpecialTopics/PediatricTherapeuticsResearch/ ucm107519.htm

Varcarolis, E. M. (2006). *Manual of psychiatric nursing care plans* (3rd ed.). St. Louis, MO: Saunders, Elsevier.

Varcarolis, E. M., & Halter, M. J. (2010). *Foundations of psychiatric mental health nursing: A clinical approach* (6th ed.). St. Louis, MO: Saunders, Elsevier.

Weyth Pharmaceuticals. (2010). *Effexor/Effexor XR label content.* Retrieved from http://www. wyeth.com/content/showlabeling.asp?id=100

SUGGESTED READINGS

Garzon, D. C. (2007). Childhood depression. *Advance for Nurse Practitioners, 15*(2), 35–44.

Jakopac, K. A., & Patel, S. C. (2009). *Psychiatric mental health case studies and care plans.* Sudbury, MA: Jones and Bartlett.

Kelly, J. (2007). Genetic variation may impact response to antidepressants. *NeuroPsychiatry Reviews, 8*(1), 1, 26.

Kelly, J. (June, 2007). Pain compounds depression's impact for retired NFL players. *NeuroPsychiatry Reviews, 8*(6), 1, 22.

Marcus, P. (2007). Understanding the use of genetics in psychiatry. Psychiatric Nursing Conference, New Orleans, LA.

Mental Health.com. (2010). http://www.mentalhealth.com

Mullen, J., Endicott, J., Hirschfeld, R. M., Yonkers, K., Tarcum, S., & Bullinger, A. L. (Eds.). (2004). *Manual of rating scales: For the assessment of mood disorders.* Wilmington, DE: Astrazeneca Pharmaceuticals LP.

National Institutes of Mental Health (NIMH). (2010). *Mental health medications.* Retrieved from http://www.nimh.nih.gov/health/publications/mental-health-medications/index.shtml

National Institutes of Mental Health (NIMH). (2010). *Publications about medications.* Retrieved from http://www.nimh.nih.gov/health/publications/medications-listing.shtml

psychINFO. (2010). Retrieved from http://www.psychinfo.com

Sequenced Treatment Alternatives to Relieve Depression (STAR*D). (2009). Retrieved from http://www.clinicaltrials.gov/ct/show/NCT00021528?order=1

U.S. Food and Drug Administration (FDA). (2010). *Approved drug products.* Retrieved from http://www.accessdata.fda.gov/scripts/cder/drugsatfda/index.cfm

U.S. Food and Drug Administration (FDA). (2010). *Depression—Medicines to help you.* Retrieved from http://www.fda.gov/ForConsumers/ByAudience/ForWomen/ucm118473.htm

U.S. Food and Drug Administration (FDA). (2010). *Index to drug-specific information.* Retrieved from http://www.fda.gov/Drugs/DrugSafety/PostmarketDrugSafetyInformationforPatientsand Providers/ucm111085.htm

Administration and Monitoring of Psychotropic Medications: Anticonvulsants/Anxiolytics

Sudha C. Patel

OBJECTIVES

The nursing student will be able to:
1. Explain the basic neurobiologic basis for patient treatment with anticonvulsant medications
2. Describe variations in therapeutic effects among different ethnic groups
3. Identify nursing responsibilities related to the administration of anticonvulsant medications including patient education
4. Recognize potential serious adverse effects of anticonvulsant medications

KEY TERMS

Anticonvulsants
Antimanic

See also key terms Chapter 13.

---

*A*nticonvulsants (antiepileptic drugs) have a broader spectrum of efficacy for use. These drugs are listed as mood stabilizers or antimanics under the psychotropic medications group. These drugs are effective in treating manic symptoms and stabilizing mood in bipolar disorders aside from their use in epileptic conditions. There is a growing body of evidence that use of anticonvulsants with other mood stabilizing agents such as lithium as a first line treatment in the acute episode of manic symptoms in bipolar disorders has a beneficial effect in stabilizing mood (Stahl, 2008, p. 672).

As stated in Chapter 13, for antipsychotics patients who are on anticonvulsants should have complete physical, neurologic, and mental status examinations as well as laboratory/diagnostic tests. Factors regarding ethnic populations are becoming more of a focus of attention regarding the pharmacodynamics, pharmacokinetics, and effect of P450 cytochrome enzyme systems for all medications including anticonvulsants.

Anticonvulsants may be prescribed for "off-label" use. Usually this involves the use of medication for other purposes than the FDA-approved use, but may also include doses or time frames/durations and dose schedules outside of the FDA-approved guidelines. According to Mossman (2009), "off-label prescribing is legal" and quotes material from the *Physician's Desk Reference* (PDR) explaining that once medications or products are FDA approved for marketing, they may be prescribed for patients or treatments "that are not included in approved labeling," and that federal statutes do "not limit or interfere with the authority of a health care practitioner to prescribe" approved medications or products "for any condition or disease." While this is true, it is acknowledged that healthcare providers can be found legally negligent "if their decision to use an off-label (medication, product) is sufficiently careless, imprudent (unwise), or unprofessional." The courts have also determined that off-label use does not require special informed consent different from standard informed consent (pp. 19–21). The psychiatric-mental health (PMH) nurse needs to be aware of typical use and doses of common psychotropic medications and keep current with literature, news, and scientific evidence related to psychotropic medications.

CLASSIFICATIONS/CATEGORIES

Anticonvulsants are classified as mood stabilizers in the treatment of bipolar disorders. The most commonly used anticonvulsants used as mood stabilizing agents are valproic acid (Depakote), carbamazepine (Tegretol), gabapentin (Neurontin), topiramate (Topamax), lamotrigine (Lamictal), oxcarbazepine (Trileptal), tigabine (Gabitril), and zonisamide (Zonegran).

PHARMACOLOGIC ACTIONS

Although the exact mechanism of action in the brain for anticonvulsants remains unknown, these drugs stabilize mood by providing relief from acute episodes of mania or depression or prevent them from occurring, and they do not worsen depression or mania or increase cycling. It is believed that anticonvulsants effect many actions in brain cells. These drugs have "anti-kindling" properties that help to decrease the sensitization of effected cells in the brain, making these cells less stimulated. Kindling is the process by which the brain becomes sensitized to having a chemical reaction to an event such as stress, injury, or drugs. The brain eventually seems to automatically re-spond in a dysfunctional manner in the absence of precipitating events (Stuart & Laraia, 2001, p. 592). At the cell membrane, anticonvulsants appear to act on ion channels, including sodium, potassium, and calcium channels, by reducing repetitive firing of action potentials in the nerves. This particular action specifically decreases the manic symptoms in bipolar disorders (Boyd, 2008, p. 118).

Anticonvulsants affect serum levels, as well as the following specific neurotrans-mitters in the brain:

- Norepinephrine
- GABA (gamma-aminobutyric acid) induces inhibitory action
- Dopamine
- Glutamate induces excitatory action

Carbamazepine (Tegretol)

Carbamazepine (Tegretol) is used as a first line of treatment for acute mania as well as for maintenance treatment for bipolar disorders. The typical dose of carbamazepine to treat acute mania is 600 to 1800 mg per day (Sadock & Sadock, 2008, p. 224). Peak plasma levels occur within 2 to 6 hours after administration, and peak therapeutic ef-fects occur within 10 days of administration. The therapeutic serum levels of carbam-azepine are from 8 to12 mcg/mL (Keltner, Schwecke, & Bostrom, 2007, p. 260). Carbamazepine is available in chewable form in doses of 100 mg, 200 mg; in sustained release tablets with doses of 100 mg, 200 mg, 400 mg; in sustained release capsules in doses of 100 mg, 200 mg, 300 mg; and in suspension form in a dose of 100 mg/5 mL (Wilson, Shannon, & Shields, 2009, p. 237).

Carbamazepine is a typical drug that absorbs in a different manner in relation to its makeup. The liquid form of this medication is absorbed more quickly than the tablet form, and it seems that food does not interfere in the absorption process. It is impor-tant to know that high doses affect the peak plasma levels causing risks for side-effects; therefore, carbamazepine should be given in divided doses two or three times a day. Since the liquid form of this medication is absorbed quickly, it can be given more fre-quently than tablet form. This drug is not recommended or should be used with cau-tion in clients who have heart conditions, blood disorders, bone-marrow depression, diabetic conditions, glaucoma, and generalized seizure disorder, as well as in pregnancy.

Side-effects

The most common side-effects are drowsiness, dizziness, ataxia, double vision, blurred vision, nausea, and fatigue or tiredness feelings. Less common side-effects include gastrointestinal upset and skin reactions. The most serious side-effect is agranulocytosis, in which there is a significant decrease in white blood cell count that does not return to normal. This drug can be lethal in low or higher doses (refer to the PDR or a nursing drug book for details).

Valproic Acid (Depakote, Valproat, Divalproex)

This drug has surpassed lithium in use for acute mania as it is effective not only on the manic phase of bipolar disorders, but also in schizoaffective disorders or with clients who are not responding to lithium; valproic acid is generally well-tolerated by clients. This drug also has anti-aggressive properties that help calm clients who exhibit frequent rage episodes. It is also used for long-term treatment along with other psychotropic medications. This drug is available in various forms, including regular capsules and sprinkle capsules in a 250 mg dose; delayed release tablets in 125 mg, 250 mg, 500 mg doses; sustained release tablets in a 500 mg dose; in syrup form in a 250 mg/5 mL dose; and in injection form in a 100 mg dose. Peak serum level occurs in about 1 to 4 hours. The liquid form absorbs more quickly and peaks in 15 minutes to 2 hours. Food does not reduce bioavailabilty of this drug (Boyd, 2008, p. 118).

The typical dose levels of valproic acid are 750 to 2500 mg per day. Therapeutic action occurs in 1 to 2 weeks with a goal of achieving blood levels of 50 to 120 mg/mL. This drug has little or no effect on cognition. Bioavailability of this drug is almost 100%, with 95% protein binding with a rapid onset. The therapeutic serum levels are from 50 to 115 mcg/mL (Keltner, Schwecke, & Bostrom, 2007, p. 260).

Side-effects

Common side-effects of valproic acid are gastrointestinal disturbances such as nausea, anorexia, vomiting, diarrhea, increased appetite and weight gain; neurologic disturbances such as headache, dizziness and ataxia, and tremors; and sedation. Blood disorders such as hematoma, thrombocytopenia with bruising, petechiae, and bleeding can occur. There is also transient hair loss called alopecia. The most serious adverse side-effects are pancreatitis and hepatic dysfunction, aplastic anemia, severe rash, agranulocytosis, and in rare cases cardiac problems as well as SIADH (inappropriate secretion of the diuretic hormone due to hyponatrimia (Boyd, 2008, p. 118)). Toxic symptoms may be seen within 1–3 hours of administration and include disturbances in the neuromuscular system such as dizziness, stupor, agitation, disorientation, and nystagmus; alterations in circulatory and respiratory systems such as tachycardia, hypotension or hypertension, cardiac shock, coma, and respiratory depression. Intake in higher doses can be lethal as this drug is absorbed rapidly, and gastric lavage may be ineffective depending on time of ingestion and delay in seeking help (Boyd, 2008, p. 118).

It is important to note that valproic acid can interfere in laboratory diagnostic testing, producing false positive results in the following situations: (1) positive ketenes in urine, (2) elevated AST, ALT, LDH, and serum alkaline phosphates, (3) prolonged bleeding time, and (4) altered thyroid function tests.

Gabapentin (Neurontin), Lamotrigine (Lamictal), Oxcarbazepine (Trileptal), and Topiramate (Topamax)

These drugs are relatively new and are becoming popular in the treatment of bipolar disorders. Although the safety and efficacy of these drugs has not been confirmed, use of these drugs in mixed state and rapid cycling types of bipolar disorders have been successful.

Gabapentin is used as a hypnotic agent due to its sedative effect. It also has anti-anxiety properties. It also helps in reducing craving effect of alcohol. It increases GABA activities by blocking sodium and calcium channels and inhibiting glutamate activity. Gabapentin is more effective in treating anxiety and agitation than carbamazepine or valproic acid. This drug is well absorbed but bioavailability decreases as dose is increased due to saturation of the neural amino acid membrane transport system in the gut. Gabapentin is available in tablet, capsule, and liquid solution forms. The use of gabapentin in older adults, children, and in pregnancy is contraindicated. The single dose should not exceed 1800 mg or not more than 5400 mg per day. Half life of 5–9 hours is reached in 2 days if administered three times a day. Gabapentin is not metabolized and is excreted in urine unchanged (Sadock & Sadock, 2008, p. 481). Gabapentin is available as 100–300 and 400 mg capsules and as 600 and 800 mg tablets.

Gabapentin has few or no side-effects; however, this drug should not be used in clients younger than 16 years old as it has a high risk of fostering development of Stevens-Johnson syndrome (Fontaine, 2009, p. 308). Discontinuation of this drug does not cause withdrawal symptoms, however, all anticonvulsants medications should be gradually tapered.

Lamotrigine (Lamictal) has approval (from the FDA in 2003) to be used as a prophylaxis treatment for bipolar disorders. This drug acts on the GABA system in the brain by inhibiting the firing action of neurons, blocking sodium as well as calcium channels, and inhibiting the action of glutamate. Lamotrigine can have, in rare cases, a serious side-effect that produces severe rashes within 2 to 8 weeks of starting this medication. This side-effect may also occur in clients taking lamotrigine and valproic acid in combination. The risk is higher in children for developing Stevens-Johnson syndrome (Fontaine, 2009, p. 308).

Oxcarbazepine (Trileptal) has a chemical structural formation that is similar to carbamazepine. This drug is the most commonly prescribed medication for bipolar disorders. Therapeutic serum levels are 15 to 35 mcg/mL for stabilization of mood (Keltner, Schwecke, & Bostrom, 2007). In terms of adverse effects, oxcarbazepine does not cause serious side-effects such as those associated with carbamazepine.

Topiramate (Topamax) has a mechanism of action that is similar to gabapentin. This is the only anticonvulsant that has a tendency to reduce weight. Topiramate affects CNS, GI, special senses, and overall body functions such as fatigue, speech problems, weight loss, decreased sweating, hypothermia in children, metabolic acidosis, somnolence, dizziness, ataxia, slow psychomotor activity, confusion, cognitive impairment, diminished memory, anxiety, depression, and anorexia. This drug can produce kidney stones, reduce digoxin levels, and induce acute myopia in rare cases; it can also cause glaucoma.

NURSING RESPONSIBILITIES AND IMPLICATIONS

See also Chapter 10, as well as **Table 15-1**, which follows.

Table 15-1   Specific Nursing Implications of Anticonvulsant Medications

(For other general nursing implications refer to the available nursing texts or drug books.)

Assessing therapeutic and side/ adverse effects	Specific nursing actions
1. Carbamazepine	• Refer to other nursing drug books for detailed information.
	• Assess vital signs every 8 hours, prior to medication administration, and as needed.

(continues)

Table 15-1   Specific Nursing Implications of Anticonvulsant Medications *(continued)*

Assessing therapeutic and side/ adverse effects	Specific nursing actions
	• Assess for anticonvulsant hypersensitivity syndrome (AHS). This syndrome rarely occurs; however, it can have a fatal outcome. AHS can occur any time within the first 12 weeks of initiation of anticonvulsants. The symptoms of AHS are fever, rash, and damage to internal organs, which can be treated with symptom-specific therapy. It is important for the nurse to stop the medication immediately if there are symptoms of AHS, document the assessment, and notify the physician or LIP.
	• Perform cardiovascular and neurologic assessments as well as a mental status examination on admission, every 8 hours, and as needed.
	• Assess elimination patterns and provide adequate fluid intake to prevent urinary retention or oliguria.
	• Obtain laboratory blood work for baseline data.
	• Monitor laboratory/diagnostic test results, report abnormal results to the LIP who ordered them and assess body system corresponding to abnormal test results.
	• Assess for signs of liver and other vital organ toxicity.
	• Assess for signs/symptoms of toxic syndromes and AHS.
	• Document all therapeutic and side/adverse effects.
	• Notify the LIP prescribing medication of side/adverse effects.
	• The liquid form of carbamazepine medication is absorbed more quickly than the tablet form, and food does not interfere in the absorption process.

(continues)

Table 15-1	Specific Nursing Implications of Anticonvulsant Medications *(continued)*

Assessing therapeutic and side/adverse effects	Specific nursing actions
	• It is important to know that high doses affect the peak plasma levels causing a risk for side-effects, therefore, carbamazepine should be given in divided doses such as two or three times a day; the liquid form of this medication is absorbed quickly; therefore, it can be given more frequently than tablet form. • This drug is not recommended or is to be used with caution in clients who have heart conditions, blood disorders, bone-marrow depression, diabetic conditions, glaucoma, and generalized seizure disorder, as well as in pregnancy. • Know the importance of baseline and periodical laboratory tests for CBCs, including platelets, reticulocytes, serum electrolytes, serum ion, liver functions, Bun, and a complete urine analysis.
Patient/family education (Permission must be obtained from the patient for family or friends to have information; if the patient has a guardian, permission must be obtained from the guardian for anyone else to have information.)	• Monitor for symptoms of side-effects of the carbamazepine that can occur in the beginning of the therapy. Side-effects usually seen are: drowsiness, dizziness, light headedness, ataxia, and gastric upset; however, if these symptoms persist for a longer time, notify physician or LIP for dose adjustment or further evaluation. • Hold the drug if there are signs of myelosuppression from a lab report on CBCs. • Monitor for toxicity that can occur even if serum concentrations are slightly above the therapeutic levels. • Monitor I&O for oliguria, fluid retention, and change in vital signs. • Monitor for confusion and agitation as these symptoms can be aggravated in older adults who have potential for fall injury. • Implement fall precautions such as side rails, supervise ambulation, and provide assistance during ADL.

(continues)

Table 15-1   Specific Nursing Implications of Anticonvulsant Medications *(continued)*

Assessing therapeutic and side/ adverse effects	Specific nursing actions
	• Keep clients under close medical supervision during treatment therapy.
	• Warn to discontinue medication and call physician immediately if client notices early signs of toxicity, AHS, or hematologic-related symptoms such as high fever, sore throat, unusual fatigue, and/or tendency to bruise, petechiae, or bleeding from nose and gums.
	• Avoid hazardous tasks that require alertness and coordination of mind and body due to feelings of drowsiness and dizziness as well experiencing ataxia or feeling of lack of muscle coordination during walking or picking up objects. Ataxia also has an effect on speech as well eye movements.
	• Change positions slowly and ask for help ambulating.
	• Initial sedation feeling and blurred vision will decrease as the body adjusts to the medication. If these symptoms continue/worsen report to LIP.
	• Avoid excessive sunlight due to photosensitivity reaction produced by the medication. Prevent skin sensitivity by applying sunscreen lotion with SPF of 12 or above for best results.
	• Avoid abrupt withdrawal of medication as such action can cause seizures or status epileptics.
	• Know that carbamazepine can alter the effectiveness of oral contraceptives.
	• Report immediately any cardiac symptoms (e.g., dizziness, syncope, palpitation, funny feeling in chest, difficulty breathing).
	• Explain common side-effects and ways to relieve dry mouth (e.g., increase fluid intake if not contraindicated, use ice chips, more frequent oral care, sugarless gum/candy).

(continues)

Table 15-1 Specific Nursing Implications of Anticonvulsant Medications *(continued)*	
Assessing therapeutic and side/ adverse effects	**Specific nursing actions**
	• Avoid caffeine (may increase agitation), CNS depressants including alcohol, narcotics, and other drugs (increased sedation and cardiovascular effects), CNS stimulants including drugs and amphetamine-like substances (increased cardiovascular effects, potentially life-threatening). • Teach signs of hepatoxicity and to report immediately (e.g., loss of appetite, abdominal or kidney pain, dark urine, jaundice, clay/light colored stools). • ECG/EKG testing prior to starting anticonvulsants is vital to get baseline data. • Periodic CBC, renal, liver function, and other laboratory tests will be needed including measuring therapeutic blood levels of some anticonvulsants (Keltner, Schwecke, & Bostrom, 2007, pp. 260–261). • Teach importance of nutrition and physical exercise to help balance weight gain. • Inform all healthcare providers of all medication taken.
2. Valproic acid (Depakote, Valproat, Divalproex)	• Obtain baseline data on required laboratory and other diagnostic tests. Obtain history of kidney disease, renal impairment, congenital metabolic disorder, HIV, hypoalbuminemia, and organic brain syndrome prior stating valproic acid. • Administer capsule or tablets whole and instruct patient to swallow the medication rather then chewing. For sprinkle form of medication, sprinkle entire contents of medication on soft food and ask patient to swallow without chewing the food. • Avoid use of carbonated drinks to dilute syrup form of medication as it will irritate the mucus membrane in the oral cavity. • Administer medication with food to avoid an adverse GI effect.

(continues)

Table 15-1	Specific Nursing Implications of Anticonvulsant Medications *(continued)*
Assessing therapeutic and side/ adverse effects	**Specific nursing actions**
	• Monitor for therapeutic effectiveness of the drug by monitoring serum levels of valproic acid. The therapeutic serum level of valproic acid ranges from 50 to 100 mcg/mL. • Monitor for alertness and symptoms of neural toxicity.
Patient/family education	• Remind client not to discontinue medication abruptly since, like other anticonvulsants, valporic acid can cause seizures. Client should consult physician before stopping this medication. • If client has diabetes, valporic acid can produce a false positive test for urine ketones. • Report to physician or LIP immediately if notice spontaneous bleeding or bruises in any part of the body. • Hold medication and notify physician or LIP for occurrence of rashes, jaundice, change in stool color, and vomiting or loose stools, as there is danger of fatal liver failure if these symptoms are ignored. • It is unsafe to use OTC drugs. Check with physician before using these drugs when on any anticonvulsants. • Inform dentist or doctor before any kind of surgery that client is taking valproic acid or other medications. • Carry medication identification card at all times. It needs to indicate medical diagnosis, list of medications, physician's name and contact number.
3. Gabapentin (Neurontin)	• Monitor patient for therapeutic effectiveness. The therapeutic effect may occur after several weeks following intake of gabapentin.

(continues)

Table 15-1	Specific Nursing Implications of Anticonvulsant Medications *(continued)*
Assessing therapeutic and side/adverse effects	**Specific nursing actions**
	• Monitor for safety since, like other anticonvulsants, gabapentin can cause alterations in vision, coordination, and concentration that may lead to falls or injuries during driving or performing hazardous tasks. (For other general nursing implications, refer to the available nursing texts or drug books.)
Patient and family education	• It is important to know about actual and potential side-effects as well as adverse effects of the medication. • Notify the physician or LIP of any change in neurologic or visual function, unusual bleeding or bruises in any part of the body. • Do not take gabapentin within 2 hours of intake of an antacid medication. • Be safe and do not drive or work with potentially hazardous tasks until physical status is stabilized or until drug responses are identified.
4. Lamotrigine (Lamictal)	• Monitor patient closely when on lamotrigine, as rash can develop that can lead to Stevens-Johnson syndrome, which can be fatal. Report to physician if rash is noticed. • Monitor plasma levels for therapeutic or adverse effect of lamotrigine. • Assess and document for worsening of symptoms and/or suicidal ideation. Notify physician and obtain order for withholding this medication for the safety of the patient. • Monitor for other adverse reactions or drug interactions when lamotrigine is used with other medications such as valproic acid.
Patient/family education	• If client notices rash in the skin, they should stop lamotrigine immediately and consult their physician at once.

(continues)

Table 15-1 Specific Nursing Implications of Anticonvulsant Medications *(continued)*

Assessing therapeutic and side/adverse effects	Specific nursing actions
	• Contact physician if any of the following are noticed: ataxia or muscle incardination, change in visual function such as blurred vision or diplopia, fever or flu-like symptoms, or sore throat. • Maintain safety and do not drive or perform hazardous activity. • Always protect skin from sunlight as the drug can cause sunburn. • Have regular ophthalmologic exams to detect any visual changes. • Do not stop lamotrigine abruptly as it can lead to seizure.
5. Oxcarbazepine (Trileptal)	• After initiation of oxcarbazepine, monitor patient closely for signs and symptoms of hyponatremia such as nausea, generalized weakness, headache, lethargic and confused look. • Monitor patient for any alternation in CNS, such as excessive sleepiness, fatigue, cognitive impairment, impairment in speech or language, and alteration in mobility causing imbalance and lack of coordination. • Implement fall precautions; conduct fall assessment screening weekly; document the result. • Periodically monitor serum sodium as well as thyroid function levels. • Monitor serum levels for therapeutic effectiveness.
Patient/family education	• Consult physician immediately if any of the following occur: dizziness, drowsiness, headache, weakness, double vision, nausea, vomiting, or problems with coordination. • To maintain safety, avoid use of alcohol or any CNS depressant medication. • Avoid potential hazardous activities until physiologic response of the drug is identified.

(continues)

Table 15-1	Specific Nursing Implications of Anticonvulsant Medications *(continued)*
Assessing therapeutic and side/ adverse effects	**Specific nursing actions**
	• Be careful when using oral contraceptives because the drug causes contraceptives to be ineffective; look into other methods.
6. Topiramate (Topamax)	• Monitor mental status for any cognitive impairment. Document the finding of cognitive impairment and notify physician if significant impairment is detected in cognition. • Periodically monitor lab report for CBC, Hgb, and Hct.
Patient/family education	• Like any other anticonvulsant, do not stop topiramate abruptly. • Drink at least 6–8 glasses of water each day to reduce the risk for kidney stones. • Maintain safety as topiramate can cause sedation, which can be hazardous for driving or operating machinery. • Do not use alcohol or other CNS depressants while on topiramate. • Be careful when using oral contraceptives as the drug causes contraceptives to be ineffective. Look into other alternatives.

REFERENCES

Boyd, M. A. (2008). *Psychiatric nursing: Contemporary practice* (4th ed.). Philadelphia, PA: Wolters-Kluwer Health/Lippincott, Williams, & Wilkins.

Fontaine, K. (2009). *Mental health nursing* (6th ed.). Upper Saddle River, NJ: Pearson Education, Inc.

Keltner, N. L., Schwecke, L. H., & Bostrom, C. E. (2007). *Psychiatric Nursing* (5th ed.). St. Louis, MO: Mosby/Elsevier.

Mossman, D. (2009). Why off-label isn't off base. *Current psychiatry online 8*(2). Retrieved from: www.currentpsychiatry.com/article-pages.asp?AID=7305&UID=131372

Sadock, B. J., & Sadock, V. A. (2008). *Kaplan & Sadock's concise textbook of clinical psychiatry* (3rd ed.). Philadelphia, PA: Lippincott, Williams, & Wilkins.

Stahl (2008). *Stahl's essential psychopharmacology* (3rd ed.). New York, NY: Cambridge University Press.

Stuart, G. W., & Laraia, M. T. (2001). *Principles and Practice of psychiatric nursing* (7th ed.). St. Louis, MO: Mosby, Inc.

Wilson, B. A., Shannon, M. T., & Shield, K. M. (2008). *Prentice Hall Nurse's Drug Guide 2009*. Upper Saddle River, NJ: Prentice Hall.

SUGGESTED READINGS

American Psychological Association (APA) (2007). *APA dictionary of psychology*. Washington, DC: Author.

Antai-Otong, D. (2004). *Psychiatric emergencies: How to accurately assess and manage the patient in crisis.* Eau Claire, WI: PESI HealthCare, Inc.

Antai-Otong, D. (2009). *Psychiatric emergencies: How to accurately assess and manage the patient in crisis* (2nd ed.). Eau Claire, WI: PESI HEALTHCARE, LLC.

Bezchlibnyk-Butler, K. Z., & Jeffries, J. J. (2005). *Clinical handbook of psychotropic drugs* (15th ed.). Ashland, OH: Hogrefe & Huber.

Evans, J. (Jul., 2008). All antipsychotics to get warnings about elderly. *Clinical Psychiatry News, 36*(7), 9.

Fontaine, K. L., & Fletcher, J. S. (2003). *Mental health nursing* (5th ed.). Upper Saddle River, NJ: Pearson Education, Inc.

Nihart, M. (2007). Psychopharmacology update. Psychiatric Nursing Conference, New Orleans, LA.

Nursing 2010 drug handbook: 30th anniversary edition. (2010). Philadelphia, PA: Wolters-Kluwer/ Lippincott, Williams, & Wilkins.

Townsend, M. C. (2009). *Psychiatric mental health nursing: Concepts of care in evidence-based practice* (6th ed.). Philadelphia, PA: F. A. Davis.

Varcarolis, E. M., & Halter, M. J. (2010). *Foundations of psychiatric mental health nursing: A clinical approach* (6th ed.). St. Louis, MO: Saunders, Elsevier.

Crisis Intervention Skills

CHAPTER 16

Psychiatric Emergencies

Kim A. Jakopac

Psychiatric emergencies encompass a very broad area of situations, including people in overwhelming crises or psychological distress, impulsive behavior, intentional or unintentional suicide attempts, behavior that is dangerous or violent toward others including domestic violence and abuse and rape; exacerbation of psychiatric illnesses, adverse reactions to psychiatric or other medications, medical crisis manifesting signs similar to psychiatric illnesses, acute/severe anxiety states, and alcohol/substance abuse. These situations involve alterations in thoughts, mood, and behaviors of individuals requiring immediate psychological, and in many cases medical, interventions (Sadock & Sadock, 2005, pp. 2442, 2453; APA, 2007, p. 524). General functioning may be severely impaired as well as the ability to assume personal responsibility and act competently (Boyd, 2008, p. 208) (see also sections on NMS in Chapter 13 and serotonin syndrome in Chapter 14).

Previous chapters in this text deal with crisis situations and interventions associated with depression, suicide, the manic phase of bipolar disorders, severe anxiety, hallucinations, schizophrenia, assaultive behavior, chemical dependency/dual diagnosis, and psychotropic medications. As previously stated, "Suicide is the leading cause of death in psychiatric hospitals . . . 5 to 6% occur in inpatient units" (Lynch, Howard, El-Mallakh, & Matthews, 2008, pp. 47, 50). Depression and substance abuse are two of the greatest risk factors for suicide, but people who are extremely anxious, agitated, impulsive or in a manic state; feel overwhelmed; hear voices telling them to harm themselves (psychosis); have difficulty expressing feelings of anger; have terminal illnesses; declining health; or are in chronic pain also are at high risk (Varcarolis & Halter, 2010, pp. 548–549; APA, 2007, p. 907; Sadock & Sadock, 2005, p. 3268). Many people who attempt suicide do not have a diagnosed psychiatric problem, but are in great emotional pain and just want the pain to end, similarly to people who suffer physical pain (Varcarolis & Halter, 2010, p. 548). Psychiatric emergency triage is included in both the first (2004) and second (2009) editions of *Psychiatric Emergencies: How to Accurately Assess and Manage the Patient in Crisis* by Antai-Otong. This chapter will focus primarily on crisis intervention, and subsequent chapters will focus on domestic violence and abuse and disaster situations.

According to Sadock & Sadock (2005), "decreased hospitalization pursuant to advances in clinical psychopharmacology and restrictions on reimbursement of psychiatrists for chronic care of patients has necessitated that all psychiatrists become expert in the treatment of psychiatric emergencies in general hospitals and mental health centers" (p. 2453). If this is true for physicians, it also is true for psychiatric-mental health (PMH) nurses and nurses working in general hospitals and community outpatient areas. "Violence may be the cause of the psychiatric emergency or a symptom of a patient presenting with a biological or psychological disorder that requires emergency care. Self-destructive behavior ranges from overtly suicidal behavior to subtle forms of self-inflicted harm, repeated accidents, and drug and alcohol abuse," or the violence could be caused by others, including domestic violence and abuse, or as the result of criminal acts (Sadock & Sadock, 2005, p. 2454). Psychiatric emergencies can occur in any setting, and the people involved may not be established clients. The information in this text may be adapted to any setting.

CRISIS

The term crisis may be defined as a state in which a person perceives a real or imagined obstacle to their ability to achieve important life goals or experiences significant stress (i.e., a threat to their well-being, safety, or security). "A crisis is not a pathological state, but a struggle for emotional balance" (Varcarolis & Halter, 2010, p. 544), but pathology may be a predisposing factor, or the crisis may be involved in the development of a pathologic condition. The Holmes-Rahe Social Readjustment Scale is an instrument used to measure stress-producing life events. It includes many common stressors (e.g., death of a spouse or close family member, financial changes, changes in living conditions, divorce, etc.) with a point value assigned to each life event (Lange & Shank, 2005, pp. 5, 8). The higher the score, the more stress an individual is experiencing, thus increasing the risk for physical or mental health problems. Due to internal tension and conflict, the person may feel anxious, distraught, overwhelmed, angry, shocked, grief stricken or demonstrate use of ego defense mechanisms such as denial (see Appendix A). There are various types of crisis, including situational or dispositional, maturational or developmental, adventitious or traumatic, psychopathological or psychiatric (Boyd, 2008, pp. 803–804; Townsend, 2009, pp. 206–209; Varcarolis & Halter, 2010, pp. 530–532). Crisis can occur in any setting, and the person in crisis may not be an identified or established client. This information can be adapted to any setting.

Not all circumstances develop into a full-blown crisis. "Crises tend to be time limited, generally lasting no more than a few months; the duration depends on the stressor and the individual's perception of and response to the stressor" (Townsend, 2009, p. 206). According to Varcarolis & Halter (2010), a crisis may resolve "within 4 to 6 weeks" (p. 533). Much depends on a person's coping abilities and skills; available resources including social support, mental and physical health, finances, access to what is needed, timing of intervention, and the ability to effectively use all of these to adapt. It has been said that *both* danger in the form of an overwhelming threat *and* opportunity to learn new coping skills and advance to a new level of development are present in crisis (Aguilera, 1998, p. 1; Sadock & Sadock, 2005, pp. 2458–2459; Townsend, 2009, p. 205). A crisis can happen to anyone at any time, and developing the ability to help a person through a crisis is valuable for use in any type of crisis situation. A person in crisis is vulnerable (representing danger) and usually very willing to accept help, open to new ideas, and to developing positive coping strategies (representing opportunity). A little aid, focused properly, can achieve greater results than more extensive help when that person is not so emotionally vulnerable. It can also prevent the need for more intense and costly interventions later if the crisis is not resolved.

ROLE OF THE PMH NURSE

The role of the PMH nurse is "to provide a framework of support systems that guide the patient (person) through the crisis and facilitate the development and use of positive coping skills. The nurse must be acutely aware that a person in crisis may be at high risk for suicide or homicide" (Boyd, 2008, p. 806). In previous chapters in this text on major depression, suicide, and bipolar disorder in the acute manic phase, information was provided regarding The Joint Commission (2008, NPSG.15.01.01 and NPSG.15.01.01 EP 3) requirements related to suicide risk reduction as one of the national patient safety goals in psychiatric-mental health settings, general hospitals, emergency rooms, ambulatory clinics, and other settings. Information about the availability of a crisis hotline or other resources is also required for any patients identified as being at risk for suicide (Joint Commission, Accreditation Programs, 2008). As previously stated in this chapter and Chapter 9, there are many other conditions that increase a person's risk for suicide including use of alcohol or other chemicals.

The ability to provide a necessary framework, manage care, and facilitate positive coping and skill development and use begins with careful assessment of many areas including risk for suicide or homicide, cognitive processes, and coping behaviors. Clients may also need medical interventions and physical nursing care in addition to psychosocial nursing care. The PMH nurse will need to provide emotional support, resource referrals, provide for or arrange physical care, and in some cases may need to act as a liaison among medical, psychiatric, and community agencies (see also Peplau's nurse roles in Chapter 1). The most successful overall client outcomes are resolution of the immediate crisis, the ability to function as independently as possible during the crisis time, becoming more empowered, and returning to their precrisis level of functioning, or possibly higher, with new insight and coping abilities (Aguilera, 1998, p. 24; Townsend, 2009, p. 209).

CRISIS THEORY AND THEORISTS

There are many relevant crisis theorists who have proposed theories, models, frameworks, paradigms, and interventions, including Lindemann, Caplan, Lazarus, Seyle,

Aguilera, Stuart, and Roberts. Some of their work dates back to the 1950s, but is still very useful and relevant to the PMH nurse's understanding of crisis prevention, development, intervention, and resolution. In the 1950s, Erich Lindemann focused on adaptation to time-limited crises, including catastrophic deaths and involving rapid, psychotherapeutic intervention to help people make changes in their lives to achieve a psychological sense of well-being (Lange & Shank, 2005, p. 7; Sadock & Sadock, 2005, p. 2454; Varcarolis & Halter, 2011, p. 529). In 1964, Gerald Caplan identified four phases of crisis events and use of problem-solving techniques stimulated by a threat to self-concept experienced as anxiety. If the usual coping or defense responses fail, disorganization occurs, leading to "trial-and-error" attempts to solve problems. If trial-and-error methods fail, relief is sought by withdrawing or fleeing the situation, or compromising or redefining the situation. Finally, if the problem or crisis remains unresolved, people become overwhelmed, which leads to personality disorganization, confusion, depression, suicide, or violence towards others (Lange & Shank, 2005, p. 7; Boyd, 2008, p. 803; Varcarolis & Halter, 2011, p. 532).

In 1966, Richard Lazarus focused on the psychological aspects of stress and the relationship between what is happening in the surrounding environment and people's perception or "appraisal" of what is happening. Lazarus was concerned with how people respond psychologically, while Hans Selye focused more on physiologic responses to stress occurring in three stages (Keltner, Schwecke, & Bostrom, 2007, p. 48). People become anxious as a response to how important or significant they perceive–appraise the threat is to their well-being. Lazarus saw "cognitive appraisal" and problem solving as key aspects of his proposed interactional model. Cognitive appraisals include judgments people make about situations/events and the assignment of personal meaning to these. The assigned meanings and potential effects lead to evaluation of ways to respond and include possible strategies, resources, support, personal values, and beliefs. Particular solutions may be effective, but they may conflict with personal values and belief systems. There are times when people cannot effectively cope, and this may be due to inadequate social support and resources. Preferred methods of coping may be ineffective or lead to further problems. If stressful situations or problems are not resolved, they can lead to physical or mental illness. Changing people's perceptions–appraisals and problem-solving techniques are ways to increase effective coping and intervene in crisis (Keltner, Schwecke, & Bostrom, 2007, pp. 35, 48–49).

In 1998, Donna Aguilera focused on stages of problem solving with a paradigm of balancing factors—disequilibrium vs equilibrium. Stressful events including biologic and psychosocial challenge the normal state of equilibrium causing temporary disequilibrium. Disequilibrium is uncomfortable and leads people to attempt to return to the more comfortable state of equilibrium. One or more balancing factors must be present to resolve problems, regain equilibrium, and avoid the development of a crisis. Balancing factors include realistic perception of events, adequate or adaptive coping mechanisms, and situational support. Distorted perception or the absence of other balancing factors decreases the ability to regain equilibrium, leading to continuing disequilibrium and eventually to a crisis (Aguilera, 1998, pp. 29–33; Lange & Shank, 2005, pp. 8–9; Townsend, 2009, p. 205; Varcarolis & Halter, 2010, p. 529; Medtrng.com, 2010).

Also how people view themselves and their ability to successfully master their environment influences attempts to cope with or solve problems. "According to Bandura and others (1977), the strength of the individual's conviction in his (her) own effectiveness in overcoming or mastering a problematical situation determines whether coping behavior is even attempted. People fear and avoid stressful, threatening situations that they believe exceed their ability to cope. They behave with assurance in those situations where they judge themselves able to manage, and they expect eventual success. It is the perceived ability to master that can influence the choice of coping behaviors, as well as the persistence used once one is chosen" (Aguilera, 1998, p. 39). Belief in personal efficacy and personal locus-of-control are important factors in crisis intervention and resolution not only for clients, but for healthcare professionals as well (see also Chapter 5).

In 2005, Gail Stuart proposed a stress adaption model beginning with predisposing factors, precipitating stressors, how people appraise stressors, possession of coping resources, emergence of coping mechanisms (i.e., problem, cognitive, or emotion focused) resulting in a continuum of responses with adaptive responses at one end of the continuum and maladaptive responses at the opposite end. There are also four treatment stages: crisis, acute, maintenance, and health promotion (Stuart & Laraia, 2005, pp. 65–68, 71). Also in 2005, Albert Roberts developed the following seven-stage model of crisis intervention:

- Planning and conducting crisis assessment including lethality measures
- Rapidly establishing rapport and relationship
- Identifying major problems including what precipitated the crisis
- Dealing with feelings
- Generating and exploring alternatives
- Developing a plan of action
  - Crisis resolution
- Formulating a follow-up plan and agreement

(Townsend, 2009, pp. 209–211; Varcarolis & Halter, 2011, pp. 533–540).

It is interesting how older and newer concepts and models are still applicable and can be used with the nursing process. Obviously prevention is the best strategy both in terms of human and resource costs. Recognition and early intervention is the next best strategy to help prevent acute stress disorders (ASDs); posttraumatic stress disorder (PTSD); other chronic, debilitating psychiatric or other medical illnesses; injury, or death. Common components in crisis theory include predisposing risk factors; precipitating factors (stressors or stimuli); perception of stressors, events, situations, or circumstances; resources including availability and access; coping mechanisms; adaptive or maladaptive coping responses including cognitive, psychological, emotional, spiritual, behavioral, physiologic/biologic; safety needs; and return to at least precrisis functioning or regression (see **Table 16-1**).

Table 16-1 Some Common Components in Crisis Theory	
Predisposing risk factors	May be biologic, psychological, and sociocultural in nature. Biologic predisposing factors may include physical and psychiatric-mental health conditions or illnesses; medical treatments and medications; genetics, chemical abuse/dependency, nutritional status, or exposure to toxins or allergens. Psychological predisposing factors may include personality, self-concept, self-esteem, psychological defenses, past experiences, mental health problems, emotional state, self-motivation, or locus of control/sense of control over outcome/fate. Sociocultural factors may be sex/gender, age, socioeconomic status, education, socialization experiences, social integration or relatedness, or values and belief systems.
Precipitating (stressors or stimuli) factors	May be anything that challenges, threatens, or puts demands on the person requiring additional energy, attention, and resources and producing frustration, tension, anxiety, or stress. Precipitating factors may occur in the person's internal or external environment. The number of precipitating factors and time frame including when they occur, how far apart they occur, and the duration are important variables involved in how a person responds to crisis.

(continues)

Table 16-1 Some Common Components in Crisis Theory *(continued)*	
Perception	Is defined as the process by which we become aware of objects, events, and relationships through our senses. Perception is further defined as involving the activities of observing, recognizing, and discriminating, which in turn helps us organize, interpret and give meaning to information or stimuli (APA, 2007, p. 683). How a person perceives stimuli, information, events, circumstances, situations, people, behavior, or words greatly determines the impact these all have on that person and the response they will have.
Resources	May include a wide variety of items including, but not limited to, physical, mental, and spiritual health; social support, finances, and material possessions; health insurance and other insurances; transportation, healthy environment including an absence of toxins, crime, disease; social status; and education including literacy. A person may have abundant resources, but may not be able to properly access or utilize them in ways that provide the most benefit.
Coping mechanisms	Are conscious or unconscious adjustments (adaptations) a person uses in stressful situations to decrease the level of stress or anxiety and relieve tension. Coping strategies are thoughts or actions/behavior responses a person uses consciously or unconsciously to deal with stressful, anxiety or tension producing situations or change the reaction to such situations. Coping styles are the ways or manner in which a person deals with problems or stress (APA, 2007, p. 232) such as direct or indirect. Coping mechanisms, strategies, and styles can be adaptive (healthy, positive, constructive, enhancing) or maladaptive (unhealthy, negative, destructive).

Source: Aguilera, 1998, pp. 35–37; Stuart & Laraia, 2005, pp. 65–66.

According to Humanistic Psychological Theory, which relates to human needs and motivation, Abraham Maslow included feeling and being safe as part of the basic human needs for survival. Not only did he include "shelter from harm," but also having a "predictable social and physical environment" (Boyd, 2008, pp. 60–61). When a person's actual or perceived ability to be safe is threatened, anxiety, tension, fear, or stress occurs, and the person responds in ways designed to preserve, defend, or regain that safety. If these responses are not adequate, or if resources or the access and ability to use resources effectively are not adequate, disequilibrium may occur, resulting in crisis. Crisis intervention assists the person to regain equilibrium and prevent crisis (Aguilera, 1998, pp. 1, 32–33; Lange & Shank, 2005, p. 9; Townsend, 2009, pp. 205–206). Crisis intervention techniques are used in the assessment and management of the common components of the crisis theories previously listed.

Returning to at least a precrisis level of functioning is vital, or else regression in part or all areas of life may occur. The worst client outcomes would include the development of serious, chronic, long-term mental or physical disability, suicide, or homicide (Aguilera, 1998, p. 1; Townsend, 2009, p. 205). The best client outcomes would include developing new insights, finding spiritual meaning and experiencing personal growth, learning new information, learning new adaptive coping strategies, returning to a precrisis level functioning or higher, moving forward in life more prepared for future problem solving, and the ability to help others in crisis (Townsend, 2009, p. 206).

GRIEF RESPONSES

Grief or mourning is a normal response to the death of a loved one or someone else we feel a close relationship with. It also occurs when a person experiences any significant loss that is life-changing, such as loss of or change in health due to the effects of an illness, including terminal illness. The person grieves the loss of a previous level of functioning or inability to work at all or in the same type of employment. Sudden or drastic changes in financial status, loss of a home due to fire or a natural disaster, unplanned need to relocate, or divorce can also cause grief responses. Parents not only grieve the loss of a child through death, but the loss of the future they had hoped for a child diagnosed with serious illness.

In 1969, Elisabeth Kubler-Ross proposed that individuals experience grief in stages through the process of dying. Other more recent theorists (e.g., Bowlby, Engel, Shear, Stroebe & Schut; Neimeyer, Gamino & Sewell; Parkes) have developed models of mourning that include tasks similar to what Kubler-Ross initially proposed. These stages or tasks may be applied to any situation that stimulates a grief response. Grief or mourning is thought to be "a complex, individual, culturally embedded process of accepting the death (or loss), confronting the painful experience, constructing an identity and a life in a transformed environment, and finding an enduring relationship with the deceased, based not on physical presence, but on accurate memory" (Varcarolis & Halter, 2010, p. 716). In some cases grief can precipitate a crisis situation or be a predisposing factor. People may vacillate between stages or tasks, especially in the earlier stages, and the time it takes to progress through the entire process is very individualized. The grief stages typically include the following:

- Denial/shock and disbelief, somatic distress, guilt, preoccupation
- Anger
- Bargaining
- Anticipatory grief
- Acceptance

(Christiansen, 2009, pp. 55–58; Varcarolis & Halter, 2010, pp. 716–717)

CRISIS INTERVENTION

Crisis intervention is not a replacement for long-term counseling or therapy, but uses tools that can provide relief to someone experiencing the trauma of an unexpected critical event. According to the American Nurses Association (ANA), "Crisis intervention is a short term therapeutic process that focuses on the rapid resolution of an immediate crisis or emergency using available personnel, family, and/or environmental resources" (Varcarolis & Halter, 2010, p. 529). Helping people through a crisis can be a rewarding experience, but it is also very challenging and requires special skills that are essential not only for PMH nursing, but all areas of nursing. Crisis intervention offers immediate help needed for the client to reestablish equilibrium (Aguilera, 1998, p. 1).

The legal–ethical principles of least restrictive alternative doctrine, autonomy, beneficence, fidelity, justice, nonmaleficence; and civil rights including confidentiality, bioethics, and safety concerns also apply in crisis situations (see also Chapters 9 and 13). There is an additional legal–ethical responsibility that may occur in the context of crisis intervention referred to as the legal standard of "duty-to-warn" resulting from the *Tarasoff v The Regents of the University of California* lawsuit. In that case, a male student confided to his therapist that he was going to kill a female student. He did not give her actual name, but she was easily identified. The therapist notified campus police, who detained and questioned him, but released him because he "appeared rational." He killed the female student shortly after she returned from a trip to South America. The parents successfully sued. "The duty to protect endangered third parties is now a national standard of practice, although some jurisdictions still hold that any disclosure of confidential information is a violation of the patient's rights" (Keltner, Schwecke, & Bostrom, 2007, p. 54). The nurse is responsible for documenting and reporting the information to the psychiatrist, who will make the determination of whether or not the situation meets the duty-to-warn criterion. If it does, the psychiatrist or their designee (e.g., social worker, psychologist) will notify the threatened individual.

As clear an understanding as possible must be obtained of the presenting crisis or problem in the context of the person's life to be able to work toward the best possible resolution (Sadock & Sadock, 2005, p. 2454; eHow.com—crisis intervention, 2010, crisis intervention). This may be very difficult, especially in circumstances where the person's speech does not make sense (e.g., disorganized thoughts or speech, hallucinations, delusions, acute/severe anxiety, panic, flashbacks, mania, delirium, dementia, profound depression, amnesia, influence of alcohol/substances). Safety is the highest priority. Using core skills such as the therapeutic use of self including self-awareness and avoidance of negatively influencing the situation with the nurse's own anxiety due to energy transfer or countertransference; and therapeutic communication skills including active listening (attending skills), empathy, positive regard, acceptance, being nonjudgmental, and genuineness help the PMH nurse obtain information about and understanding of the true nature of the crisis as well as the life context in which it is occurring; make decisions regarding the person's safety, and help avoid escalation of the situation (eHow.com—crisis intervention, 2010). Communication is critical and occurs on two levels: content (facts) and emotion (emotional response to facts); people typically seek connection with others when feeling fear.

Crisis intervention begins with initiating rapport in the formation of a therapeutic alliance or therapeutic nurse–client relationship by communicating that the nurse cares about the person. It is through communication, empathy, and the formation of a therapeutic alliance or therapeutic nurse–client relationship that trust can be built and used therapeutically. In crisis situations there is less time available to do this and also obtain necessary information—referred to as the "Big Picture" by Christiansen (2009)—than in other client encounters due to the urgency of the situation (p. 10).

Phases/Stages of Crisis Intervention

Crisis intervention may occur in phases or stages that lend themselves to the nursing process. During this process, if medical intervention—including medication—is required, it will need to be administered before proceeding (Lange & Shank, 2005, p. 10). The PMH nurse will not be acting alone, but in conjunction with other members of the treatment or healthcare team (see **Table 16-2** and Chapters 3–5, 7, 9, 12).

Table 16-2   Phases of Crisis Intervention

Phase 1: Assessment

- Begin to develop rapport and a therapeutic alliance/nurse–client relationship by remaining calm, communicating that you care about the person and providing comfort by therapeutic use of self, active listening, attending skills, empathy, and emotional support.

  "Hi. My name's _____. I'm a nurse. You sound upset. I want to help you. What's going on?"

  "You sound like you are hurting."

  "It's okay to cry."

  "Everybody messes up sometimes."

  "Anger is a normal emotion."

  "Fear is a normal emotion."

  Note: *If an interpreter is needed, you must wait until the interpreter arrives to begin an interview unless it is obvious that* **emergency medical treatment is needed immediately.**

- Obtain a *brief, clear* description of the crisis situation or event and when it occurred (clarification of information will occur throughout the assessment and in Phase 3 as needed).

  "It sounds like a difficult situation. How are you feeling?"

  "When did it start?"

  "Then what happened?"

  "What do you think triggered this?"

  Note: *If there are minor children, disabled, or elderly family members this person is providing care for, are they with someone safe, or do you have to contact a social worker to evaluation the situation?*

- Determine how life-threatening the situation is and the need for medical intervention.

  "You sound really sad" or "You said you 'just can't handle it anymore.' Are you thinking about suicide?"

  "Are you thinking of harming someone?"

  "Do you have any medical or mental health conditions?" or "Are you under a doctor's care for any reason?"

- **Avoid** giving false reassurances such as "Everything will be all right." If the result is not "all right" the client will be angry and stop trusting you. **Instead,** reiterate your desire to listen and help.

  "I care about you and will listen." or "I want to help you."

(continues)

Table 16-2	Phases of Crisis Intervention *(continued)*

- Guide the client through the assessment process, which may at times require being direct or firm to help the client focus/refocus.

  "Stay with me."

  "Tell me more about..."

  "What about...?"

  "I'm here."

  "Yes, go on...".

  Note: During the assessment the nurse may need to repeat requests for information and directions in a calm, firm voice as many times as needed like a "broken record"—specific information to be able to treat/intervene, send emergency services.

- What is the client's perception of what is happening? Keep focused on one thing at a time.

  "What do you think is happening?"

  "What do you think caused him to act that way?"

  "How has this been affecting your life?"

- Assess the client's mental and physical status including predisposing risk factors.

  "How has the rest of your life been going?" or *"How has your health been?"*

- Assess the potential for suicide/homicide including thoughts, plans, means, lethality of means, access, and ability or lack of ability to contract at least verbally not to act. (Also, if the person in crisis is calling rather than being physically present, ask if they are alone or if someone else is there/nearby.) (see also Chapter 9).

  "Have you thought about harming yourself or someone else?"

  "What is happening that makes suicide (homicide) look like a solution?"

  "Help is available. Let us help you."

  "Do you have a plan to harm yourself or someone else?"

  "Would you tell someone if you were thinking of killing yourself?"

  "Do you have access to a gun, knives, ropes, pills?"

  "Can you refrain from acting on your thoughts or plans?"

  Note: *If unable to contract at least verbally not to harm self or others, then initiate 1:1 observation/COs, remove potentially harmful objects/contraband, and report to physician, document.*

  Note: *If the person is threatening or planning to harm someone else, a psychiatrist should be notified immediately to determine who to warn—duty to warn/Tarosoff ruling.*

(continues)

Table 16-2   Phases of Crisis Intervention *(continued)*

- Are there any precipitating (stressors, stimuli) factors?

  "What do you think triggered these feelings/reactions?"

  "Has anything else happened to you recently?"

  "What changed?"

  "What led to walking out on your spouse?"

  "What do you think was 'the last straw'?"

- What caused the person to seek help at this time rather than wait (or what is different this time)?

  "What led (caused) you to seek help now?" or *"What's different now?"*

- What is this person's ability to cope; what coping strategies has he/she been using and their effect?

  "What do you usually do to cope?"

  "How have you been coping with this? Is it working?"

- Assess if chemical abuse/dependency is involved.

  "How much are you drinking?"

  "What drugs have you been using to cope?"

  "When did you last use alcohol, drugs, or prescription pain pills to cope?"

- What is the person's perception of their own personal strengths and limitations (i.e., positive vs. negative qualities)?

  "What do you think your personal strengths are? How can you use these now?"

  "Do you think you have limitations?"

- Do they have past experience dealing with similar situations that they can draw on now?

  "Has something like this ever happened to you before? What did you do?"

  "How have you handled crisis before? What worked then?"

- Does this person have a social support system?

  "Is there someone you can call?"

  "Do you want me to call someone for you?"

  "Do you have any family, friends, neighbors, spiritual advisor, church members in the area?"

  "Who do you turn to for support?"

  "Who do you feel close to or comfortable talking to?"

  "Who do you ask for advice when you need it?"

(continues)

Table 16-2   Phases of Crisis Intervention *(continued)*

- Are there any additional cultural or spiritual factors that need to be considered?

    "Is there any spiritual/religious or cultural factors we should be aware of when providing treatment or help?"

    "Are you able to find comfort or strength from your spiritual or cultural beliefs?"

- Are there any legal problems, charges that have a bearing on this situation?

- What other resources does this person have?

    "Do you have a safe place to live?"

    "Do you have enough food and water?"

    "Are your utilities (electric, gas, phone) working?"

    "Do you have a job or are you unemployed?"

    "Do you have transportation to home, work, doctor visits, grocery store, etc.?"

    "Do you have health insurance?"

- Does this person have access to their resources and the ability to fully utilize them or need assistance with this?

    "Are you in contact with your family or other support people?"

    "Did you bring any identification, your purse or wallet with you?"

    "Did you drive yourself here or do you need a ride back home?"

    "Is there someone you can stay with after you leave here?"

    "Do you know how to contact your health insurance company? Do you have to have someone call for precertification for treatment? Do you know how to use your medical card?"

- What was the person's precrisis level of functioning?

    "How were you functioning before this happened?"

    "Were you able to take care of your personal, family, work/school responsibilities?"

- Are there any obstacles to successful crisis resolution and if so, how can these be circumvented (e.g., language barriers, literacy problems, lack of basic resources, unstable psychiatric or other medical illnesses, cultural factors including meaning/word connotation, spiritual/religious factors)?

- Document.

- Analysis of the information obtained is performed and possible nursing diagnoses identified.

(Aguilera, 1998, pp. 29–31, 35–38; Boyd, 2008, p. 810; Christiansen, 2009, pp. 8–22; Townsend, 2009, p. 209; Varcarolis & Halter, 2010, pp. 532–536; GP-Training.net, 2010; eHow.com—crisis intervention, 2010.)

(Phase 1 corresponds to Stages I–III of Roberts's Seven-Stage Crisis Intervention Model)

(continues)

Table 16-2   Phases of Crisis Intervention *(continued)*

Phase 2: Planning

In the planning phase, appropriate nursing diagnoses are chosen (refer to NANDA–I Diagnoses Used in Psychiatric Disorders in O'Brien, Kennedy, and Ballard, 2008, pp. 552-557; Jakopac & Patel, 2009, pp. 241–242, 251–252, 261, 273–274; Townsend, pp. 212–217; Varcarolis & Halter, 2010, pp. 542–544). Client centered outcomes/goals and interventions are also part of the planning phase.

Outcomes/goals for the client include:

- Remain safe
- Demonstrate an ability to form a therapeutic alliance with the PMH nurse
- Accept offered assistance
- Engage in problem-solving activities
- Explore possible alternations in perceptions and thinking patterns
- Collaborate in the formation of and commit to a plan
- Achieve resolution of the immediate crisis
- Be able to function as independently as possible during the crisis time
- Utilize resources, including support system, effectively
- Return to their precrisis level of functioning, or possibly higher
- Gain new insight
- Learn and begin to use new adaptive coping strategies
- Become more empowered
- Follow through with plan of action and referrals
- Become better equipped to deal with future problems or crises

Other more specific outcomes/goals will depend on the nature of the crisis (Aguilera, 1998, pp. 24, 31; Townsend, 2009, pp. 209-210; eHow.com—crisis intervention, 2010).

(Phase 2 corresponds to Stage III of Roberts's Seven-Stage Crisis Intervention Model)

Phase 3: Interventions/Implementation

- Continue to develop rapport and the therapeutic alliance/nurse–client relationship.
- Acknowledge and facilitate verbalization of feelings.
- Clarify information the client is providing as needed, including gently clarifying medical information they are receiving rather than allowing fantasy or false hope that will undermine trust when the situation does not resolve in ways the client wanted it to.

(continues)

Table 16-2   Phases of Crisis Intervention *(continued)*

- Support the person's ability to decide and act independently while providing emotional support.
- If needed provide more direct assistance (e.g., making phone calls, contacting support people, arranging transportation, physical care, basic needs, arranging for transfer to specific facilities or units for additional care) if the person's ability to function is compromised or impaired by the crisis event, psychiatric or other medical illness, or chemical abuse/dependency.
- Use short, simple sentences, especially in situations where the client is experiencing or unable to concentrate related to feelings of being extremely overwhelmed, impulsivity, suicidal or homicidal thoughts, severe anxiety, panic, depersonalization, derealization, psychosis, mania, severe depression or other symptoms of psychiatric or medical illnesses.
- Engage the client in problem solving and alternative approaches *to the extent the person is able; sometimes this is not possible due to severe anxiety states, panic, psychosis, and additional intervention including relaxation or distraction techniques, or medication may be needed before attempting this.*

"Let's work together."

"What else do you think can be done?"

"Let's take a look at some other possible options."

"Are you aware of any community resources that could be useful?"

"Do you have enough resources to try that?"

"Is there someone you can stay with?"

"Who else would be willing to help you with this?"

- Assist the client to examine errors in perceptions and thinking patterns; assist in confronting reality if ineffectively using ego defense mechanisms such as depression, which is not effective in crisis resolution. However, this is done *to the extent the person is able; sometimes this is not possible due to severe anxiety states, panic, psychosis, and additional intervention including relaxation or distraction techniques or medication may be needed before attempting this.*

"You may feel as if you are all alone, but we are here to help you."

"I know right now you feel as if you won't be able to get through this, but in time your ability to cope will get better."

"Could there be another explanation for the person's behavior?"

"What else could be happening?"

"Do you have enough information to support what you think is going on?"

"What makes you think this person no longer loves you?"

"What leads you to believe that your partner is cheating on you?"

"Is it possible that your view of what's going on isn't quite right?"

"Is it possible that things happened a little differently than what you remember?"

(continues)

Table 16-2   Phases of Crisis Intervention *(continued)*

- In early escalation stages of anger or agitation, interventions may include repeating a willingness to listen and respect; encouraging verbalization of feelings, agreeing with the client as long as the client is not threatening to harm themselves or others, maintaining an open, nonthreatening body posture; providing additional personal space, avoiding physically (standing in directly in front of the client or blocking the exit) or psychologically (making demands vs suggestions or limit setting) cornering the client.

- Consistently set limits on unacceptable, destructive, or aggressive behavior while reinforcing that the PMH nurse and others are there to help the client.

- Explore availability of resources including social support system/network. (If the client is not initially willing to involve family, clarify their reasons and if appropriate attempt to help the client see the advantage of their involvement; if not, explore other social support such as friends, neighbors, community and religious organizations, etc.).

- Make a plan in collaboration with this person. **Note:** *The plan will need to be congruent or agree with the client's values and belief systems, and take into account cultural and spiritual factors to be fully implemented and successful. Otherwise the client will not be fully able to carry it out.*

- Obtain a firm commitment from the person to follow through with the agreed upon plan.

- Assist as needed with mobilization of resources including social support system/network.

- Explore new coping strategies.

- Teach/provide information on new coping strategies and allow time to attempt these as appropriate before the client is discharged from the setting.

- Provide information for referral services.

- Arrange follow-up appointment(s)—time frames will depend on the nature of the crisis from 24 hours to 1 week or 1 month later.

- Document using individual facility or organization forms.

- Report to local/state agencies as required by individual states (e.g., childhood abuse is required to be reported in all 50 states; elder abuse is required in the majority of states and recommended in the remaining states).

(Aguilera, 1998, p. 31; Wilder & Sorensen, 2001, pp. 52–58, 72–79; Keltner, Schwecke, & Bostrom, 2007, pp. 104–108, 126, 134–137; Boyd, 2008, p. 810; Townsend, 2009, p. 210, 258–259; eHow.com—crisis intervention, 2010)

(Phase 3 corresponds to Stages IV–VI of Roberts's Seven-Stage Crisis Intervention Model)

(continues)

Table 16-2   **Phases of Crisis Intervention** *(continued)*

Phase 4: Evaluation

During this phase initial progress toward planned outcomes is analyzed and interventions adjusted if needed. Outcomes may also need to be adjusted as information is clarified, if the client's mental or physical condition changes, and as the collaborative plan is implemented. If the client is not suicidal or homicidal: is not compromised by exacerbations of psychiatric or other medical conditions or problems related to chemical abuse/dependency; and has the necessary social support and other resources including housing to return home, they will be discharged from the setting. If the client requires inpatient admission or transfer to another facility or program for treatment, then that will be the disposition and included in the documentation. When leaving the care setting and returning to home, the client should have all of the following:

- Maintained or returned to an adequate level of safety
- Information for referral services (see Box 16-1)
- Follow-up appointment(s)
- Information on new adaptive coping strategies
- Clear (verbalized) understanding of plan to follow or reinforcement needed
- Instructions to return to the care setting/emergency department/clinic or who else to contact if the crisis situation becomes worse (usually telephone hotline phone numbers, 911/emergency contact information, community agencies, safe houses).
- Documentation including the disposition of the client (i.e., discharge to home with whom, admitted where and report given to whom; transferred to another facility and report given to whom; follow-up appointment arranged with whom, or client agrees to call if unable to arrange before being discharged). In addition, all the above-mentioned information in the previous items in this bulleted list should be entered in the facility/organization's charting/recordkeeping system.

The evaluation phase may extend to include the follow-up visit/care so that better evaluation of the interventions and plan can be made over time and continuity of care maintained (Townsend, 2009, p. 211; Varcarolis & Halter, 2010, p. 540).

(Phase 4 corresponds to Stage VII of Roberts's Seven-Stage Crisis Intervention Model)

Basic Telephone Crisis Intervention

Telephone crisis intervention presents even more of a challenge because the PMH nurse does not have visual cues from the caller that are present with someone face to face. Most of communication is nonverbal, which means much valuable information from facial expressions (affect) and body language is not available during the interaction. However, voice tone and inflection are helpful both when listening to the caller and when responding to them. This type of intervention may occur in three phases (see also phases I–IV in Table 16-2):

1. Stabilization—assessment of the person and the problem
   a. *Calmly, but assertively* obtain information and give clear directions.
      Many times the person in crisis is out of control or feels they are losing control and needs reassurance that someone is attempting to reestablish control.
   b. Show empathy and interest in the person in crisis. Even on the telephone this comes through in your voice and words (see Chapter 4 and questions in phases I and III of Table 16-2).
   c. Keep verbal interaction flowing in a logical sequence so the caller can follow you.
   d. Obtain enough information to quickly assess and analyze the situation. If the person resists giving information, do not try to force them to.
   e. Get the name, address, and phone number of the caller. *Note: If the caller is hesitant to provide this information, reinforce your desire to help, but you need this information to provide/send help. If they continue to resist and there is risk for suicide or homicide, quietly get the attention of another nurse or staff member to try to have the call traced while you continue to attempt to persuade the caller to remain calm and provide the information.*
   f. Use therapeutic communication techniques to communicate empathy, genuineness, support, and willingness to help.
   g. "I" statements may be useful depending on the situation: "I get the feeling that . . ."; "I'm wondering . . ."; "I sense that . . ." when the caller sounds hesitant or it is evident that there is more information or "more to the story" that they are not freely expressing.

2. Assessment and planning—risk of danger: plan and determine therapeutic and safe interventions
   a. The goal is not to deliver therapy, but to help alleviate some of the immediate stress or perceived threat.
   b. Information including resources, personal strengths, and coping ability is obtained if possible.
   c. If the person has adequate resources including emotional/social support and positive coping skills, interventions will be more focused on mobilizing those resources and encouraging the use of coping skills.

3. Intervention
   a. Repeat requests for information and directions in a calm, firm voice as many times as needed, like a "broken record."
   b. Facilitate expression of feelings unless the person needs to leave the area immediately for safety.
   c. Provide directions in clear, simple language using short sentences.
   d. Make use of the person's personal strengths and positive coping skills.
   e. *If appropriate* (i.e., the person is calm enough, no immediate danger to self or others), instruct the person to call 911 (ambulance, police, fire department, on-call counselor/psychiatrist, crisis teams in larger cities) or go to the nearest hospital.
   If it is not appropriate for the person to place the call (e.g., too overwhelmed, is suicidal or has attempted suicide; is homicidal or has attempted homicide; is being threatened; or is unwilling to do so and the situation is an emergency); is unable to or unwilling to call 911/emergency services, then place the call yourself.
   f. If possible, stay on the line to continue talking to the person in a calm, clear, reassuring manner while another nurse/staff member contacts 911/emergency services. Otherwise you may have to call the person back after calling 911/emergency services to check on them and let them know help is on the way, but will need a contact number to do so.
   g. If there is contact information available regarding a family member, contact the family member and inform them of the action taken.
   h. Make referrals and provide information on community resources (see **Box 16-1**).
   i. If appropriate make follow-up appointments.
   j. Document interactions and disposition (e.g., referrals given, emergency services contacted, agreement to contact crisis hotlines, call back/return if situation becomes worse or occurs again).

(Aguilera, 1998, pp. 29–32; Christiansen, 2009, pp. 1–14; GP-Training.net, 2010; NOVA, 2010; AAETS, 2010; *Crisis intervention*—MentalHealthCE.com, 2010).

Children/Adolescents

Children/adolescents by nature are impulsive, have no or limited life experience, limited problem-solving skills, and may engage in risky behaviors, all of which can result in volatile, dangerous situations. They are greatly influenced by their peer group and

BOX 16-1   Referrals

Clients will need referrals for general and specific needs depending on the type of crisis. Information should be given in writing (or download information to cell phones/portable information devices) because clients are too overwhelmed to remember while trying to cope with the situation. If they initially refuse the information, tell them the information is always available if they change their mind (see also Chapter 17).

- Local community resources for basic needs (e.g., housing/shelter, homeless shelters, food, clothing, transportation, help with utility bills)
- Local community support groups including substance abuse support groups
- Crisis hotline telephone numbers:
  Suicide Prevention: 1-800-273-TALK (8255) or 1-800-749-COPE (2673) or 1-800 SUICIDE
      (784-2433)
  Child Abuse/Neglect Hotline: 1-800-422-4453
  Youth Crisis Runaway Hotline: 1-800-621-4000 or 1-800-448-4663
  Education Crisis Hotline for Teachers: 1-800-957-0532
  Parents Anonymous Hotline: 1-800-348-5437 (National)
  National Domestic Violence Crisis Line 1-888-411-1333 or 1-800-799-SAFE (7233) or
      1-800-787-3224 (TTY)
  Pregnancy Hotline: 1-800-395-4357
  Elderly Abuse Hotline: 800-259-4990
  Adult Protective Services: 1-800-898-4910 to report abuse, neglect, exploitation, or extortion
- Suicide prevention: website: www.suicidepreventionlifeline.org
- Elder abuse website: http://www.preventelderabuse.org/
- Local community legal aid
- Medical physician follow-up appointment
- Psychiatrist follow-up appointment
- Counseling/psychotherapy follow-up appointment with a psychologist, APRN, or social worker for individuals and families
- Chemical abuse/dependency follow-up appointments with addictionologist and chemical dependency counseling
- Local college campus counseling resource information for college students
- Local/state/national community organizations including:
  Catholic Charities: www.catholiccharitiesusa.org
  The Salvation Army: 1-800-725-2769 (National), www.salvationarmyusa.org
  United Way agencies: 1-877-923-2114
  Goodwill Industries
  Second Harvest Food Banks
  Local churches
  Operation Blessing: 1-800-436-6348 (National)

(continues)

State unemployment agencies

Council on Aging: 1-877-340-9100 (National) services: Meals on site, meal delivery, prescription service, personal care, homemaker, transportation

- Volunteers of America: 1-800-899-0089 for a variety of services including basic needs
- National Organization for Victim Assistance (NOVA): http://www.trynova.org/victiminfo/
- CyberbullyNOT: Student Guide to Cyberbullying: http://new.csriu.org/cyberbully/docs/cbstudentguide.pdf
- For situations involving military veterans:

Military Counseling Services: 1-800-342-9647 (National)

United States Department of Veterans Affairs: https://vip.vba.va.gov/portal/VBAH/Home

United States Army Center for Health Promotion and Preventive Medicine (USACHPPM): http://chppm-www.apgea.army.mil/dhpw/Population/combat.aspx

school environment. Young children have limited use of vocabulary and are less able to comfort themselves. Use of play therapy techniques and art supplies to draw, paint, or sculpt feelings can help the PMH nurse gain better understanding of the situation and individuals' feelings and perceptions.

Adolescents may feel they have no one to talk to, have difficulty trusting adults, and feel intense emotions including anger or fear, but have difficulty expressing or dealing with strong feelings. They may have difficulty with problem solving and engage in self-destructive behavior including alcohol and drug use, promiscuity, self-mutilation, and reckless driving—if old enough to drive—to express strong emotions vs doing so verbally. Communicating that you genuinely want to help them is an important step in developing rapport and a therapeutic alliance with these clients. They are sensitive to someone "faking" interest. Adolescents may also be more able to express themselves using art supplies or role play.

When dealing with legal minors, the PMH nurse will need to include parents or guardians, who may be able to provide more information, may not understand their child/adolescent's intense reactions, may need education, and also may need emotional support and empathy. Grief responses/reactions may be triggered by the death of a pet, or loss of a friend due to moving/relocation or death. The PMH nurse may also need to involve social services, child protective services, family counseling, planned parenthood, and pregnancy hotlines (refer to individual state regulations regarding legal minors and teen pregnancy). Referral information is included in Box 16-1 (see also Chapters 4 and 17).

Elderly

Although elderly clients have more life experience, they have decreased physical re-serves and are more likely to have suffered many losses, including outliving spouses and other family members and friends, retirement, decreased finances, and loss of in-dependence. Transportation may be a problem. Predisposing factors in the develop-ment of crises for this population more frequently include exacerbations of medical illnesses, poor nutrition, poverty, and abuse or neglect. Crisis interventions are fo-cused as much on the medical aspects as the psychiatric. More time is needed to as-sess elderly clients due to the medical aspects and need for more frequent breaks to avoid overtiring them. Clients presenting with symptoms of delirium or dementia, in-cluding Alzheimer's type, provide even more of a challenge to provide for their safety needs. Adult children and guardians may be involved as well, may have medical power of attorney or medical proxy, and may be able to provide more information. Local area agencies on aging, the national council on aging, elder abuse hotline and protec-tive services and websites (see Box 16-1) can provide assistance and information (see also Chapters 4 and 17).

Critical Incident Stress Debriefing (CISD)

Critical incident stress debriefing (CISD) or management is a strategy that provides structured time for sharing thoughts and feelings following highly stressful events or "endeavors" including violence, suicide, and hostage situations, where "small over-sights or omissions may result in serious, or perhaps tragic outcomes. . . . Critical in-cidents are those events that overwhelm an individual's ability to cope. They are psychologically traumatic, causing emotional turmoil, cognitive problems and behav-ioral changes" (Everly & Mitchell, 2010). These situations can be extremely emotion-ally and spiritually distressing, and debriefing is thought to be one way of helping prevent the development of acute stress disorders or PTSD in people who provide crisis intervention. CISD is also viewed as part of self-care. Not all crisis intervention situations are experienced as critical incidents, but there are times when rare events "overwhelm the normal coping abilities of even the most experienced professional." Common symptoms experienced by crisis intervention personnel fall into the follow-ing categories:

- Physical—insomnia, nausea, loss of appetite, elevated vital signs, lightheaded-ness, headaches, muscle weakness
- Cognitive—distractibility, disorientation, flashbacks, recurrent intrusive im-ages, nightmares, distortion of facts

- Affective—depression, sadness, anxiety, feeling overwhelmed, guilt, anger, fear, shame, negative/pessimistic attitude, emotional numbness
- Behavioral—constricted or blunted affect, social isolation, distancing from others, exaggerated startle reflex, hyper-vigilance, use of substances, possible phobic behaviors
- Spiritual–existential—questioning one's own competence, questioning career choice, questioning one's faith, questions about the afterlife, questioning the purpose of life

CISD has been used by the military for years and more recently has been available for healthcare professionals, crisis volunteers, hotline volunteers, first responders, ambulance–paramedics, policemen, firemen, teachers and other school employees, natural disaster relief volunteers, and even students effected by violence or shootings in their schools. Professionals leading the CISD receive formal training. There is more than one model, but most employ the following steps or phases that occur in separate meetings for each phase:

- Introductory phase—CISD team members identified, reasons for meeting explained, overview of debriefing process, guidelines established, reassurance of confidentiality, questions answered
- Fact or "reconstruction" phase—participants in the crisis intervention situation discuss what happened from their perspective and explain their involvement
- Thought or "cognitive" phase—first thoughts about the incident discussed
- Reaction phase—discussion of the worst parts or most painful/emotional events of the situation
- Symptom phase—symptoms experienced during the crisis, at the scene, and following the initial experience
- Teaching or "psychoeducational" phase—acknowledgment of symptoms expressed as normal; anticipatory guidance given regarding future symptoms including stress management techniques
- Reentry phase—material discussed is reviewed, questions answered, new topics introduced, reassurance given, referral sources provided as well as encouragement, support, and appreciation

(Varcarolis & Halter, 2010, pp. 539–540; Medtrng.com, 2010)

In addition to CISD, there are other recommended strategies for recovery following critical incidents:

- Stay connected to others to avoid temptation to isolate
- Reduce noise levels at home

- Protect private time and space to avoid increased anxiety or feeling overwhelmed
- Try to return to as normal a daily schedule as possible to help in the normalization process
- Try to eat even small amount even if not hungry to maintain energy and avoid becoming ill
- Try to maintain normal sleep pattern and habits to help with general coping ability and decrease stress
- Avoid caffeine and other stimulating products that lead to CNS stimulation and increased stress responses; avoid alcohol to avoid interference with the normal relaxation response
- Talk openly with others and do not be ashamed to ask for help
- Let loved ones know that you experienced a traumatic event (without breaking confidentiality) and let them know what they can do for you
- Seek assistance for prolonged symptoms/reactions

(Medtrng.com, 2010)

Even when crisis intervention does not result in situations needing CISD, PMH nurses should regularly attend to self-care to protect their own mental, spiritual, and physical health to avoid becoming burned out or suffering from vicarious traumatization from absorbing stress and negative energy from crisis situations.

REFERENCES

Aguilera, D. (1998). *Crisis intervention theory and methodology* (8th ed.). St. Louis, MO: Mosby.

American Academy of Experts in Traumatic Stress. Retrieved from www.aaets.org

American Psychological Association (2007). *APA dictionary of psychology*. Washington, DC: Author.

Antai-Otong, D. (2004). *Psychiatric emergencies: How to accurately assess and manage the patient in crisis.* Eau Claire, WI: PESI Healthcare.

Antai-Otong, D. (2009). *Psychiatric emergencies: How to accurately assess and manage the patient in crisis* (2nd ed.). Eau Claire, WI: PESI Healthcare.

Assessing needs-10 questions to answer. (2010). Retrieved from http://www.gptraining.net/training/communication_skills/consultation/assessing_needs.htm and http://www.gp-training.net/training/communication_skills/consultation/bathe.htm

Bandura, A. (1977). Self-efficacy: Toward a unifying theory of behavioral change. *Psychological Review, 84*(2): 191–215.

Bandura, A. (1977). Self-reinforcement: The power of positive personal control. In P. G. Zimbardo & F. L. Ruch (Eds.), *Psychology and life* (9th ed.). Glenview, IL: Scott Foresman.

Boyd, M. A. (2008). *Psychiatric nursing: Contemporary practice* (4th ed.). Philadelphia, PA: Wolters-Kluwer Health/Lippincott, Williams, & Wilkins.

Christiansen, K. (2009). *The crisis intervention manual* (2nd ed.). Reseda, CA: Zero Point Communications.

Crisis intervention: Assessment & practice strategies (Section 2, Track #2)—Interviewing in crisis intervention, stage I. (2010). Retrieved from: http://www.mentalhealthce.com/courses/contentCRI/ (click "trkCR102).

Everly, G. S., & Mitchell, J. T. (2010). *A primer on critical incident stress management.* International Critical Incident Stress Foundation. Retrieved from http://www.icisf.org

How to intervene in a crisis situation. (2010). Retrieved from http://www.ehow.com/how_2138570_ intervene-crisis-situation.html

How to use the six steps of effective intervention. (2010). Retrieved from http://www.ehow.com/ how_5239330_use-six-steps-effective-intervention.html

Improving triage techniques: A guide for clinicians undertaking telephone consultations. Retrieved from http://www.gp-training.net/training/communication_skills/consultation/telephone_triage2.htm

Jakopac, K. A., & Patel, S. C. (2009). *Psychiatric mental health case studies and care plans.* Sudbury, MA: Jones and Bartlett.

Joint Commission. (Dec., 2008). *Suicide risk reduction.* Retrieved from http://www.jointcommission. org/AccreditationPrograms/BehavioralHealthCare/Standards/09_FAQs/NPSG/Focused_risk_ assessment/NPSG.15.01.01/Suicide+risk+reduction.htm

Keltner, N. L., Schwecke, L. H., & Bostrom, C. E. (2007). Psychiatric nursing (5th ed.). St. Louis, MO: Mosby, Elsevier.

Lange, S. P., & Shank, S. I. (2005). *Managing psychiatric crisis.* Lakeway, TX: National Center of Continuing Education, Inc.

Lynch, M. A., Howard, P. B., El-Mallakh, P., & Matthews, J. M. (2008). Assessment and management of hospitalized suicidal patients. *Journal of Psychosocial Nursing, 46*(7), 45–51.

Medtrng.com: Medical training resources. (2010). *Suicide prevention and awareness.* Retrieved from http://www.medtrng.com/suicideprevention/index.htm

National Organization for Victim Assistance (NOVA). (2010). Retrieved from www.try-nova.org and http://www.trynova.org/victiminfo

O'Brien, P. G., Kennedy, W. Z., & Ballard, K. A. (2008). *Psychiatric mental health nursing: An introduction to theory and practice.* Sudbury, MA: Jones and Bartlett.

Sadock, B. J., & Sadock, V. A. (2005) *Kaplan & Sadock's comprehensive textbook of psychiatry* (8th ed.). Philadelphia, PA: Lippincott, Williams, & Wilkins.

Stuart, G. W., & Laraia, M. T. (2005). *Principles and practice of psychiatric nursing* (8th ed.). St. Louis, MO: Mosby, Elsevier.

Townsend, M. C. (2009). *Psychiatric mental health nursing: Concepts of care in evidence-based practice* (6th ed.). Philadelphia, PA: F. A. Davis.

Varcarolis, E. M., & Halter, M. J. (2010). *Foundations of psychiatric mental health nursing: A clinical approach* (6th ed.). St. Louis, MO: Saunders, Elsevier.

Wilder, S. S., & Sorensen, C. (2001). *Essentials of aggression management in health care.* Upper Saddle River, NJ: Prentice Hall, Inc.

CHAPTER 17

Crisis Intervention in Domestic Violence and Abuse

Kim A. Jakopac

The nursing student will be able to:
1. Define and provide examples of domestic violence and abuse
2. Recognize signs and symptoms of people who may be in domestic violence or abuse situations
3. Identify the role of the psychiatric-mental health (PMH) nurse when dealing with victims or survivors of domestic violence and abuse
4. Discuss the needs and legal rights of victims or survivors of violence and trauma
5. Apply crisis theory and utilize crisis intervention strategies when working with victims or survivors of domestic violence and abuse
6. Assist victims or survivors of domestic violence and abuse to develop a domestic violence safety plan
7. Provide appropriate referrals and resource information for victims or survivors of domestic violence and abuse
8. Discuss special considerations regarding children/adolescents and elderly clients

KEY TERMS

Abuse
Battering
Cyberbullying
Cycle of violence
Family violence
Hate crimes
Incest
Intergenerational transmission

Intimate partner violence (IPV)
Neglect
Rape
Sexting
Sexual harassment
Shaken baby syndrome
Stalking
Workplace violence

Definitions of *domestic violence and abuse* have been put forth by many sources and relate to the type and source of violence and abuse: "an ongoing, debilitating experience of physical, psychological, and/or sexual abuse in the home, associated with increased isolation from the outside world and limited personal freedom and accessibility to resources." (Townsend, 2009, p. 730) (see also Chapter 16).

The American Academy of Family Physicians defines family violence as "intentional intimidation, abuse or neglect of children, adults or elders by a family member, intimate partner or caretaker, in order to gain power and control over the victim" (Varcarolis & Halter, 2010, p. 585).

The Centers for Disease Control and Prevention (CDC) define intimate partner violence (IPV) as "physical, sexual, or psychological harm by a current or former partner or spouse. This type of violence can occur among heterosexual or same-sex couples and does not require sexual intimacy" (CDC, 2010). IPV is noted to be on the increase among teen dating partners (Boyd, 2008, p. 848).

Violence in many forms occurs for multiple reasons across all socioeconomic, ethnocultural/racial, and sexual/gender boundaries. It is a pattern that becomes more frequent and severe over time; a "reign of force and terror" (Fontaine, 2009, p. 580). It has been estimated that one-half of all Americans have experienced violence in their families and that 5 of every 10 people will be exposed to a major trauma in their lifetime. Violence is increasingly the cause of childhood injuries (Varcarolis, Carson, & Shoemaker, 2006, p. 507; Fontaine, 2009, pp. 580, 634). Every year 10 million Americans are abused by a family member. Fewer than 10% of all cases involve an abuser who is mentally ill. The majority of abusers look "normal," and are charming and persuasive. Millions of cases of violence and abuse occur each year as well as thousands of deaths. We usually think of victims as being female and abusers as being male, but there are a significant number of victims who are male and are too embarrassed to report abuse or seek help. Many people suffer in silence, fearing retaliation or death, while others cling to promises of change. Victims leave situations temporarily an average of six to seven times before leaving for good (Varcarolis, Carson, & Shoemaker, 2006, p. 507; Fontaine, 2009, pp. 580, 634). The term *survivor* is also used to acknowledge "the recovery and healing process that follows victimization" (Varcarolis & Halter, 2010, p. 589). Statistics are difficult to accurately assess due to differences in collecting data, reporting from state to state, and unwillingness of victims to come forward. More resources are needed for prevention efforts.

Violence and abuse occur in different ways. Abuse is defined as actions that can result in serious harm or death (Varcarolis & Halter, 2010, pp. 584–587) and involves many types, including the following:

- Physical (including battering) abuse
- Sexual abuse
- Social isolation
- Economic abuse–withholding financial support; exploiting money/resources
- Emotional and/or verbal intimidation or threats (including using "male privilege" or the children to control the victim)
- Torture/Ritual abuse/Mind control

(Keltner, Schwecke, & Bostrom, 2007, p. 622; Fontaine, 2009, p. 581; Varcarolis & Halter, 2010, p. 585)

Neglect is defined as failure to provide or act on a person's behalf resulting in medical, mental, developmental, or social problems or illness (Varcarolis & Halter, 2010, pp. 584–587). Types of neglect include:

- Physical
- Emotional
- Medical
- Educational—generally applies to children younger than 11 years
- Abandonment

(Fontaine, 2009, p. 581)

Violence and abuse that occurs in the context of a relationship with an intimate partner/significant other, spouse/domestic partner, family/domestic, sibling or according to age involving minor children and the elderly is then further defined as previously stated. Other forms of violence and abuse occur whether or not there is a relationship due to rape/sexual assault, stalking, sexual harassment or in the workplace. Some forms of abuse (e.g., emotional or verbal) are harder to prove, but nevertheless are harmful and destructive to a person's self-concept and psychological well-being. Unfortunately, the abuser/perpetrator/victimizer frequently is someone the victim knows or trusts and is someone they are dependent upon for nurturing and basic care. Power and control over the victim are the main issues for the abuser.

Cyberbullying, also known as Internet harassment or electronic aggression, is a more recent form of violence and abuse. The CDC has begun to focus more recently on cyberbullying and defines it as "any kind of aggression perpetrated through technology—any type of harassment or bullying (teasing, telling lies, making fun of someone, making rude or mean comments, spreading rumors, or making threatening or aggressive comments) that occurs through email, a chat room, instant messaging, a website (including blogs), or text messaging" (CDC, 2009). The peak time for this type of activity seems to be in the middle school years. School systems are being urged to address this issue as well as traditional bullying, alcohol and drug use with help from the CDC guidelines. While more research needs to be done regarding the effects of cyberbullying, potential effects include victims being more likely to use alcohol and drugs, skip school, receive detention, experience face-to-face victimization (bullying at school or after school), change schools, become depressed, or commit suicide or murder as extreme responses. There is growing concern due to the availability of and access to electronic devices for even very young children. Legal consequences for this type of violence and abuse are becoming increasingly more strict.

ROLE OF THE PMH NURSE

As previously stated in Chapter 16, the role of the PMH nurse is "to provide a framework of support systems that guide the patient (person) through the crisis and facilitate the development and use of positive coping skills. The nurse must be acutely aware that a person in crisis may be at high risk for suicide or homicide" (Boyd, 2008, p. 806). These clients frequently need medical intervention and physical nursing interventions for physical injuries as well as psychosocial nursing care. Referrals, including community resources and follow-up care, are vital, but healthcare professionals may be more prone to focus on the victim's immediate medical care needs (Alexy, 2009). The victim's children will also need to be included when providing intervention, referrals, and follow-up care. The crisis theories, models, frameworks, paradigms, and interventions previously mentioned in Chapter 16 also apply in domestic violence and abuse crisis situations. Initially, victims may need more direct assistance due to a period of disorganization immediately following the incident during which they may have difficulty thinking rationally, trusting others, and making decisions (Townsend, 2009, p. 741). The PMH nurse will need to practice self-care to be effective in their role. There may be situations where critical incident stress debriefing is appropriate and necessary (see Chapter 16).

The ability to provide a necessary framework, manage care, and facilitate positive coping skill development and use begins with careful assessment of many areas, including risk for suicide or homicide, cognitive processes, coping behaviors, and safe living arrangements. The PMH nurse will need to provide emotional support, resource referrals, provide for or arrange physical care, and in some cases may need to act as a liaison between medical and psychiatric service providers. The most successful overall client outcomes are resolution of the immediate crisis, the ability to function as independently as possible during the crisis time, becoming more empowered, and a return to their precrisis level of functioning, or possibly higher, with new insight and coping abilities (Aguilera, 1998, p. 24; Townsend, 2009, pp. 209, 739).

RISK FACTORS

As previously stated, violence and abuse occur across all socioeconomic, ethnocultural/racial, and sexual/gender boundaries. Risk factors include cultures and families where aggression is accepted and used to solve problems; occurrence of intergenerational transmission; continued media exposure to violence or portrayal of women as second-class citizens; gender bias; organic brain syndromes/cerebral disorders that may predispose people to be aggressive or violent; multiple life stressors; limited outlets or resources for stress management; lack of impulse control; poor parenting skills and problem-solving abilities; lack of parental social support and social isolation; parental lack of knowledge and expectations beyond what is developmentally possible; and pregnancy. Abused pregnant women are twice as likely to delay prenatal care until the third trimester of pregnancy for many reasons including fear that the violence and abuse will be discovered; that they will be denied transportation to the healthcare provider's office by the abuser; or that the abuser may not want the baby and when they find out that she is pregnant will increase the level of violence and abuse. There are situations where the violence or abuse does not start until after people have been dating for awhile or after the legal marriage of cohabiting individuals. In other situations such as date or acquaintance rape, the people involved have just met (Keltner, Schwecke, & Bostrom, 2007, p. 626; Fontaine, 2009, pp. 583–587; Marcus, 2009; Townsend, 2009, pp. 727–729; Varcarolis & Halter, 2010, p. 589).

CYCLE OF VIOLENCE

In 1979, Walker described a predictable pattern or cycle of violent behavior that abusers/perpetrators/victimizers seem to use to control their partners (Varcarolis & Halter, 2010, p. 585) (see **Figure 17-1**). The cycle continually repeats unless there is intervention. The cycle is similar in battering behavior and occurs in three phases: (1) tension building, (2) eruption of violence/incident, and (3) honeymoon (Keltner, Schwecke & Bostrom, 2007, p. 624; Boyd, 2008, p. 853; Townsend, 2009, pp. 730–731; Varcarolis & Halter, 2010, p. 585).

During the tension building phase, the abuser takes or establishes control by emotional or psychological methods. Accusations, demands, verbal abuse, and degradation occur. The abuser monitors all of the victim's activities including social contact, phone calls, and mail; and socially isolates the victim from family and friends so that the victim will have to totally depend on the abuser. The tension builds until it becomes unbearable. In some cases the victim may provoke something to happen to "get it over with," being unable to bear the tension any longer.

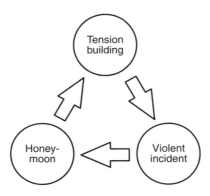

FIGURE 17-1   Cycle of violent behavior.

During the eruption of violence/incident phase, actual violence and injury occur. It may be precipitated by a triggering event. The last phase has been given the name "honeymoon" because the abuser not only apologizes for the violence, but shows loving behavior towards the victim, buys gifts, and makes promises including a promise to change their behavior. The victim remembers the behavior in the honeymoon phase and clings to false hope that the violence and abuse will never happen again. Unfortunately, the cycle begins again and again until the victim has enough resources, support, and intervention to break the cycle or injuries are fatal.

There is also a wheel of power and control that identifies types of physical and psychological abuse. The wheel includes behaviors such as making threats towards the victim or the children; intimidation using gestures, facial expressions, voice tone or volume; actions such as destruction of property; using male privilege by treating the victim as a servant and making all the major decisions without any input or regard for the victim's needs or wishes; socially isolating the victim; emotional/verbal abuse including minimizing or denying behavior, and blaming the victim for causing the violence/abuse; economic and sexual abuse (Keltner, Schwecke, & Bostrom, 2007, p. 622; Boyd, 2008, p. 845).

There are many reasons why people stay in abusive relationships, including:

- Maintaining a state of emotional denial as a coping mechanism (ego defense mechanism)
- Lack of ways to financially support themselves and their children
- Lack of other resources including alternate housing
- Lack of social support

- Believing the abuse is somehow their own fault
- Believing that as long as the abuser directs the violence toward the victim, they will not harm the children
- Fear of retaliation and greater violence if they try to leave or have the abuser arrested
- Having been threatened with loss of or never being allowed to see the children if they leave
- Guilt about failure of the relationship
- Poor self-image
- Believing no one else will ever love them
- Depression
- Fear of tarnishing the family's image/social embarrassment
- Belief that the abuser needs them and will finally change as promised
- Influence of intergenerational transmission
- Cultural/religious factors
- Difficulty navigating the legal system
- Loving the abuser in spite of everything

Victims leave situations an average of six to seven times before leaving for good. (Keltner, Schwecke, & Bostrom, 2007, p. 623; Boyd, 2008, pp. 852–853).

SIGNS AND SYMPTOMS

Healthcare professionals do not always think to ask about the possibility of violence and abuse if the client does not mention it. More recently, screening questions such as asking if the client feels safe in their own home are being included on general health assessment forms. It is being suggested that screening should be performed not only during the last trimester of pregnancy, but also at least once in each trimester. More focus is also needed on follow-up and referral services (Alexy, 2009). The CDC offers assessment and screening tools for assessing intimate partner violence (IPV) and sexual violence (SV) victimization, as well as other harmful situations, in clinical/healthcare settings at http://www.cdc.gov/NCIPC/pub-res/ipv_and_sv_screening.htm. Signs and symptoms of adult violence and abuse include:

- Frequent ER visits/hospitalizations for "accidental" injuries
- Explanations given for injuries that do not match or support, or actually conflict with the type or intensity of injury
- Blackened eyes, facial bruising or fractures, other broken bones including skull fractures, burns, symmetrical vs asymmetrical injuries, "twisting" type injuries,

multiple bruises or injuries at various stages of healing, abdominal trauma or rupture of abdominal organs

- Living in inadequate or unsafe housing
- Little or no control over their financial situation
- Socially isolated with no other social support except for the abuser
- Ill or injured, but having sought no medical/dental/psychiatric attention or having delayed such action
- Displaying fear, anxiety, withdrawal, extreme passivity or shame when the abuser is present; may try unsuccessfully to act calm, unafraid, or brave
- Appearing confused or in shock
- The abuser being unwilling to allow, or being suspicious of, any healthcare providers spending time alone with victim
- The abuser answering all questions, even those directed to the victim, or being evasive or refusing to answer certain questions
- The abuser being overly helpful (e.g., insisting on helping the victim change into a hospital gown, go to the bathroom rather than allow staff to be alone with the victim)
- That if the victim comes alone for treatment, they may not wait to receive complete treatment or follow through with discharge recommendations fearing the abuser may find out the victim sought help and now someone else knows about the situation

(Keltner, Schwecke, & Bostrom, 2007, p. 626; Fontaine, 2009, pp. 583–587)

SIGNS OF INCREASED DANGER FOR THE VICTIM

There are signs that indicate increased danger for the victim of domestic violence and abuse (Keltner, Schwecke, & Bostrom, 2007, p. 627). The PMH nurse should include these in the assessment as well as in client teaching:

- The number of incidents of violence has increased over the past year.
- There has been an increased severity of violence over the past year (e.g., threatened with or used a weapon).
- Abuser attempts to or actually strangles victim.
- Victim is forced to have sex with the abuser.
- Abuser uses alcohol/drugs to control the victim.
- Abuser abuses alcohol/drugs themselves.
- Abuser threatens to kill the victim, the children, or themselves.

- Victim believes the abuser is capable of killing them, the children, or the abuser themselves.
- Victim thinks about or attempts suicide/homicide.

RAPE/SEXUAL ASSAULT

As previously stated regarding violence and abuse, accurate statistics are difficult to assess due to differences in collecting data, reporting from state to state, and unwillingness of victims to come forward. This is true of rape/sexual assault as well. The perpetrator may threaten to kill the victim or the victim wants to forget what happened, move on with their life, and avoid going through the additional trauma of legal prosecution.

Signs and symptoms of rape trauma syndrome are similar to acute stress disorders (ASDs) and posttraumatic stress disorder (PTSD) (see Chapter 7) and include:

- Nightmares
- Inability to trust others
- Anxiety and fear
- Distrust/suspicion of everyone
- Guilt, blaming self for this happening
- Worthlessness, decreased self-esteem
- Isolation, decreased socialization
- Emotional distancing and numbing
- Decreased motivation
- Problems with most relationships

(Keltner, Schwecke, & Bostrom, 2007, p. 612; Townsend, 2009, p. 737)

After the incident, the victim may appear outwardly calm due to a delayed response to the rape or be in extreme denial that the rape/sexual assault ever took place. Victims may appear uncooperative during assessment/examination due to trying to regain a sense of emotional control over the situation.

CRISIS INTERVENTION

As previously stated in Chapter 16, crisis intervention is not a replacement for long-term counseling or therapy, but uses tools that can provide temporary relief to someone experiencing the trauma of an unexpected critical event. According to the American Nurses Association (ANA), "Crisis intervention is a short term therapeutic process that focuses on the rapid resolution of an immediate crisis or emergency using available personnel, family, and/or environmental resources" (Varcarolis & Halter, 2010, p. 529).

The same legal–ethical principles of least restrictive alternative doctrine, autonomy, beneficence, fidelity, justice, nonmaleficence, civil rights including confidentiality, bioethics, "duty to warn," and safety concerns also apply in crisis situations (see Chapters 12, 13, and 16). Additionally, nurses are required by law to report (mandatory reporting) suspected child abuse in all 50 states. Regarding elder abuse, nurses are required by law in 43 states (and it is recommended in the remaining states) to report suspected elder abuse. The PMH nurse usually reports information to the psychiatrist/physician present and the nursing supervisor, and documents assessment information including photographs of injuries. Local child and elderly protection services are contacted by the person designated in the organization/facility to do so (e.g., physician, nursing supervision). The nurse should also refer to individual state laws and the facility/organization's policies and forms. Adult victims should give permission for photographs to be taken and are legally able to choose not to prosecute the perpetrator. However, evidence should be collected and documented with the same strict procedures in case the victim changes their mind regarding legal prosecution.

Also, as previously stated in Chapter 16, crisis intervention begins with initiating rapport in the formation of a therapeutic alliance or therapeutic nurse–client relationship by communicating that the nurse cares about the person. It is through communication, empathy, and the formation of a therapeutic alliance or therapeutic nurse–client relationship that trust can be built and used therapeutically. Victims need to hear that any type of violence and abuse is not their fault and they acted as they did to try to survive. When interviewing/assessing someone who needs a translator, it is recommended that the nurse *avoid* allowing family members to translate because they may be the perpetrator or have reasons to caution the victim not to report the violence and abuse (see also Chapter 16). As clear an understanding as possible must be obtained of the presenting crisis or problem in the context of the person's life to be able to provide safety and work toward the best possible resolution (Sadock & Sadock, 2005, p. 2454; eHow.com—crisis intervention, 2010).

Phases/Stages of Crisis Intervention

The phases/stages of crisis intervention, as well as basic telephone crisis intervention, were presented in Chapter 16. As previously stated, if medical intervention, including medication, is required, this will need to be administered before proceeding (Lange & Shank, 2005, p. 10). The PMH nurse will not be acting alone, but in conjunction with other members of the treatment or healthcare team (see **Table 17-1**). Victims of violence and abuse should be interviewed/assessed separately because they may deny or not report violence or abuse when family members or friends are present (see Chapters 3–5, 7, 9, and 12).

Table 17-1   Phases of Crisis Intervention

Phase 1: Assessment

- Begin to develop rapport and a therapeutic alliance/nurse—client relationship by remaining calm, communicating that you care about the person, and providing comfort by therapeutic use of self, active listening, attending skills, empathy, and emotional support.

  "Hi. My name's _____. I'm a nurse. You sound upset."

  "I want to help you. I'm glad you came in today."

  "What's going on?"

  "It's not your fault."

  "I'm sorry you've been treated (hurt) this way."

  "No one deserves to be treated this way."

  "You did what you had to do to survive."

  "Do you feel like talking about what happened?"

  "You sound like you are hurting."

  "It's okay to cry."

  "Anger is a normal emotion."

  "Fear is a normal emotion."

- Determine how life-threatening the situation is and the need for medical intervention.

  "You sound really sad" or "You said you 'just can't handle it anymore.' Are you thinking about suicide?"

  "Are you thinking of harming someone?"

  "Do you have any medical or mental health conditions?" or "Are you under a doctor's care for any reason?"

- **Avoid** giving false reassurances such as "Everything will be all right." If the result is not "all right" the client will be angry and stop trusting you. **Instead** reiterate your desire to listen and help.

  "I care about you and will listen." or "I want to help you."

- Guide the client through the assessment process, which may at times require being direct or firm to help the client focus/refocus.

  "Stay with me."

  "Tell me more about…"

(continues)

Table 17-1   Phases of Crisis Intervention *(continued)*

"What about...?"

"I'm here."

"Yes, go on ..."

Note: *During the assessment the nurse may need to repeat requests for information and directions in a calm, firm voice as many times as needed—like a "broken record"—specific information to be able to treat/intervene, send emergency services.*

- What is the client's perception of what is happening? Keep focused on one thing at a time.

  "What do you think is happening?"

  "What do you think caused him to act that way?"

  "How has this been affecting your life?"

- Assess the client's mental and physical status including predisposing risk factors.

  "How has the rest of your life been going?" or "How has your health been?"

- Ask about the location and safety of children or other people living with the victim who may depend on the victim for care. Contact a social worker to evaluate the situation and intervene if the victim is unsure about the safety of other family members/dependents.

- Assess signs of increased danger for the victim.

- Assess the potential for suicide/homicide including thoughts, plans, means, lethality of means, access, and ability or lack of ability to contract at least verbally not to act (also if the person in crisis is calling rather than being physically present, ask if they are alone or if someone else is there/nearby) (see also Chapters 9 and 16).

- Take photographs of injuries for documentation. Injuries may have healed before cases go to court, and these will be needed as evidence along with diagnostic test results. Adults need to give permission for photographs to be taken of them.

- If the victim says they need to leave, attempt to persuade them to stay as long as they can for treatment and provide referral information including safe houses/shelters, crisis hotline telephone number; legal information regarding how to obtain a restraining order/protection from abuse (PFA) order; how to develop a domestic safety plan; the cycle of violence; and basic needs. If the victim does leave early, tell them they can come back if they change their mind.

  Note: *The victim may only be able to take information written on as small a piece of paper as possible to avoid it being found by the abuser. Instruct the victim to place the crisis hotline telephone information in the lining of a shoe or hem of clothing to conceal it. If the victim refuses the information, tell them it is always available if they change their mind. The victim may be afraid or in denial of the reality of the situation.*

- Document, including need to contact the social worker regarding the victim's children/dependents, refusal of treatment, and contact of children/elderly protective services.

(continues)

Table 17-1   Phases of Crisis Intervention *(continued)*

• Analysis of the information obtained is performed and possible nursing diagnoses identified.

(Aguilera, 1998, pp. 29–31, 35–38; Boyd, 2008, p. 810; Christiansen, 2009, pp. 8–22; Townsend, 2009, p. 209; Varcarolis & Halter, 2010, pp. 532–536; eHow.com—crisis intervention, 2010)

(Phase 1 corresponds to Stages I–III of Roberts's Seven-Stage Crisis Intervention Model)

Phase 2: Planning

In the planning phase, appropriate nursing diagnoses are chosen (refer to NANDA–I Diagnoses Used in Psychiatric Disorders in O'Brien, Kennedy, and Ballard (2008), pp. 552–557; Jakopac & Patel, 2009, pp. 241–242, 251–252, 261, 273–274; Townsend, (2009) pp. 212–217; Varcarolis & Halter, 2010, pp. 542–544). Client centered outcomes/goals and interventions are also part of the planning phase.

Outcomes/goals for the client include:

• Remain safe as well as the safety of other family members directly involved
• Demonstrate an ability to form a therapeutic alliance with the PMH nurse
• Accept offered assistance
• Engage in problem-solving activities
• Explore possible alternations in perceptions and thinking patterns
• Collaborate in the formation of and commit to a plan including a domestic safety plan
• Achieve resolution of the immediate crisis
• Be able to function as independently as possible during the crisis time
• Utilize resources, including support system, effectively
• Return to their precrisis level of functioning, or possibly higher
• Gain new insight
• Learn and begin to use new adaptive coping strategies
• Become more empowered
• Follow through with plan of action and referrals
• Become better equipped to deal with future problems or crises

Other more specific outcomes/goals will depend on the nature of the crisis. (Aguilera, 1998, pp. 24, 31; Townsend, 2009, pp. 209–210; eHow.com—crisis intervention, 2010).

(Phase 2 corresponds to Stage III of Roberts's Seven-Stage Crisis Intervention Model)

(continues)

Table 17-1   Phases of Crisis Intervention *(continued)*

Phase 3: Interventions/Implementation

- Continue to develop rapport and the therapeutic alliance/nurse–client relationship.
- Provide emotional support.
- Acknowledge and facilitate verbalization of feelings.
- Provide physical interventions and assist with medical care and diagnostic tests if needed.
- Help empower the victim by providing information, giving choices, and treating them as a partner rather than dependent and powerless.
- Identify the victim's strengths and use these to assist to help self.
- Clarify information the client is providing as needed, including gently clarifying medical information they are receiving rather than allowing fantasy or false hope which will undermine trust when the situation does not resolve in ways the client wanted it to.
- Support the person's ability to decide and act independently while providing emotional support.
- If needed provide more direct assistance (e.g., making phone calls, contacting support people, arranging transportation, physical care, basic needs, arranging for transfer to specific facilities or units for additional care) if the person's ability to function is compromised or impaired by the crisis event, psychiatric or other medical illness, or chemical abuse/dependency.

    Note: The victim initially may not think there is anyone they can call because of the social isolation created by the abuser. The nurse can gently suggest that other people may be more willing to help the victim than they realize and ask them to think about who can be called. A safe place to stay and not being alone are essential at this time.

- In cases of rape/sexual assault, contact the local Sexual Assault Nurse Examiner (SANE) and local rape counselor.

    Note: If the area does not have a SANE nurse, the PMH nurse will assist the physician in the examination and collection of evidence including specimens for STDs, HIV, and pregnancy testing. Most ER/EDs have rape kits that include all materials needed for collection, drapes, bags, tags, etc. The victim's clothing including undergarments will need to be collected. Victims of rape/sexual assault may have showered and thrown away the clothing they were wearing at the time of the incident. A full examination is still performed and the same process of data collection conducted because with improved testing/equipment it is possible to detect more evidence than in the past. Ask about the possibility of retrieving the items thrown away.

    Note: Once evidence collection has begun, the person collecting it cannot leave until it has been completed or else the chain of evidence will be broken and the evidence will not be able to be used in court or may be discredited (Townsend, 2009, pp. 780–782).

- Assist with medical intervention including initiation of treatment for STDs.

(continues)

Table 17-1 Phases of Crisis Intervention *(continued)*

- Use short, simple sentences especially in situations where the client is experiencing or unable to concentrate related to feelings of being extremely overwhelmed, impulsivity, suicidal or homicidal thoughts, severe anxiety, panic, depersonalization, derealization, psychosis, mania, severe depression or other symptoms of psychiatric or medical illnesses. Engage the client in problem solving and alternative approaches to the extent the person is able; sometimes this is not possible due to severe anxiety states, panic, psychosis, and additional intervention including relaxation, distraction techniques or medication may be needed before attempting this.

- Assist the client to examine errors in perceptions and thinking patterns; assist in confronting reality if ineffectively using ego defense mechanisms such as depression which is not effective in crisis resolution. However, this is done *to the extent the person is able; sometimes this is not possible due to severe anxiety states, panic, psychosis; and additional intervention including relaxation, distraction techniques or medication may be needed before attempting this.*

- Teach what normal responses to expect following this type of experience and when to seek help.

- Teach assertiveness techniques.

- Consistently set limits on unacceptable, destructive or aggressive behavior while reinforcing that the PMH nurse and others are there to help the client.

- Explore availability of resources including social support system/network (if the client is not initially willing to involve family, clarify their reasons and if appropriate attempt to help the client see the advantage of their involvement; if not, explore other social support such as friends, neighbors, community and religious organizations, etc.).

- Provide information on how to develop a domestic safety plan (http://www.aardvarc.org/dv/plan.shtml).

  Note: *The plan will need to be congruent or agree with the client's values and belief systems, and take into account cultural and spiritual factors to be fully implemented and successful. Otherwise the client will not be fully able to carry it out.*

- Assist as needed with mobilization of resources including social support system/network.

- Explore new coping strategies.

- Teach/provide information on new coping strategies and allow time to attempt these as appropriate before the client is discharged from the setting.

- Provide information for referral services.

- Teach the importance of nutrition, rest, exercise, and keeping as normal a schedule as possible to help with recovery.

(continues)

Table 17-1   Phases of Crisis Intervention *(continued)*

- If the victim decides to leave an abusive partner, teach that they are still in danger and ways to remain safe such as going to a safe house/women's shelter, telling only a trusted person where they are going, filing a police report, obtaining a restraining order/protection from abuse (PFA) order, developing a domestic safety plan, and checking into self-defense classes. Victims are in the most danger during the violence *and* immediately after they leave the situation. The nurse should inform them of this while providing information on how to remain safe.

- Arrange follow-up appointment(s)— time frames will depend on the nature of the crisis from 24 hours to 1 week or 1 month later.

- Obtain a firm commitment from the person to follow through with the agreed upon referrals, follow-up care and domestic safety plan.

- Document using individual facility or organization forms.

- Report to local/state agencies as required by individual states (e.g., childhood abuse is required to be report in all 50 states; elder abuse is required in the majority of states and recommended in the remaining states). Local child and elderly protection services are contacted by the person designated in the organization/facility to do so (e.g., physician, nursing supervision).

- Offer to call local police if victim wants to pursue legal action.

(Aguilera, 1998, p. 31; Wilder & Sorensen, 2001, pp. 52–58, 72–79; Keltner, Schwecke, & Bostrom, 2007, pp. 104–108, 126, 134–137; Boyd, 2008, p. 810; Townsend, 2009, p. 210, 258–259; eHow.com—crisis intervention, 2010)

(Phase 3 corresponds to Stages IV–VI of Roberts's Seven-Stage Crisis Intervention Model)

Phase 4: Evaluation

During this phase initial progress toward planned outcomes is analyzed and interventions adjusted if needed. Outcomes may also need to be adjusted as information is clarified, if the client's mental or physical condition changes, and as the collaborative plan is implemented. If the client is not suicidal or homicidal; is not compromised by exacerbations of psychiatric or other medical conditions or problems related to chemical abuse/dependency; and has the necessary social support and other resources including housing to return home, they will be discharged from the setting. If the client requires inpatient admission or transfer to another facility or program for treatment, then that will be the disposition and included in the documentation. When leaving the care setting and returning to home, the client should have all of the following:

- Maintained or returned to a adequate level of safety
- Information for referral services. (see Table 17-2)
- Follow-up appointment(s) and prescriptions for medication including STD treatment
- Information on new adaptive coping strategies
- Clear (verbalized) understanding of plan to follow or reinforcement needed

(continues)

Table 17-1 Phases of Crisis Intervention *(continued)*

- Instructions to return to the care setting/emergency department/clinic or who else to contact if the crisis situation becomes worse (usually telephone hotline phone numbers, 911/emergency contact information, local ER/ED, community agencies, safe houses).

- Documentation including the disposition of the client (e.g., discharge to home with whom; admitted where and report given to whom; transferred to another facility and report given to whom; follow-up appointment arranged with whom or client agrees to call if unable to arrange before being discharged). In addition, all the above-mentioned information in the previous items in this bulleted list should be entered in the facility/organization's charting/recordkeeping system.

The evaluation phase may extend to include the follow-up visit/care so that better evaluation of the interventions and plan can be made over time and continuity of care maintained (Townsend, 2009, p. 211; Varcarolis & Halter, 2010, p. 540).

(Phase 4 corresponds to Stage VII of Roberts's Seven-Stage Crisis Intervention Model)

RECOVERY FROM VIOLENCE AND ABUSE

Recovery from any type of violence and abuse is influenced by factors such as the duration and degree of severity of the violence, availability of resources, and the type of intervention. Recovery is generally believed to occur in three stages: (1) impact or initial disorganization, (2) recoil or the struggle to adapt, and (3) reorganization or reconstruction (see **Box 17-1**). In each of these stages, reactions and behaviors occur as the victim or survivor begins the process of recovery. These stages may also apply to victims or survivors of various crimes and disasters.

BOX 17-1 Stages of Recovery from Trauma

Impact
Lasting from a few minutes to a few days or longer if the trauma is ongoing

- Includes initial disorganization, confusion, shock, denial, fear that can be paralyzing, horror, shame, guilt, anger, helplessness, powerlessness; symptoms of ASD including intrusive memories, flashback nightmares, emotional detachment or numbing; dissociation may also occur
- For some victims reactions may be delayed and they may appear calm, rational

(continues)

BOX 17-1   Stages of Recovery from Trauma *(continued)*

Recoil
Lasting from weeks to months

- Struggle to adapt as the emotional stress continues; need for temporary dependence and support; may appear and act normal; activity helps suppress fears, sadness, and anger
- Later in this phase may want to talk about what happened
- Gradual awareness of the full event this incident has on their life

Reorganization
Lasting from months to years

- Reconstruction of their life
- Review what happened
- Question own actions and why the event happened, justify or assign blame to self, others or both
- Still remember the trauma, but the associated emotions diminish
- Grief over losses resolves slowly
- Regain a sense of control and the ability to protect themselves
- Lingering nightmares
- Lingering frustrations, disillusionment
- Negative feelings subside as the survivor reengages in activities and life
- If the survivor does not effectively reorganize they may develop PTSD

Source: Keltner, Schwecke, & Bostrom, 2007, pp. 605–606.

CHILDREN/ADOLESCENTS

Children/adolescents who are difficult to parent due to temperament, congenital problems, or chronic illness, or who are the product of an unwanted pregnancy are at greater risk for violence and abuse (Varcarolis & Halter, 2010, p. 589). In order to gain cooperation in cases of sexual abuse, the perpetrator frequently buys gifts or threatens the child/adolescent with harm to their siblings, pets, or a parent if they reveal their "secret."

The Child Abuse Prevention and Treatment Act (CAPTA) "identifies a minimum set of acts or behaviors that characterize maltreatment" of children (Townsend, 2009, p. 732). Asking questions about how the family shows anger, being touched in areas that are covered by a bathing suit, being asked to keep secrets from a parent, along with the use of play therapy and art supplies can help with interview/assessment. Victims of violence and abuse should be interviewed/assessed separately because they may deny or not report violence or abuse when family members or friends are present. Previously mentioned information on the phases of crisis intervention will also apply to children/adolescents (see also Chapters 3-5 and 16). Nurses are required by law in all 50 states to report suspected child abuse—see also previous information regarding reporting and documenting in the Crisis Intervention section of this chapter. Referrals and community resources for these situations should include child protective services, social services, and psychoeducation including anger management, parenting classes, normal child growth and development, and stress management as well as counseling (see **Table 17-2**).

Table 17-2   Referrals

Clients will need referrals for general and specific needs depending on the type of crisis. Information should be given in writing, on a piece of paper small enough to be concealed in the lining of a shoe or the hem of their clothing (or download information to cell phones/portable information devices), because clients are too overwhelmed to remember while trying to cope with the situation or if the abuser finds it and suspects the victim may leave, the violence will escalate. If they initially refuse the information, tell them the information is always available if they change their mind (see also Chapter 16).

- Domestic Violence Safety Plan: http://www.aardvarc.org/dv/plan.shtml
- Local women's shelters/safe houses
- Victim Services Domestic Violence (Safe Horizons): http://www.safehorizon.org/
- Local rape crisis counseling information
- Local community domestic violence and abuse and rape resource information
- Local college campus violence and abuse/rape resource information for college students
- Local community legal aid; Retraining Orders/Protection From Abuse (PFAs) Orders
- Rape and Domestic Violence Aid and Resource Collection; Federal/State: http://www.aardvarc.org
- National Organization for Victim Assistance (NOVA): http://www.trynova.org/victiminfo
- For victims in denial or increasing awareness, the following quiz may be helpful in helping present reality:

  Relationship Quiz: Am I in an Abusive Relationship?: http://www.aardvarc.org/dv/abusequiz.shtml

(continues)

Table 17-2   Referrals *(continued)*

- Crisis hotline telephone numbers:

  Child Abuse/Neglect Hotline: 1-800-422-4453

  Youth Crisis Runaway Hotline: 1-800-621-4000 or 1-800-448-4663

  Parents Anonymous Hotline: 1-800-348-5437 (National)

  National Domestic Violence Crisis Line 1-888-411-1333 or 1-800-799-SAFE (7233) or 1-800-787-3224 TTY

  Pregnancy Hotline: 1-800-395-4357

  Elderly Abuse Hotline: 1-800-259-4990

  Adult Protective Services: 1-800-898-4910 to report abuse, neglect, exploitation or extortion

  Suicide Prevention: 1-800-273-TALK (8255) or 1-800-749-COPE (2673) or 1-800 SUICIDE (784-2433)

- MaleSurvivor: http://www.malesurvivor.org

- Medical physician follow-up appointment

- Psychiatrist follow-up appointment

- Counseling/psychotherapy follow-up appointment with a psychologist, APRN, or social worker for individuals and families

- Chemical abuse/dependency follow-up appointments with addictionologist and chemical dependency counseling

- Elder abuse website: http://www.elderabuse.org

- Volunteers of America: 1-800-899-0089 for a variety of services including basic needs

- David Baldwin's Trauma Information Pages focus on trauma and symptoms including PTSD: http://www.trauma-pages.com

- CyberbullyNOT: Student Guide to Cyberbullying: http://new.csriu.org/cyberbully/docs/cbstudentguide.pdf

- Threats Online: Student Guide to Cyberthreats: http://new.csriu.org/cyberbully/docs/ctstudentguide.pdf

- For situations involving military veterans:

  Military Counseling Services: 1-800-342-9647 (National)

  United States Department of Veterans Affairs: https://vip.vba.va.gov/portal/VBAH/Home

  United States Army Center for Health Promotion and Preventive Medicine (USACHPPM): http://chppm-www.apgea.army.mil/dhpw/Population/combat.aspx

Referrals for males who perpetrate violence and abuse:

- Men Can Stop Rape. Helping men who rape: www.mencanstoprape.org

Violence and abuse may be suspected if parents, guardians or caretakers exhibit the following behavior (see **Table 17-3**):

- Changes information given regarding the cause of injuries, gives conflicting information or refuses to give an explanation
- Has a history of child abuse
- Has an authoritarian style of parenting
- Uses harsh physical discipline
- Describes the child as "evil"
- Overtly rejects the child
- Constantly belittles, berates, shames, blames or threatens the child
- Is unconcerned about or indifferent to the child's needs
- Refuses offers of help for the child's illness or problems
- Is apathetic or depressed
- Exhibits irrational or bizarre behavior
- Uses alcohol or drugs
- Leaves the child or children unattended or in the care of siblings not much older
- Is overly protective of the child and severely limits contact with other children, especially children of the opposite sex
- Is secretive and isolative
- Is jealous and controlling of other family members
- Has problems with impulse control or loses temper easily

(Townsend, 2009, pp. 732–733; Varcarolis & Halter, 2010, p. 588; Frisch & Frisch, 2011, p. 730)

Table 17-3 Signs and Symptoms of Child Abuse and Neglect	
• Is socially withdrawn, isolated, frightened or aggressive	• Child feels little or no attachment to, affection for, or sense of belonging to the parent/caregiver or opposite (is afraid of parent/caregiver)
• Demonstrates extremes of behavior such as extreme passivity, is overly compliant, is demanding or aggressive	

(continues)

Table 17-3   Signs and Symptoms of Child Abuse and Neglect *(continued)*

- Acts inappropriately adult (e.g., parents other children) or inappropriately infantile (e.g., frequently head-banging or rocking back and forth)
- Is developmentally delayed emotionally or physically
- Has attempted suicide
- Has inadequate clothing or material goods for situation/weather/climate
- Is malnourished, dehydrated; begs for or steals food
- Has poor hygiene—lice, scabies
- Has inadequate or unsafe housing
- Is ill, but no medical/dental/psychiatric attention has been sought on behalf of the child
- Injuries do not "match" the explanation given—broken bones, skull fractures, intracranial or intraocular bleeding, burns, symmetrical vs asymmetrical injuries; multiple injuries but at various stages of healing; abdominal trauma or rupture of abdominal organs
- Excessive absences from school; change in school performance
- Failure to thrive physically, emotionally, psychologically, intellectually, socially; lags behind on developmental testing
- Has had frequent ER visits/hospitalizations for "accidental" injuries
- There is much resistance from parent/caregiver to examining the child without their presence

- Has an obvious need for special education services, but not provided
- Is left alone for long periods of time when not old enough to be responsible for self (or siblings)
- Has frequent urinary, genital, or throat infections; evidence of injuries to urethra, vagina, or rectum
- Had an STD or becomes pregnant before age 14 years of age
- Reports being molested, inappropriately touched, or having sex with an adult
- Has difficulty walking or sitting
- Engages in sexually provocative behavior
- Vocabulary/knowledge related to sex far above developmental level, unusually sophisticated or bizarre
- Has problems with nightmares or bed wetting
- Suddenly refuses to participate in physical activities or change for gym/physical education class
- Suddenly refuses to go/afraid of a baby sitter, relative, family friend
- Sets fires
- Bullies or is abusive toward, or sexually molests other children
- Has attempted to or actually run away

Source: Keltner, Schwecke, & Bostrom, 2007, pp. 611–612; Townsend, 2009, pp. 732–733; Frisch & Frisch, 2011, pp. 731–733.

ELDERLY

The APA suspects that the number of elderly people who are victims of violence, abuse, and neglect "may be far higher and that for every case reported, five go unreported" (Varcarolis & Halter, 2010, pp. 586–587). Increased physical, mental, and financial demands on caregivers cause increasing caregiver stress and strain. Intergenerational transmission and adult children caring for formerly abusive parents also add to the potential for violence and abuse toward the elderly (Varcarolis & Halter, 2010, p. 589).

The violence or abuse may be physical, emotional, psychological, financial, or even sexual. Proper nutrition, fluids, and medical and psychiatric care may be withheld. The abuser may need the elderly person's financial income to survive and may feel "trapped" in the situation and express it inappropriately towards the victim. Age-related screening tools are more available according to Frisch & Frisch (2011), such as a screening tool developed by researchers in Canada, the Elder Abuse Suspicion Index (EASI) (see **Table 17-4**).

Table 17-4   Signs and Symptoms of Elder Abuse or Neglect

- Shows obvious signs/symptoms of malnutrition or dehydration (e.g., substantial weight loss, poor skin turgor, sunken appearance to eyes, muscle weakness, lethargy, difficulty concentrating, low blood sugar)
- Has poor hygiene, strong body odor, or odor of urine/feces
- Has infestations—lice, scabies
- Has skin breakdown, decubiti
- Has inadequate clothing or material goods for situation/weather/climate
- Is socially withdrawn or apathetic
- Is easily startled
- Adamantly refuses to say anything against their caregiver in spite of facts pointing to neglect/abuse

- Has difficulty concentrating, but not due to illnesses such as diagnosed dementia/Alzheimer's
- Has difficulty swallowing or speaking
- Has contractures of extremities
- Has limited range of motion (ROM)
- Injuries do not "match" the explanation given—broken bones, skull fractures, intracranial or intraocular bleeding, burns, symmetrical vs asymmetrical injuries; multiple injuries but at various stages of healing; abdominal trauma; signs of sexual assault
- Is taking medications not justified by medical or psychiatric conditions; appears over-medicated
- Allows family member/caregiver to answer any questions even when questions are directed to the elder client

(continues)

Table 17-4 Signs and Symptoms of Elder Abuse or Neglect *(continued)*	
• Is fearful of contradicting family member/caregiver • Physically withdraws when approached as if expecting to be hurt • Is overly concerned about "offending" anyone • Is unable to answer questions related to financial matters when intellectually able to do so	• Has poor environmental/living conditions–major repairs to building structure needed (e.g., roof, foundation), piled up garbage, infestations, blocked stairways, lack of necessary assistive devices, locks on refrigerator or cupboards

Source: Keltner, Schwecke, & Bostrom, 2007, pp. 611–612; Boyd, 2008, p. 866; Fontaine, 2009, pp. 584–585; Varcarolis & Halter, 2010; pp. 586–587; Frisch & Frisch, 2011, pp. 731–735.

Nurses are required by law in 43 states (and it is recommended in the remaining states) to report and document suspected elder abuse—see also previous information regarding reporting and documenting in the Crisis Intervention section of this chapter (see also Chapters 3-5 and 16). Victims of violence and abuse should be interviewed/ assessed separately because they may deny or not report violence or abuse when family members or friends are present. Elderly clients may need to be admitted for a short hospital stay until safe, suitable living arrangements can be made (see Table 17-2 for referral information).

REFERENCES

An Abuse, Rape and Domestic Violence Aid and Resource Collection. (2010). Retrieved from http://www.aardvarc.org

Aguilera, D. C. (1998). *Crisis intervention theory and methodology* (8th ed.). St. Louis, MO: Mosby, Inc.

Alexy, E. M. (Mar./Apr., 2009). Intimate partner violence. Presentation at Psychiatric Nursing Conference, Nashville, TN.

Boyd, M. A. (2008). *Psychiatric nursing: Contemporary practice* (4th ed.). Philadelphia, PA: Wolters/ Kluwer/Lippincott, Williams, and Wilkins.

Centers for Disease Control and Prevention (CDC). (2010). *Intimate partner violence:* Definitions. Retrieved June 27, 2010 from: http://www.cdc.gov/ViolencePrevention/intimatepartner violence/definitions.html

Centers for Disease Control and Prevention (CDC). (2010). *Intimate partner violence and sexual violence victimization assessment instruments for use in healthcare settings.* Retrieved from http://www. cdc.gov/NCIPC/pub-res/ipv_and_sv_screening.htm

Centers for Disease Control and Prevention (CDC). (2009). *Issue Brief for Educators and Caregivers US*. Retrieved from www.cdc.gov/ncipc/dvp/YVP/electronic_agression_brief_for_parents.pdf

Christiansen, K. (2009). *The crisis intervention manual* (2nd ed.). Reseda, CA: Zero Point Communications.

CyberbullyNOT: Student Guide to Cyberbullying. (2009). Retrieved from http://new.csriu.org/cyberbully/docs/cbstudentguide.pdf

David Baldwin's Trauma Information Pages. (2010). Retrieved from http://www.trauma-pages.com

Elderabuse.org. (2010). Retrieved from http://www.elderabuse.org

Fontaine, K. L. (2009). *Mental health nursing* (6th ed.). Upper Saddle River, NJ: Pearson Education, Inc.

Frisch, N. C., & Frisch, L. E. (2011). *Psychiatric mental health nursing* (4th ed.). Clifton Park, NY: Delmar/Thomas Learning, Inc.

How to intervene in a crisis situation. (2010). Retrieved from http://www.ehow.com/how_2138570_intervene-crisis-situation.html

Jakopac, K. A., & Patel, S. C. (2009). *Psychiatric mental health case studies and care plans*. Sudbury, MA: Jones and Bartlett.

Keltner, N. L., Schwecke, L. H., & Bostrom, C. E. (2007). *Psychiatric nursing* (5th ed.). St. Louis, MO: Mosby, Elsevier.

Lange, S. P., & Shank, S. I. (2005). *Managing psychiatric crisis*. Lakeway, TX: National Center of Continuing Education, Inc.

Louisiana Domestic Violence Crisis Support Resources. (2009). Retrieved from http://www.aardvarc.org/dv/states/ladv.shtml

Marcus, P. (Mar./Apr., 2009). Neurobiology of violence. Presentation at Psychiatric Nursing Conference, Nashville, TN.

Male survivors: Overcoming sexual victimization of boys & men. (2010). Retrieved from http://www.malesurvivor.org

Men Can Stop Rape. *Helping men who rape.* (2010). Retrieved from http://www.mencanstoprape.org

National Organization for Victim Assistance (NOVA). (2010). Retrieved from www.try-nova.org and http://www.trynova.org/victiminfo

O'Brien, P. G., Kennedy, W. Z., & Ballard, K. A. (2008). *Psychiatric mental health nursing: An introduction to theory and practice*. Sudbury, MA: Jones and Bartlett.

Relationship Quiz: Am I In An Abusive Relationship? (2010). Retrieved from http://www.aardvarc.org/dv/abusequiz.shtml

Sadock, B. J., & Sadock, V. A. (2005). *Comprehensive textbook of psychiatry* (8th ed.). Philadelphia, PA: Lippincott, Williams, and Wilkins.

Threats Online: Student Guide to Cyberthreats. (2009). Retrieved from http://new.csriu.org/cyberbully/docs/ctstudentguide.pdf

Townsend, M. C. (2009). *Psychiatric mental health nursing* (6th ed.). Philadelphia, PA: F. A. Davis.

Varcarolis, E. M., Carson, V. B., & Shoemaker, N. C. (2006). *Foundations of psychiatric mental health nursing: A clinical approach* (5th ed.). St. Louis, MO: Saunders/Elsevier.

Varcarolis, E. M., & Halter, M. J. (2010). *Foundations of psychiatric mental health nursing: A clinical approach* (6th ed.). St. Louis, MO: Saunders/Elsevier.

Victim Services Domestic Violence (Safe Horizons). (2010). Retrieved from http://www.safe horizon.org

United States Department of Veterans Affairs. (2010). Retrieved from https://vip.vba.va.gov/ portal/VBAH/Home

United States Army Center for Health Promotion and Preventive Medicine (USACHPPM). (2010). Retrieved from http://chppm-www.apgea.army.mil/dhpw/Population/combat.aspx

Wilder, S. S., & Sorensen, C. (2001). *Essentials of aggression management in health care.* Upper Saddle River, NJ: Prentice-Hall, Inc.

SUGGESTED READINGS

Bell, C. C. (June, 2007). Bullying and school violence. *Clinical Psychiatry News, 35*(6), 36.

Centers for Disease Control and Prevention (CDC) Podcast. (2009). Retrieved from Cyberbullying www2a.cdc.gov/podcasts/player.asp?f=7306

Dharmapala, D., Garoupa, N., and McAdam, R. (Sept., 2006). *The just world bias and hate crime statutes.* Retrieved from http://www.law.virginia.edu/pdf/olin/0607/mcadams.pdf

Fontaine, K. L., & Fletcher, J. S. (2003). *Mental health nursing* (5th ed.). Upper Saddle River, NJ: Pearson Education, Inc.

HRSA Department of Education. (2009). *Stop Bullying Now.* Retrieved from http://www.stop bullyingnow.hrsa.gov/HHS_PSA/pdfs/SBN_Tip_23.pdf

Kalman, I. (2009). *Bullies to buddies: A psychological solution to bullying.* Retrieved from www.Bullies2 Buddies.com

Muller, E., & Dowling, M. (2008). Mental health consequences of child sexual abuse. *British Journal of Nursing, 17*(22), 1428–1433.

National Institute of Mental Health (NIMH). (2010). Retrieved from http://www.nimh.nih. gov/index.shtml

Paulk, D. (Oct., 2004). How to recognize child abuse and neglect. *The Clinical Advisor,* 43-49.

Stuart, G. W., & Laraia, M. T. (2005). *Principles and practice of psychiatric nursing* (8th ed.). St. Louis, MO: Mosby, Elsevier.

The Center for Safe and Responsible Internet Use. (2009). Retrieved from http://csriu.org/

U. S. Department of Justice Office of Juvenile Justice and Delinquency Prevention. (2009). Retrieved from www.ojjdp.ncjrs.org/ and http://ojjdp.ncjrs.org/programs/index.html

Varcarolis, E. M. (2006). *Manual of psychiatric nursing care plans* (3rd ed.). St. Louis, MO: Saunders/ Elsevier.

Wood, S. J., & Isenberg, M. A. (July, 2001). Adaptation as a mediator of intimate abuse and traumatic stress in battered women. *Nursing Science Quarterly, 14*(3), 215–221.

CHAPTER 18

Crisis Intervention in Disasters

Kim A. Jakopac

OBJECTIVES

The nursing student will be able to:
1. Define and provide examples of types of disaster
2. Identify the role of the PMH nurse in disaster situations
3. Recognize common, age-related responses of survivors of natural disasters
4. Identify high risk groups for developing more serious responses including stress disorders
5. Apply concepts of crisis intervention, nursing process, and psychological first aid
6. Discuss primary, secondary, and tertiary prevention planning measures

KEY TERMS

Acute stress disorder (ASD)   Psychological triage
Disaster   Terrorism
Psychological first aid

Definitions of *disaster* have been put forth by many agencies. Events that overwhelm community resources and threaten the safety and ability to function of individuals living in the community are considered to be disasters. These events may be caused by nature or be man-made, but all result in destruction and devastation of property and life, as well as some degree of psychological trauma (Townsend, 2009, p. 211). Terrorism is a specific type of man-made disaster perpetrated by an individual or specific group using premeditated acts of violence that are politically motivated and perpetrated against civilians or private citizens (Fontaine, 2009, p. 651) (see also Chapter 16).

SIGNIFICANT RISK FACTORS

Significant risk factors affecting the impact of disasters on individuals and communities include:

- Lower socioeconomic rank
- Environmental (e.g., buildings and infrastructure, geographic environment)
- Adequate, accessible basic resources including food, water, shelter, clothing, medical and mental health care, transportation
- General wellness of the population
- Percentage of the population that is very young or very old
- Cultural aspects
- Anticipation, preplanning, and preparation for future disasters

(Townsend, 2009, p. 211)

An individual's psychosocial, cognitive, and biologic responses to disasters may be evident immediately or be delayed. Not only are people directly involved affected by disasters, but also others who are related to them, know them personally, or experienced the event through media contact. Factors affecting a survivor's ability to cope include the level of involvement in the event (i.e., directly or indirectly; themselves or significant others), degree of personal threat, and the ability to ask for and receive help. Many people find comfort being with and talking to family members, close friends, spiritual advisors, and mental health and medical health care professionals (Fontaine, 2009, p. 658; CDC, 2010).

HIGH-RISK GROUPS

High-risk groups for developing more severe stress responses and stress disorders including acute stress disorder (ASD) and posttraumatic stress disorder (PTSD) include:

- Primary/directly impacted survivors and anyone fearing for their life
- First responders—EMTs, paramedics, ambulance drivers
- Policemen
- Firemen
- Support providers
- Anyone with prior exposure to psychological or physical trauma
- Anyone with prior history or current psychiatric or other medical illnesses
- Survivors with poor or no supportive relationships/support system

- Children/adolescents—lack life experiences, coping skills, and sensitivity to disruptions in their physical and social environment or daily schedule
- Elderly

(Fontaine, 2009, p. 652; Townsend, 2009, p. 211)

ROLE OF THE PMH NURSE

According to Fontaine (2009), "nurses are in the forefront of planning and providing care in the event of mass trauma....Whether at the disaster site, in a community triage area, the emergency room, or a general hospital, nurses should be prepared to provide intervention strategies that address the particular needs of people during different stages of the crisis" (p. 651). As previously stated in Chapter 16, the role of the psychiatric-mental health (PMH) nurse is "to provide a framework of support systems that guide the patient (person) through the crisis and facilitate the development and use of positive coping skills. The nurse must be acutely aware that a person in crisis may be at high risk for suicide or homicide" (Boyd, 2008, p. 806). Identifying survivors needing more intense psychiatric intervention and those at high risk for developing stress disorders and other psychiatric disorders is vitally important.

Survivors of disasters need psychosocial crisis interventions and frequently need medical intervention as well as physical nursing interventions for physical injuries. Interventions may have to be carried out in makeshift settings depending on what is available. Multiple age groups and massive numbers of people may be affected simultaneously. It will take longer to achieve client outcomes of resolution of the immediate crisis, the ability to function as independently as possible during the crisis time, become more empowered, and return to a precrisis level of functioning, or possibly higher, with new insight and coping abilities (Aguilera, 1998, p. 24; Townsend, 2009, p. 209). The PMH nurse will need to be able to integrate interventions as part of the interdisciplinary emergency response team.

RESPONSES TO DISASTERS AND RECOVERY

Responses to disasters are complex and can affect the survivor's entire well-being. As previously mentioned, response may be immediate or delayed and influenced by how directly the survivor was involved in the actual disaster. Responses may also be influenced by the age of the survivor and cultural influences on perception and processing of the event, but there is not much empirical research available, especially for children. Most survivors experience fear, "visual memories," and a decreased sense of safety. Effects across the life span are varied (Fontaine, 2009, pp. 653-655; American Academy of Pediatrics Work Group on Disasters, 2010). The responses are considered to be normal unless they progressed to signs of ASD or PTSD.

Infants and Preschool Children

- Infants—sleep pattern disruption
- More easily startled; increased reaction to loud noises
- Increased clinging behaviors, whining, fear of the dark
- Requiring more comforting, reassurance
- More irritable and aggressive; more tantrum behavior
- Regressive behaviors—wanting a bottle after able to drink from a cup, toileting problems
- Reenactment of event through play and in art work
- Fear of toys/objects that remind them of details of the event (e.g., toy planes, trucks)

Stressed, anxious parents may have been transmitting their feelings to their infants/children.

School-age Children and Adolescents

- If directly affected by injury or loss, demonstration of signs of ASD or PTSD (increased in girls)
- Not feeling safe
- Increased problems concentrating
- Transient confusion
- Experience of long-term anxiety
- Difficulty with their own self-soothing behaviors
- Guilt for surviving if lost family members or friends
- More risk-taking behavior and display of hostility from adolescents
- Children's responses by gender:
  - Boys—take longer to recover; display more aggressive, antisocial, and violent behaviors
  - Girls—are more distressed, verbal about emotions, ask more questions, and have more frequent thoughts about the disaster

Adults

- Not feeling safe
- Anxiety
- Tearfulness
- Difficulty sleeping and nightmares
- Flashbacks of the event
- Anger
- Guilt
- Emotional numbness or distancing
- Helplessness, hopelessness
- Problems concentrating
- Social self-isolation
- Profound sadness
- Physical/somatic symptoms

The phases of recovery: impact, recoil, and reorganization (see Box 17-1), apply to survivors of disasters, as well as the information on grief responses in Chapter 16.

Coping Behaviors and Psychological Responses

- Talking to others
- Turning to spirituality/religion
- Involvement in group activities
- Involvement in contributing to helping others

(Fontaine, 2009, p. 652)

Additional Coping Behaviors

- Perceived sense of control over events demonstrated by:
  - Being immersed in the media coverage, at times to point of neglecting responsibilities
  - Denying the event happened
  - Becoming detached from the event
  - Avoiding any discussion of the event
- *Inappropriate or ineffective* behaviors:
  - Loss of ability to care about what happened to themselves or others

- Remaining in denial
- Continuing periods of irritability, mood swings, difficulty concentrating, or crying

(Fontaine, 2009, p. 652)

PSYCHOLOGICAL OUTCOMES

"Psychological outcomes over time were significantly related to variations in the use of specific coping strategies directly post-event (9/11 terrorists attacks). The strongest predictor of psychological outcomes over time were coping strategies used shortly after the attacks" (Fontaine, 2009, p. 658)

- Seeking social support
- Self-distraction
- Acceptance
- Denial
- Self-blame
- Behavioral disengagement

Significantly more distress was reported by survivors who used self-blame, denial, self-distraction, sought social support, or disengaged from coping efforts. A significantly lower amount of distress was reported by survivors who began to use coping strategies immediately after the event. Survivors who used disengagement as a coping strategy reported increased stress and PTSD (Fontaine, 2009, p. 658).

PLANNING CARE FOR PEOPLE AFFECTED BY TERRORISM/DISASTER

- Preventing risk of developing serious mental illness/dysfunction
- Primary prevention—measures to decrease the effect of the event
- Secondary prevention—measures to meet immediate needs of individuals and communities
- Tertiary prevention—measures to provide care for as long as is needed

Implementing Primary Prevention Measures

- Community education, disaster plans
- Individual family disaster preparedness kits
- Teaching signs/symptoms of stress reactions and how to comfort infants/children/adolescents

- Strengthening social networks
- Desired outcome—will develop specific disaster plans and identify community resources they can use

Implementing Secondary Prevention Measures

- Providing for basic needs including shelter, food, information, medical care for injuries, emotional support/coping strategies/relaxation techniques, care for existing psychiatric disorders/medical disorders
- Desired outcome—will verbalize feelings of safety.

Implementing Tertiary Prevention Measures

- Need for help may continue for an indefinite amount of time.
- Providing medical, mental health services; individual/family/group support services and psychotherapy; spiritual support
- More permanent housing if temporarily relocated
- Continued education and information on coping strategies, empowerment strategies to increase feelings of control over situation and promote healing
- Desired outcome—will attend community programs, therapy, and verbalize increased feelings of control over situation.

Evaluation needs to occur on all levels by individuals and communities (Fontaine, 2009, pp. 656–658; SAMSHA, 2010)

CRISIS INTERVENTION

As previously stated in Chapters 16 and 17, crisis intervention is not a replacement for long-term counseling or therapy, but uses tools that can provide relief to someone experiencing the trauma of an unexpected critical event. According to the American Nurses Association (ANA), "Crisis intervention is a short term therapeutic process that focuses on the rapid resolution of an immediate crisis or emergency using available personnel, family, and/or environmental resources" (Varcarolis & Halter, 2010, p. 529) (see legal–ethical information in Chapters 12, 13, and 16).

Crisis intervention in disaster also includes concepts and techniques of *psychological first aid*. Psychological first aid consists of techniques used to help survivors of disasters handle intense emotional reactions that are a result of intense fear, apprehension, or uncertainty (see **Table 18-1**).

Table 18-1 Psychological First Aid Techniques	
Communicate calmly	• Sit or stand using the L-stance (chair or shoulder 90° to the other person's shoulder). • Maintain open body posture. • Lean forward. • Make eye contact. • Relax.
Communicate warmth	• Use an empathetic tone. • Smile. • Use open and welcoming gestures. Allow the person you are talking with to dictate the personal distance between you.
Establish a relationship	• Introduce yourself if they do not know you. • Ask the person what they would like to be called. • Do not shorten their name or use their first name without their permission. • With some cultures, it is important to always address the person as "Mr." or "Mrs."
Use concrete questions to help the person focus	• Use focused, closed-ended questions. • Briefly explain why you are asking the question.
Come to an agreement on something	• Establish a point of agreement that will help solidify your relationship and gain their trust. • Active listening will help you find a point of agreement.
Speak to the person with respect	• Use words like please and thank you. • Do not make global statements about the person's character. • Lavish praise is not believable. • Use positive language.
Promote safety	• Help people meet basic needs for food and shelter, and obtain emergency medical attention. • Provide repeated, simple, and accurate information on how to get these basic needs.
Promote calm	• Listen to people who wish to share their stories and emotions, and remember that there is no right or wrong way to feel. • Be open, empathetic, and compassionate even if people are being difficult.

(continues)

Table 18-1	Psychological First Aid Techniques *(continued)*
	• Offer accurate information about the disaster or trauma and the relief efforts underway in order to help victims understand the situation.
Promote connectednes	• Help people contact friends and loved ones. • Keep families together. Keep children with parents or other close relatives whenever possible.
Promote self-efficacy	• Give practical suggestions that steer people toward helping themselves. • Engage people in meeting their own needs.
Promote help	• Find out the types and locations of government and nongovernment services and direct people to those services that are available.
Behaviors to avoid	• Criticizing existing services or relief activities in front of people in need of these services. • Forcing people to share their stories with you, especially very personal details, in order to accept shelter or obtain emergency medical attention; offer and suggest rather than force. • Using overly simple responses, false hope or clichés such as "everything will be OK" or "at least you survived." • Telling people what you think they should be feeling, thinking, or how they should have acted earlier. • Telling people why you think they have suffered by alluding to personal behaviors or beliefs of victims. • Making promises that may be difficult to keep or may not be kept.
Potential Agitated Behaviors and How to Respond	
Challenges or questions authority	• Answer the question calmly. • Repeat your statement calmly.
Refuses to follow directions	• Do not assert control. Let the person attempt to gain control of themselves. • Remain professional. • Restructure your request in another way. • Give the person time to think about your request.

(continues)

Table 18-1 Psychological First Aid Techniques *(continued)*	
Loses control and becomes verbally agitated	• Give additional personal space. • Maintain open body posture while standing in an L-stance (shoulder 90° to the other person's shoulder). If initially you were sitting, stand up slowly, but avoid standing directly in front of the person so that you do not appear threatening to them. • Reply calmly. • State that you may need assistance to help them.
Becomes threatening	• If the person becomes threatening or intimidating and does not respond to your attempts to calm them, seek immediate assistance.

Source: SAMHSA, 2010 [http://mentalhealth.samhsa.gov/Disasterrelief/pubs/manemotion.asp].

Phases/Stages of Crisis Intervention

The phases/stages of crisis intervention, as well as basic telephone crisis intervention, were presented in Chapters 16 and 17. The survivor may have basic needs for water or food and need to be taken to a quiet, safe area to talk (see **Table 18-2**).

Again, the PMH nurse will not be acting alone, but as part of a multidisciplinary emergency team to provide services and support team efforts including helping with psychological triage of survivors. It is important to know scope of practice, and professional and personal limitations in order to ask for assistance when needed and provide safe interventions. Approaches may have to be modified due to makeshift settings (see also Chapters 3-5, 7, 9, and 12). For recommended referral services, see **Table 18-3**.

Psychological first aid for crisis responders and critical incident stress debriefing (CISD) are ways in which to mitigate stress for healthcare personnel and decrease the development of serious stress disorders such as ASD or PTSD, other anxiety disorders, or depression. Reinforcing the importance of practicing self-care, signs and symptoms to watch for, and need to seek help are important to keep crisis responders able to perform at the best level possible and avoid problems themselves.

Preplanning before disasters occur, clearly defining roles and procedures, frequently rotating crisis responders between high-stress areas, low-stress areas, and break times; establishment of separate areas where crisis responders can meet their

Table 18-2   Phases of Crisis Intervention

Phase 1: Assessment

(See also Table 16-2 and Table 17-1 for more information on crisis intervention, and Table 18-1 for psychological first aid techniques.)

- Assist with psychological triage by:
  - Determining how close physically and emotionally the survivor was to the disaster.
  - Remembering that subjective impressions of danger can be just as or more critical than actual exposure.
  - Knowing that children/adolescents are influenced by the reactions of adults to the disaster.
  - Referring to high-risk groups previously mentioned.
  - Assessing for signs of ASD.
- Survivors who are confused, disoriented, dissociating, remaining silent rather than responding to questions (shock, disbelief, emotional numbing), hysterical, suicidal/homicidal, psychotic, with a history of psychiatric disorders or chemical dependency, or history of prior exposure to trauma should be high priority for intervention.
- Screening/assessment tools for children/adolescent impacted by disasters:
  - The Child Behavior Checklist for 4 to 18 year olds
  - The Pediatric Emotional Distress Scale (PEDS)
  - Impact of Events Scale
  - Reaction Index
  - Children's PTSD Inventory
- Provide as quiet an area as possible for assessment.
- Begin to develop rapport and a therapeutic alliance/nurse–client relationship by remaining calm, communicating that you care about the person, and providing comfort by therapeutic use of self, active listening, attending skills, empathy, and emotional support.

  "Hi. My name's _____. I'm a nurse. What is your name?"

  "Are you hurt?" or "Were you injured? Point to where you were injured."

  "Where were you when the _____ (event) happened?"

  "It's okay to cry."

  "Anger is a normal emotion."

  "Fear is a normal emotion."

  "Do you feel like talking about what happened?"

  "What are you feeling?"

(continues)

Table 18-2   Phases of Crisis Intervention *(continued)*

- Obtain a *brief, clear* description of the crisis situation or event and when it occurred (clarification of information will occur throughout the assessment and in Phase 3 as needed).

  "When did it start?"

  "Take your time."

  "Then what happened?"

  Note: *If you meet with resistance or it is obvious the survivor is having difficulty mentally processing information, do not force the survivor to tell their story (see Table 16-1 and 16-2).*

  Note: *If there are other people the survivor is concerned about, offer to help them make phone calls and enlist the help of other crisis responders to locate these people. Avoid giving false hope/reassurance that they probably are okay.*

- Perform a brief mental status exam, assess for suicidal/homicidal thoughts, and determine the need for medical intervention.

- **Avoid** giving false reassurances such as "Everything will be all right." If the result is not "all right" the client will be angry and stop trusting you. **Instead** reiterate your desire to listen and help.

  "I/we care about you and will listen." or "I/we want to help you."

- Guide the client through the assessment process, which may at times require being direct, firm, or gentle to help the client focus/refocus. Adapt your approach to the individual survivor's response.

  "Stay with me."

  "Tell me more about . . ."

  "What about . . . ?"

  "I'm here."

  "Yes, go on . . ."

- What is the client's perception of what is happening? Keep focused on one thing at a time, but do not force the survivor to provide information.

  "What do you think is happening?"

  "What do you think caused him to act that way?"

  "How has this been affecting your life?"

- What is this person's ability to cope and what coping strategies do they usually use?

  "What do you usually do to cope?"

- Provide information on coping strategies.

(continues)

Table 18-2   Phases of Crisis Intervention *(continued)*

- Does this person have a social support system?

  "Is there someone you can call?"

  "Do you want me to call someone for you?"

  "Do you have any family, friends, neighbors, spiritual advisor, church members in the area?"

  "Who do you usually turn to for support?"

  "Who do you feel close to or comfortable talking to?"

  "Who do you ask for advice when you need it?"

- Are there any additional cultural or spiritual factors that need to be considered?

  "Are there any spiritual/religious or cultural factors we should be aware of when providing treatment or help?"

  "Are you able to find comfort or strength from your spiritual or cultural beliefs?"

- What other resources does this person have?

  "Do you have a safe place to stay?"

  "Do you have enough food, water, ice?"

  "Are your utilities (electric, gas, phone) working?"

  "Do you have a job or are you unemployed?"

  "Do you have transportation to home, work, doctor visits, grocery store, etc.?"

  "Do you have health insurance?"

- Does this person have access to their resources and the ability to fully utilize them or need assistance with this?

  "Have you been able to contact anyone—your family or other support people?"

  "Did you have any identification, your purse or wallet with you?"

- What was the person's precrisis level of functioning?

  "How were you functioning before this happened?"

  "Were you able to take care of your personal, family, work/school responsibilities?"

- Are there any obstacles to successful crisis resolution and if so, how can these be circumvented (e.g., physical injuries, lack of basic resources, problems with utilities, problems communicating with the outside world beyond the disaster area, language barriers, literacy problems, unstable psychiatric or other medical illnesses, cultural factors including meaning/word connotation, spiritual/religious factors)?

(continues)

Table 18-2 Phases of Crisis Intervention *(continued)*

- Document.
- Analysis of the information obtained is performed and possible nursing diagnoses identified.

(Aguilera, 1998, pp. 29–31, 35–38; Boyd, 2008, p. 810; Christiansen, 2009, pp. 8–22; Townsend, 2009, p. 209; Varcarolis & Halter, 2010, pp. 532–536; eHow.com—crisis intervention, 2010)

(Phase 1 corresponds to Stages I–III of Roberts's Seven-Stage Crisis Intervention Model)

Phase 2: Planning

In the planning phase appropriate nursing diagnoses are chosen (refer to NANDA–I Diagnoses Used in Psychiatric Disorders in O'Brien, Kennedy, and Ballard, 2008, pp. 552–557; Jakopac & Patel, 2009, pp. 241–242, 251–252, 261, 273–274; Townsend, 2009, pp. 212–217; Varcarolis & Halter, 2010, pp. 542–544). Client centered outcomes/goals and interventions are also part of the planning phase.

Outcomes/goals for the client include:

- Remain safe
- Demonstrate an ability to form a therapeutic alliance with the PMH nurse
- Accept offered assistance
- Family members are kept together
- Provide basic life needs (e.g., safe shelter, food, water, medicines), mental health and medical care
- Engage in adaptive coping behaviors
- Engage in problem-solving activities
- Explore possible alternations in perceptions and thinking patterns
- Collaborate in the formation of and commit to a plan
- Achieve resolution of the immediate crisis
- Be able to function as independently as possible during the crisis time
- Utilize resources, including support system, effectively
- Return to their precrisis level of functioning, or possibly higher
- Gain new insight
- Learn and begin to use new adaptive coping strategies
- Become more empowered
- Follow through with plan of action and referrals
- Become better equipped to deal with future problems or crises

(continues)

Table 18-2   Phases of Crisis Intervention *(continued)*

Other more specific outcomes/goals will depend on the nature of the crisis. (Aguilera, 1998, pp. 24, 31; Townsend, 2009, pp. 209–210; eHow.com—crisis intervention, 2010)

(Phase 2 corresponds to Stage III of Roberts's Seven-Stage Crisis Intervention Model)

Phase 3: Interventions/Implementation

- Continue to develop rapport and the therapeutic alliance/nurse–client relationship.
- Acknowledge and facilitate verbalization of feelings.
- Engage the survivor in stress management techniques such as deep breathing and spiritual support.
- Teach/provide information on new coping strategies and allow time to attempt these as appropriate before the client is discharged from the setting.
- Teach importance of reestablishing a daily routine/schedule to help normalize their life and the lives of their children.
- Clarify information the client is providing as needed, including gently clarifying medical information they are receiving rather than allowing fantasy or false hope that will undermine trust when the situation does not resolve in ways the client wanted it to.
- Support the person's ability to decide and act independently while providing emotional support.
- Refer to psychological first aid techniques in Table 18-1.
- If needed provide more direct assistance (e.g., making phone calls, contacting support people, arranging transportation, physical care, basic needs, arranging for transfer to specific facilities or units for additional care) if the person's ability to function is compromised or impaired by the crisis event, psychiatric or other medical illness, or chemical abuse/dependency.
- Use short, simple sentences especially in situations where the client is experiencing or unable to concentrate related to feelings of being extremely overwhelmed, impulsivity, suicidal or homicidal thoughts, severe anxiety, panic, depersonalization, derealization, psychosis, mania, severe depression or other symptoms of psychiatric or medical illnesses.
- Engage the client in problem solving and alternative approaches to the extent the person is able; sometimes this is not possible due to severe anxiety states, panic, psychosis and additional intervention including relaxation or distraction techniques, or medication may be needed before attempting this.

"Let's work together."

"What else do you think can be done?"

"Let's take a look at some other possible options."

"Do you have enough resources to try that?"

(continues)

Table 18-2   Phases of Crisis Intervention *(continued)*

"Is there someone you can stay with?"

"Who else would be willing to help you with this?"

- Assist the client to examine errors in perceptions and thinking patterns; assist in confronting reality if ineffectively using ego defense mechanisms such as depression, which is not effective in crisis resolution. However, this is done *to the extent the person is able; sometimes this is not possible due to severe anxiety states, panic, psychosis and additional intervention including relaxation or distraction techniques, or medication may be needed before attempting this.*

"You may feel as if you are all alone, but we are here to help you."

"I know right now you feel as if you won't be able to get through this, but in time your ability to cope will get better."

"You may think you could have done something more to avoid being in this situation, but it sounds like you did all you could."

- In early escalation stages of anger or agitation, interventions may include repeating a willingness to listen and respect; encouraging verbalization of feelings; agreeing with the client as long as the client is not threatening to harm themselves or others; maintaining an open, nonthreatening body posture; providing additional personal space; and avoiding physically (standing in directly in front of the client or blocking the exit) or psychologically (making demands vs suggestions or limit setting) cornering the client (see also Table 18-1).

- Consistently set limits on unacceptable, destructive or aggressive behavior while reinforcing that the PMH nurse and others are there to help the client (see also Table 18-1).

- Explore availability of resources and assist with provision of basic needs.

- Provide information related to the disaster as accurately as you can.

- Make a plan in collaboration with this person.

    Note: *The plan will need to be congruent or agree with the client's values and belief systems, and take into account cultural and spiritual factors to be fully implemented and successful. Otherwise the client will not be fully able to carry it out.*

- Obtain a firm commitment from the person to follow through with the agreed upon plan.

- Assist as needed with mobilization of resources including social support system/network.

- Teach normal reactions to crisis as well as signs of ASD and PTSD to watch for and when to seek professional help.

- Provide information for referral services.

- Arrange follow-up appointment(s)—time frames will depend on the nature of the crisis from 24 hours to 1 week or 1 month later.

(continues)

Table 18-2 Phases of Crisis Intervention *(continued)*

- Document.

(Aguilera, 1998, p. 31; Wilder & Sorensen, 2001, pp. 52–58, 72–79; Keltner, Schwecke, & Bostrom, 2007, pp. 104–108, 126, 134–137; Boyd, 2008, p. 810; Townsend, 2009, p. 210, 258–259; eHow.com—crisis intervention, 2010)

(Phase 3 corresponds to Stages IV–VI of Roberts's Seven-Stage Crisis Intervention Model)

Phase 4: Evaluation

During this phase initial progress toward planned outcomes is analyzed and interventions adjusted if needed. Outcomes may also need to be adjusted as information is clarified, if the client's mental or physical condition changes, and as the collaborative plan is implemented. If the survivor is not suicidal or homicidal; is not compromised by exacerbations of psychiatric or other medical conditions or problems related to chemical abuse/dependency; and has the necessary social support and other resources including housing to return home or temporary shelter, they will be discharged from the setting. If the survivor requires inpatient admission or transfer to another facility or program for treatment, then that will be the disposition and included in the documentation. When released the survivor should have all of the following:

- Maintained or returned to a adequate level of safety
- Information for referral services (see Table 18-3)
- Been reunited with family members if possible
- Follow-up appointment(s)
- Information on new adaptive coping strategies
- Clear (verbalized) understanding of plan to follow or reinforcement needed
- Instructions to go to a care setting/emergency department/clinic or who else to contact if the crisis situation becomes worse (usually telephone hotline phone numbers, 911/emergency contact information, community agencies, shelters/temporary housing).
- Documentation including the disposition of the survivor (e.g., released to home/shelter/ temporary housing with whom, admitted where and report given to whom; transferred to a psychiatric or medical facility and report given to whom; follow-up appointment arranged with whom or client agrees to call if unable to arrange before being discharged. In addition, all the above-mentioned information in the previous items in this bulleted list should be entered in the facility/organization's charting/recordkeeping system. The evaluation phase may extend to include the follow-up visit/care so that better evaluation of the interventions and plan can be made over time and continuity of care maintained (Townsend, 2009, p. 211; Varcarolis & Halter, 2010, p. 540). Follow-up care may need to be rendered in a more stable environment away from the direct disaster area.

(Phase 4 corresponds to Stage VII of Roberts's Seven-Stage Crisis Intervention Model)

Table 18-3   Referrals

Survivors will need referrals for general and specific needs depending on the type of disaster. Information should be given in writing (or downloaded to cell phones/portable information devices) because clients are too overwhelmed to remember while trying to cope with the situation. If they initially refuse the information, tell them the information is always available if they change their mind (see also Chapter 17).

- Crisis hotline telephone numbers:
  - Disaster Support Line (crisis counseling): 1-888-524-3578
  - SAMHSA Disaster Relief Information: 1-877-SAMHSA7
  - Suicide Prevention: 1-800-273-TALK (8255) or 1-800-749-COPE (2673) or 1-800 SUICIDE (784-2433)
  - SAMHSA National Helpline: 1-800-662-HELP (4357) (English and Español); 1-800- 487-4889 (TDD); Workplace Helpline: 1-800-WORKPLACE (967-5752) and http://www.workplace.samhsa.gov

- Suicide prevention website: www.suicidepreventionlifeline.org

- American Red Cross: 1-866-438-4636; www.redcross.org

- CDC: Emergency Preparedness and Response

- Coping with a disaster or traumatic event: Information for individuals & families; http://www.emergency.cdc.gov/mentalhealth

- Disaster Help: www.disasterassistance.gov
  - Information and links related to the relief efforts

- FEMA: 1-800-621-3362; www.fema.gov

- National Flood Insurance Program: www.floodsmart.gov

- Mental Health Services Locator: www.mentalhealth.samhsa.gov/databases

- National Mental Health Information Center (NMHIC): www.mentalhealth.samhsa.gov

- National Clearinghouse for Alcohol and Drug Information (NCADI): 1-800-729-6686 (English and Español); 1-800-487-4889 (TDD); www.ncadi.samhsa.gov

- National Organization for Victim Assistance (NOVA): www.try-nova.org and http://www.trynova.org/victiminfo

- Banking Information: 1-877-275-3342; www.fdic.gov (for lost records, ATM cards, etc.)

(continues)

Table 18-3   Referrals *(continued)*

- Local/state/national community organizations including:

  Catholic Charities: www.catholiccharitiesusa.org

  The Salvation Army: 1-800-725-2769 (National), www.salvationarmyusa.org

  United Way agencies: 1-877-923-2114

  Goodwill Industries

  Second Harvest Food Banks

  Local churches

  Operation Blessing: 1-800-436-6348 (National)

  State unemployment agencies

  Council on Aging: 1-877-340-9100 (National) services: Meals on site, meal delivery, prescription service, personal care, homemaker, transportation

- Volunteers of America: 1-800-899-0089—variety of services including basic needs

- Environmental Protection Agency Hotline for hazardous waste pick-up: 1-800-401-1327

- National Archives: 1-866-272-6272 or www.archives.gov

  - Provides guidelines for preserving and caring for your flood-damaged photos, books, papers, etc.

basis needs and rest away from survivors/work areas; and partnering less experienced crisis responders with more experienced personnel all help to decrease stress for those providing crisis interventions and help prevent serious complications (SAMHSA, 2010).

REFERENCES

Aguilera, D. (1998). *Crisis intervention theory and methodology* (8th ed.). St. Louis, MO: Mosby.

American Academy of Pediatrics Work Group on Disasters. (2010). *Psychosocial issues for children and families in disasters: A Guide For The Primary Care Physician*. Retrieved from http://mental health.samhsa.gov/publications/allpubs/SMA95-3022/default.asp

Boyd, M. A. (2008). *Psychiatric nursing: Contemporary practice* (4th ed.). Philadelphia, PA: Wolters-Kluwer Health/Lippincott, Williams, & Wilkins.

Centers for Diseases Control and Prevention (CDC). (2010). *Emergency preparedness and response*. Retrieved from http://www.emergency.cdc.gov/disasters/earthquakes/mentalhealth.asp

Christiansen, K. (2009). *The crisis intervention manual* (2nd ed.). Reseda, CA: Zero Point Communications.

Fontaine, K. L. (2009). *Mental health nursing* (6th ed.). Upper Saddle River, NJ: Pearson Education, Inc.

How to intervene in a crisis situation. (2010). Retrieved from http://www.ehow.com/how_2138570_intervene-crisis-situation.html

Jakopac, K. A., & Patel, S. C. (2009). *Psychiatric mental health case studies and care plans*. Sudbury, MA: Jones and Bartlett.

Keltner, N. L., Schwecke, L. H., & Bostrom, C. E. (2007). Psychiatric nursing (5th ed.). St. Louis, MO: Mosby, Elsevier.

National Clearinghouse for Alcohol and Drug Information (NCADI). (2010). Retrieved from ncadi.samhsa.gov

National Mental Health Information Center (NMHIC). (2010). Retrieved from www.mental-health.samhsa.gov

National Organization for Victim Assistance (NOVA). (2010). Retrieved from www.try-nova.org and http://www.trynova.org/victiminfo

O'Brien, P. G., Kennedy, W. Z., & Ballard, K. A. (2008). *Psychiatric mental health nursing: An introduction to theory and practice*. Sudbury, MA: Jones and Bartlett.

SAMSHA's National Mental Health Information Center. (2010). *A guide to managing stress in crisis response profession*. Retrieved from http://store.samhsa.gov/product/SMA05-4113

Substance Abuse and Mental Health Services Administration (SAMHSA). (2010). *Psychological first aid for first responders: Tips for emergency and disaster response workers*. Retrieved from http://mentalhealth.samhsa.gov/Disasterrelief/pubs/manemotion.asp

Substance Abuse and Mental Health Services Administration (SAMHSA). (2010). Division of Workplace Programs. Retrieved from http://www.workplace.samhsa.gov

Townsend, M. C. (2009). *Psychiatric mental health nursing: Concepts of care in evidence-based practice* (6th ed.). Philadelphia, PA: F. A. Davis.

Varcarolis, E. M., & Halter, M. J. (2010). *Foundations of psychiatric mental health nursing: A clinical approach* (6th ed.). St. Louis, MO: Saunders, Elsevier.

Wilder, S. S., & Sorensen, C. (2001). *Essentials of aggression management in health care*. Upper Saddle River, NJ: Prentice Hall, Inc.

SUGGESTED READINGS

American Academy of Experts in Traumatic Stress. (2010). Retrieved from www.aaets.org

Brock, S. E. (2006). Psychological triage: Preventive psychological interventions (EDS 246b). Seminar in Preventive Psychological Intervention School Crisis Intervention.

Department of Health and Human Services (DHHS). (2005). *DHHS Publication No. SMA 4113: A guide to managing stress in crisis response professions*. Retrieved from http://mentalhealth.samhsa.gov/publications/allpubs/SMA-4113/default.asp

Everly, G. S., & Mitchell, J. T. (2010). *A primer on critical incident stress management*. Retrieved from the Internal Critical Incident Stress Foundation and the International Society for Traumatic Stress Studies at www.icisf.org

How to use the six steps of effective intervention. (2010). Retrieved from http://www.ehow.com/how_5239330_use-six-steps-effective-intervention.html

Living Works Education. (2010). ASIST: *Applied suicide intervention skills training*. Retrieved from http://medtrng.com/suicideprevention

Mental Health Services Locator. (2010). Retrieved from www.mentalhealth.samhsa.gov/databases

Minnesota Department of Health (MDH). (2010). *Behavioral health web*. Retrieved from www.health.state.mn.us/mentalhealth/mhep.html

Mohr, W. K. (2009). *Psychiatric-mental health nursing: Evidence based concepts, skills, and practices* (7th ed.). Philadelphia, PA: Wolters Kluwer/Lippincott, Williams, & Wilkins.

Sadock, B. J., & Sadock, V. A. (2005) *Kaplan & Sadock's comprehensive textbook of psychiatry* (8th ed.). Philadelphia, PA: Lippincott, Williams, & Wilkins.

Sedlacek, B. (2003). Psychiatric emergencies. Seminar at PESI Healthcare, LLC.

Stuart, G. W., & Laraia, M. T. (2005). *Principles and practice of psychiatric nursing* (8th ed.). St. Louis, MO: Mosby, Elsevier.

UNIT V

Appendices

Ego Defense Mechanisms

Defense mechanism	Definition	Example
Compensation	When a person exaggerates or overemphasizes one trait or ability to cover up or make up for feeling inferior, inadequate or limited by/about another trait or ability	Writes expressive poetry and wins awards, but has difficulty verbalizing feelings directly to people.
Conversion	Physical symptoms/expression of unconscious emotional or intra-psychic conflicts, but there is no organic basis for the symptoms	Sudden onset of paralysis, blindness, seizures unrelated to injuries or disease process.
Denial	Refusing or failing to admit an unacceptable event, idea or behavior	A woman sets a place for dinner for her husband after being told he has just been killed. A person with chemical dependency problems believes they can control their consumption of substances. Refusing to acknowledge obvious physical limitations and insisting on continuing to perform certain duties or engage in certain activities. Refusing to admit to having chest pain or impending heart attack when it is obvious to others that this is what is happening.

(continues)

Defense mechanism	Definition	Example
Displacement	Discharging or directing feelings and actions toward a less threatening object or person that are really meant for something or someone else	An employee yells at children or kicks a dog because they are angry with the boss, but fears being fired if they express themselves directly to the boss.
Fixation	Remaining "stuck" in a developmental stage rather than progressing to the next stage	A husband totally depends on his wife for most of his activities of daily living even though physically capable of taking care of himself.
Identification	Integrating or modeling attributes of someone that are desired or admired in someone else you respect	A client tells the psychologist that he wants to go back to school to become a psychologist. A shy adolescent dresses exactly like the teacher.
Introjection	Incorporating attitudes, beliefs, and values of another person as one's own	A client expresses the same attitudes of the group psychotherapy leader.
Intellectualization	Using logical, rational explanations and avoiding affective or feeling components	A person talks about a relative's death in technical terms and how it was a merciful, but avoids talking about how they feel about the death.
Projection	Blaming or attributing to others unacceptable or unethical feelings, emotions or thoughts rather than admit to having them	Accusing someone else of cheating on them when they are having thoughts about wanting to cheat on their partner.
Rationalization	Attempting to justify one's actions, or substituting socially acceptable or fictitious reasons for how one really feels about situations or outcomes	Rather than admit to illness, a person may say they did not wish to attend an event or had a prior engagement.
Reaction formation	Substituting behavior, desires or verbal responses for the exact opposite of how one truly feels	A person tells everyone how wonderful their sister is and goes out of their way to please her, but truly does not like her and hates being with her.

(continues)

Defense mechanism	Definition	Example
Regression	Returning to patterns of behavior or a stage of development that is less anxiety-provoking or more comfortable	A 4 year old wants to drink from a baby bottle after the birth of new sibling. A child who was previously toilet trained begins wetting the bed.
Repression	Involuntary forgetting of painful events, ideas or psychological conflicts	An adult survivor of sexual abuse doesn't remember what actually happened, but may feel dislike towards someone who reminds them of the perpetrator.
Sublimation	Redirecting socially unacceptable urges into socially acceptable behaviors	A person plays sports or exercises to channel aggressive tendencies. A person starts a support group rather than give in to cravings to use drugs.
Suppression	Refusing to think about situations or acknowledge feelings related to situations that are anxiety provoking	When asked about their feelings about a recent divorce, the client states they are not ready to talk about it and do not want to think about it.
Undoing	Engaging in actions or thoughts in an attempt to atone for or cancel out prior actions that may have been harmful to someone else or that feel psychologically threatening.	A person takes on a second job and pays for the damage done to a neighbor's car they damaged in an accident.

Sources: American Psychological Association (APA). (2007). *APA dictionary of psychology,* pp. 498–499. Washington, DC: Author; Keltner, N. L., Schwecke, L. H., & Bostrom, C. E. (2007). *Psychiatric nursing* (5th ed.), 37. St. Louis, MO: Mosby, Elsevier; O'Brien, P. G., Kennedy, W. Z., & Ballard, K. A. (2008). *Psychiatric mental health nursing: An introduction to theory and practice,* p. 10. Sudbury, MA: Jones and Bartlett.

Erickson's Psychosocial Developmental Stages

Stage/task/age	Description
Trust vs mistrust (infancy; 0 to 1 year)	Development of basic trust as a critical building block. Trust develops from a consistent, nurturing relationship with a caregiver (e.g., mother or other parental figure) and consistent meeting of basic needs. Mistrust develops if basic needs are not met or are inconsistently met. Positive outcomes/resolution of this stage include trust, faith, hope, and optimism.
Autonomy vs shame and doubt (early childhood; 1 to 3 years)	In this stage the child learns to "hold on and let go." Successful autonomy or independence comes from activities such as walking, climbing, and toilet training. Forced dependence and belittling lead to shame and doubt. Positive outcomes/resolution of this stage include self-control and willpower.
Initiative vs guilt (preschool; 3 to 6 years)	In this stage the child explores their environment for all possible physical learning experiences. Heightened physical activity and imagination characterize this stage. An early development of a sense of right and wrong (i.e., a conscience) and appropriate social behaviors occurs as well as guilt. Competes with peers. Positive outcomes/resolution of this stage include direction and purpose.

(continues)

Stage/task/age	Description
Industry vs inferiority (school age; 8 to 12 years)	In this stage the child works on completing purposeful activities/projects and learning new skills. Identification with teachers and imagining themselves in different occupational roles also occurs. Feelings of inferiority, inadequacy, and stifling of creativity may occur when expectations are too high or when the child perceives an inability to meet the standards of others. The positive outcome/resolution of this stage is competence.
Ego identity vs role confusion (adolescence; 12 to 18 years)	In this stage the adolescent deals with rapid physical, social, and emotional changes. Development of emotional stability. Preoccupation with how they are perceived by others, especially peers, and how they perceive the self. Tests/tries on adult roles. Confusion occurs as a result of problems integrating all the changes that occur. Positive outcomes/resolution of this stage include fidelity and devotion.
Intimacy vs isolation (young adulthood; 18 to 30 years)	In this stage the adult learns to form significant loving, intimate relationships with peers, colleagues, lovers. Isolation can result if the adolescent was unable to trust that it is safe to share themselves in a mutually giving relationship. Positive outcomes/resolution of this stage include affiliation and love.
Generativity vs stagnation (middle adulthood; 30 to 65 years; may vary depending on the reference centering around the 40s and 50s)	In this stage the adult learns to nurture children, sacrifice for others, collaborate on work projects, attend to parental/societal responsibilities and/or become involved in creative pursuits. Stagnation occurs when the adult becomes so self-absorbed that it interferes with creativity. Positive outcomes/resolution of this stage include caring and production.
Ego integrity vs despair (older adulthood; 65 years to death)	In this stage the adult is aware of time moving on, accepts themselves and their past including both what has occurred and what has not occurred; is comfortable with previous life stages, has feeling of satisfaction. Despair occurs when the focus is on what might have happened, but did not. The positive outcome/resolution of this stage is wisdom.

Sources: Keltner, N. L., Schwecke, L. H., & Bostrom, C. E. (2007). *Psychiatric nursing* (5th ed.), pp. 39–40. St. Louis, MO: Mosby, Elsevier; O'Brien, P. G., Kennedy, W. Z., & Ballard, K. A. (2008). *Psychiatric mental health nursing: An introduction to theory and practice,* p. 463. Sudbury, MA: Jones and Bartlett; Sadock, B. J., & Sadock, V. A. (2003). *Kaplan & Sadock's synopsis of psychiatry* (9th ed.), p. 212. Philadelphia, PA: Lippincott, Williams, & Wilkins.

Freud's Stages of Psychosexual Development

Stage/age	Description
Oral (birth to 18 months)	Main source of pleasure from mouth, lips, and tongue. Dependent on mother (caregiver) to meet needs and provide care. Feelings of dependency develop; trust. Successful resolution results in a sense of trust in self and others; being able to give and receive attention/love without excessive dependence or envy.
Anal (18 months to 3 years)	Focus is on muscle control necessary to control defecation and urination. Expulsion of feces gives a sense of relief. Learns to postpone gratification by postponing defecation/urination (muscle control) and subsequent relief. Strives for independence and separation from parents. Successful resolution results in personal autonomy, independence, personal initiative without guilt, lack of ambivalence, and capacity for willing cooperation without excessive willfulness or self-defeat.
Phallic (3 to 6 years)	Develops awareness of genital area. Sexual and aggressive feelings associated with functioning of sexual organs. Foundation for emerging sexual gender identity. Masturbation. Fantasy. Oedipus or Electra Complex. Successful resolution results in a sense of mastery over internal processes and impulses as well as external environment. Curiosity without embarrassment, initiative without guilt. Internal source of regulation is the Superego derived mainly from parental figures.

(continues)

Stage/age	Description
Latency (6 to 12 years)	Sexual development dormant. Focus of energy on cognitive and intellectual development. Further maturation of the Ego and Superego. Greater control over instinctual impulses. Problems may occur due to a lack of inner development of control or overcontrol. Successful resolution results in patterns of adaptive functioning, sense of industry, capacity for mastery of concepts and objects that allow ability to function autonomously. Sense of industry, initiative without guilt or sense of inferiority. Provides basis for being a mature adult who finds satisfaction in work and love.
Genital (12 years to early adulthood)	Physiologic maturation and intensification of hormonal drives including libido. Conflicts of previous stages reemerge, providing another opportunity to resolve them to achieve a mature adult sexual identity. Ultimate separation from dependence and attachment to parents. Establishment of mature sexual relationships with opposite sex. Successful resolution results in mature personality, capacity for full and satisfying sexual relationships; consistent sense of identity; capacity for self-realization; meaningful participation in areas of love, work, creativity; productive and satisfying, meaningful values and goals.

Sources: Fontaine, K. L. (2009). *Mental health nursing* (6th ed.), p. 13. Upper Saddle River, NJ: Pearson Education, Inc; Sadock, B. J., & Sadock, V. A. (2005). *Kaplan & Sadock's comprehensive textbook of psychiatry* (8th ed.), volume 1, pp. 725–729. Philadelphia, PA: Lippincott, Williams, & Wilkins.

Piaget's Intellectual/Developmental Stages and Kohlberg's Stages of Moral Reasoning

Piaget's Stages of Cognitive (Intellectual) Development

Stage/age	Defining characteristics
Sensorimotor (birth to 2 years)	Gains refined conceptualization of space (internal & external); uses body senses to explore environment; learns to anticipate an experience by constructing a model of each experience; results in new skills including object permanence; internal challenge of constructing new schemes to fit old and new experiences into a universal uniform reality; adjustment (accommodating) to new functions allows cognitive ability to broaden.
Preoperational (2 to 7 years)	Development of intuition; able to anticipate experiences with consequences; symbolic thought, but "illogically and eccentrically unable to perceive themselves as separate from others in their environment"; inner world with magical thinking.
Concrete operational (7 to 11 years)	Ability to think logically/rationally and in an organized way. Magical thinking is replaced by more realistic worries about school, health, dying, and social relationships.

(continues)

Stage/age	Defining characteristics
Formal operations (11 to 19 years)	Development of abstract thought, "imaginary audience phenomenon," leading to thought of everyone being able to watch them; language an important "tool" now that they are able to use hypothetical and deductive reasoning; propositional thought. Ability to think about potential results of own actions and other possible factors that could affect the outcome. Able to think about possible solutions to a problem before trying them out.

Kohlberg's Stages of Moral Reasoning

Stage	Defining characteristics
Preconventional/Preschool period	Decisions or actions based on avoiding punishment or obtaining reward.
Conventional morality	Understanding of the concepts of authority and mutual benefit so decisions or actions based on these.
Principled morality	General "internalized" moral principles. Decisions or actions based on internal sense of right or wrong; because "it's the right thing to do."

Sources: O'Brien, P. G., Kennedy, W. Z., & Ballard, K. A. (2008). *Psychiatric mental health nursing: An introduction to theory and practice,* p. 463. Sudbury, MA: Jones and Bartlett; Sadock, B .J., & Sadock, V. A. (2005). *Kaplan & Sadock's comprehensive textbook of psychiatry* (8th ed.), volumes 1 and 2, pp. 725–729, 3025–3027. Philadelphia, PA: Lippincott, Williams, & Wilkins.

Interpersonal Process Recording Form

**Client's Statements/
Responses**
(include both verbal and
nonverbal communication)

**Analysis of Client's
Communication**
(include themes)

**Nurse's Statements/
Responses and Identified
Therapeutic Communication
Technique**

(continues)

Client's Statements/ Responses (include both verbal and nonverbal communication)	Analysis of Client's Communication (include themes)	Nurse's Statements/ Responses and Identified Therapeutic Communication Technique

Source: Keltner, N. L., Schwecke, L. H., & Bostrom, C. E. (2007). *Psychiatric nursing* (5th ed.), pp. 112–113. St. Louis, MO: Mosby, Elsevier.

Stress Management/Self-Care Exercises

Positive affirmations (place these positive affirming statements where you can see them every day)

- "I will treat myself with gentle respect."
- "I will flow with the times."
- "I can practice new ways of being."
- "I can create new beliefs."
- "I seize the moment as it arrives."
- "I honor my experience and personal truth."
- "I can release and let go."
- "I can let go of stress and worry."
- "I create my life and my being."
- "What I do is good enough."
- "I am good enough."
- "I feel good about the way I do my job."
- "I will connect with my Higher Power and see where that connection leads me."
- "I can live a comfortable life."
- "I know there are things I can control and things I cannot. Let it go."
- "I am a positive and valuable contributor to my relationships."
- "I am a confident and positive person."
- "I am sure of my ability to do what is necessary to improve my life."
- "I have compassion for myself and the way my life has developed."
- "I am deserving of all the good things in my life."

(continues)

- "I create health by expressing love, understanding and compassion."

(Lim, 2010)

Simple meditation

- Sit in a comfortable position, either in a chair or on the floor, with your back and head straight.
- You can "warm up" with a couple of deep breaths, ujjayi pranayama, or nadi shodhana.
- Close your eyes. Breathe through your nose.
- Focus on your breath—cool air in, warm air out. If the mind wanders, gently bring it back to the breath. That's it. Start with a 5–10-minute meditation and work your way up to 15, 20, 30 minutes or more.
- A variation that may make things a little easier at the beginning is to count your breaths. Count up to four and then repeat, over and over. You can add an "and" between counts to fill up the space between breaths. It goes like this: inhale (1)—exhale (and)—inhale (2)—exhale (and) . . . and so on up to four.

(The Yoga Site, 2010)

Simple self-hypnosis technique

Recognize that to be hypnotized is to enter a trance state. You will be very focused, but will also be aware of what is happening around you.

- Sit in a comfortable chair or recline on a couch in a quiet place. Be sure that your clothes are loose and comfortable and the temperature is not too warm or cool.
- Turn down the lights so that it's not too bright. It doesn't need to be dark.
- Relax. You can have your eyes open or closed, whichever is most comfortable for you.
- Let yourself go loose. Feel every muscle go limp. Feel your mind slow down. Good.
- Breathe deeply and hold it. Feel all of your stress and worries sucked from your body and your head into your lungs. Blow them out slowly and watch them swirl away from you.

(continues)

- Notice the different colors of each concern. See them float away and dissolve in the air. You are feeling more and more relaxed with every breath.

- Feel your heart. It is strong and slow. You can feel it beating, slowly, slowly. Each time you exhale, your body relaxes more. You are calm and safe. You can feel your heart. It's beating so slowly.

- Feel your toes. They feel empty and light. They want to float away. That lightness is spreading up your legs, through your hips and into your back. Your body is so empty. You can see through it.

- Feel your arms. They feel empty. Your shoulders are empty. Your neck is empty. Your head is floating, weightless. You feel so calm.

- Feel liquid begin to fill your body through your navel. It's deep blue. It feels cool and comfortable. Watch it fill up your body. Cool blue. When you are full, you will feel calm and completely at ease.

- Now open your eyes and sit up. Your cool, blue feeling will stay with you.

(eHow.com—self-hypnosis, 2010)

Basic guided imagery (with or without soft music in the background for at least 10 minutes)

- Choose a comfortable chair to sit on, preferably one without arms.

- Sit back while placing your feet flat on the floor.

- Roll your shoulders back; then let your arms dangle at your side.

- Sink into the chair and close your eyes.

- Relax, let yourself *feel* loose.

- Take a slow deep breath in to the count of 5 and let it out slowly to the count of 5. Do this 2 more times—in . . . and out . . .

- Choose to envision a familiar, safe, comfortable or happy place (e.g., a beach, a forest, a lake, a cottage, a boat/canoe, a favorite room in a home, a favorite vacation spot, etc.).

(continues)

- What do you first see when you arrive there? (e.g., colors, shapes, objects, surroundings)
- What do you smell? (e.g., the ocean, a lake, pine scent, leaves, food cooking, etc.)
- What do you hear? (e.g., water lapping at the shore, birds calling/singing, chipmunks or squirrels scampering about, people talking/laughing, etc.)
- What sensations do you feel? (e.g., warmth of the sun, sand under your feet, water, a cool breeze, pebbles, leaves, or pine needles crunching under your feet, etc.)
- Feel your muscles relax.
- Stay in this imagined place as long as you need to or change it to another place.
- When you are ready to come back to the room you are in, take another slow deep breath in to the count of 5 and let it out slowly to the count of 5. Do this 2 more times—in . . . and out . . .
- Open your eyes.

Sources: Dayton, T. (1992). *Daily affirmations for forgiving and moving on: Powerful inspiration for personal change*. Deerfield, FL: Health Communications, Inc; Edleman, C. L., & Mandle, C. L. (1998). *Health promotion throughout the lifespan* (4th ed.), pp. 342–344. St. Louis, MO: Mosby, Inc; Frisch, N. C., & Frisch, L. E. (2011). *Psychiatric mental health nursing* (4th ed.), pp. 889–892. Clifton Park, NY: Delmar/Cengage Learning, Inc; eHow.com. (2010). *How to Do Self-Hypnosis*. Retrieved from http://www.ehow.com/how_7949_self-hypnosis.html; Lim, Evelyn. (2010). *List of Positive Daily Affirmations*. Retrieved from http://hubpages.com/hub/List-Of-Positive-Daily-Affirmations; The Yoga Site. (2004). Meditation. Retrieved from http://www.yogasite.com/meditation.htm

Glossary

Abstract thinking: The ability to understand and state the meaning of concepts and proverbs, and think using symbols; includes the ability to recognize a deeper meaning than the obvious, surface meaning.

Abuse: Actions that can result in serious harm or death; involves many forms.

Acute stress disorder: The immediate psychological aftermath (30 days or less) of exposure to a traumatic stress including symptoms of anxiety, fear, sleep pattern disturbance or nightmares, intrusive memories, emotional distancing or numbing, social isolation, difficulty trusting others, hypervigilance, relationship problems, and decreased motivation. This disorder is included in DSM-IV-TR diagnoses.

Adaptive behavior: Behavior that allows or helps a person positively, appropriately, and effectively adjust to a new situation, environment or level of development; includes coping skills. Thought patterns (cognitive theory vs behavioral theory or cognitive–behavioral theory) can also be adaptive.

Addictionologist: A psychiatrist who specializes in the treatment of people with chemical abuse/dependency addiction and disorders. The psychiatrist obtains additional education and clinical experience in this area of specialty. The treatment of people with chemical abuse/dependency addiction and disorders is included in the education and clinical experience of all psychiatrics, but they can then choose to further specialize in this area and develop further expertise.

Adventitious or traumatic crisis: Unplanned, unexpected, large-scale events including accidents, natural disasters, crimes of violence, or terrorism.

Affect: The outward manifestation of a person's feelings, tone, or mood. Affect and emotion are commonly used interchangeably.

Agonist: Medications or drugs that both have a high affinity (attraction) and produce a pharmacologic effect at a cell receptor site. The response produced is predictable.

Agranulocystosis: A severe abnormally low number of white blood cells limiting the body's ability to fight off infection. If the body's defenses are severely depleted, there is risk of death from overwhelming infection.

Akathesia: Extreme restlessness, inability to sit still, and/or a subjective report of internal restlessness. Frequently an adverse effect (extrapyramidal effect) of antipsychotic medications.

Akinesia: Decrease in motor movement or muscle weakness; complaints of fatigue or becoming tired easily with physical activity. Loss of voluntary muscle movements, but not due to paralysis; medication side-effect.

Alternative: In this text the term is used for therapies, herbal supplements, and other methods of treatment used in place of Western medicine.

Ameliorating: Improving.

Anergia: Extreme lack of energy or fatigue.

Anhedonia: An inability to enjoy hobbies, activities, or experiences that usually provide pleasure or joy; seen in clients with diagnoses of major depression and schizophrenia.

Antagonist: Medication or drugs that have an affinity or attraction to a cell receptor site, but counteract the action of other medications, drugs, or substances at the receptor. Antagonists may compete with agonists to bind to the cell receptor (competitive) causing an opposing effect, or bind to a site near the cell receptor site and change the way the receptor responds (noncompetitive), making it inactive.

Anticholinergic: Blockage of acetycholine receptors resulting in inhibition (slowing or stopping) of nerve impulse transmission. Medications that have this action compete with the neurotransmitter acetycholine for receptor sites at synaptic junctions or gaps.

Antidepressants: Class of psychotropic medications used in the treatment of mood disorders (e.g., major depression).

Antipsychotics: Medications referred to in the past as "major tranquilizers or neuroleptics" and classified as "traditional, conventional, or first generation" or "atypical, second generation antipsychotics (SGAs) or novel." Traditional antipsychotics are also classified by degree of potency (e.g., low, moderate, high) or chemical composition (e.g., phenothiazines, butyrophenones, thioxanthenes).

Anxiety: Somatic symptoms of tension and a mood state of apprehension; anticipation of catastrophe or impending danger. Apprehension, tension, or uneasiness from anticipation of danger, the source of which is largely unknown or unrecognized. Origin of anxiety is primarily intrapsychic. Anxiety may turn into pathology when it interferes with daily functioning in life.

Anxiety disorders: Types of psychiatric disorders where there is constant and overwhelming anxiety that can interfere in an individual's daily functions in life. It crosses from normal anxiety into the territory of anxiety disorders.

Apathetic/Apathy: Decrease in or lack of feeling, emotion, interest, or concern. Frequently seen with diagnoses of major depression or schizophrenia.

Aplastic anemia: Failure of the bone marrow to produce or generate cells resulting in deficiency of all formed blood elements including RBCs, WBCs, and platelets. Also known as bone marrow suppression. Common causes include neoplastic diseases, ionizing radiation, toxic chemicals, some antibiotics, and some other medications.

Appearance: Physical presentation including how old the client looks compared with their reported biologic age, posture, manner of dress, hygiene, grooming, obvious signs of IV drug use (needle tracks), general nutrition, and eye contact.

Assault: A deliberate threat to a person's physical or mental safety or the fear of physical contact or harm to mental security.

Assessment: The act of obtaining, gathering, classifying, analyzing, and documenting information related to the client. This is the first step of the nursing process.

Asthenia: Loss of strength or energy, weakness.

Attachment: The quality of the emotional bond between an infant and parents/caregivers that provides the foundation for the infant's future relationships. Secure attachment develops from appropriate, consistent responses to the infant's attachment behaviors of calling, clinging, crying, following, or protesting when a parent leaves. The infant also seeks comfort from a parent in unfamiliar surroundings, but explores the environment when the parent is present. Lack of exploring along with clinging when the parent is present, intense protest, hostility, or even indifference when the parent leaves all indicate problems with developing a secure attachment.

Attending skills: See **Therapeutic listening skills**.

Attention: The amount of conscious effort used to focus on an activity, task, or experience; concentration.

Autonomic nervous system: A part of the central and peripheral nervous systems that controls involuntary body functions. It is divided into two parts: sympathetic and parasympathetic. In the past it was thought to function separately from the central nervous system and given the name "autonomic" as a result.

Autonomy: The principle of acknowledging the rights of others to make their own decisions and exercise self-determination. In bioethics this principle includes a client's right to refuse treatment, including medication.

Battering: A pattern of behavior used by a person who believes they are entitled to control another person. This pattern of behavior is used to establish power and control over another person through fear and intimidation, often including the threat or use of physical violence.

Battery: Intentionally touching someone in an inappropriate or socially unacceptable way without the person's consent; intentionally violating another person's physical security. The person does not have to be aware that battery has occurred.

Behavior modification: The reinforcement or strengthening of positive, adaptive, healthy behaviors and application of consequences of negative, maladaptive, unhealthy behaviors.

Beneficence: The principle of having a duty to act for the benefit of or promote the good of others. In bioethics this principle includes measures to keep a client safe, help the client deal with anxiety or psychosis, and advocacy.

Bereavement: Grieving over a death of a person or a pet.

Bioethics: The study of specific ethical beliefs or moral values and questions related to health care. Bioethics include five basic principles: beneficence, autonomy, justice, fidelity, and veracity.

Biopsychosocial: Pertaining to biologic, psychological, and social information, assessment, or domains.

Bipolar I: A mood disorder consisting of two phases: depressed phase and manic phase. The manic phase in Bipolar I disorder lasts for 1 week.

Bipolar II: There is a presence of one or more major depressive episodes, and presence of at least one hypomanic episode instead of manic episode. And causes significant distress and impairment in daily functioning. See also **Bipolar I**. The signs and symptoms of Bipolar II disorder (hypomania) are the same, but of less intensity and duration. The manic phase in Bipolar II disorder lasts for 4 days.

Bizarre: Strange, odd, unexpected, out of the ordinary; frequently seen in the behavior of clients experiencing psychosis.

Blackouts: An early sign of alcoholism. Blackouts are a form of amnesia for events that occurred during the drinking period. The person has no memory of this time period even though they may function "normally."

Blocking: See **Thought blocking**.

Blood-brain barrier: Walls of capillaries in the central nervous system that separate brain cells from the bloodstream. This barrier prevents or slows the rate of any substance (e.g., medications, toxins, microorganisms) entering the central nervous system.

Boundaries: In psychiatric-mental health nursing, boundaries are psychological limits that protect the client and the nurse. Boundaries set realistic limits on behavior, communication, and interaction.

Catatonic/Catatonia: Decreased reactivity or unresponsiveness to one's environment. It may be displayed as severe muscle rigidity or bizarre postures. In some cases there is extreme restlessness and purposeless movements (catatonic excitement).

CBT (cognitive behavioral therapy): According to the theory this therapy is based upon, a person's perceptions/beliefs/values result in certain emotions that are followed by behaviors or actions. The goal of this type of therapy is to change faulty or illogical thinking, the emotions that accompany this type of thinking, and the behaviors that follow. Irrational beliefs and inappropriate rules for living are examined and replaced by more logical, appropriate ones.

Central nervous system (CNS): One of two main divisions of the body's nervous system, consisting of the brain and spinal cord. It is the main network for controlling and coordinating functions of the entire body and processes information to and from the peripheral nervous system (PNS).

Circumstantial/Circumstantiality: Pattern of speech that is indirect and delayed in reaching its goal because of irrelevant detail or parenthetical remarks. The speaker does not lose the point, as is characteristic of loosening of associations, and clauses remain logically connected, but to the listener it seems that the end will never be reached. Compare with tangentiality.

Clang association: A type of speech in which the sound of a word rather than its meaning gives the direction to subsequent association. May occur in schizophrenia or mania.

CNS. See **Central nervous system.**

Cognition: Thinking, knowing, perceiving; closely associated with judgment.

Cognitive behavioral therapy. See **CBT.**

Cognitive distortion: Errors that occur in thinking or perceiving that lead a person to arrive at false conclusions. The person makes decisions, experiences emotions, and behaves in ways based upon these errors and false conclusions. These errors do not meet criteria for delusional thinking or hallucinations.

Collaboration: An interpersonal process, act, or relationship where two or more people work together showing cooperation and sensitivity to each other's needs.

Complementary: In this text the term is used for therapies, herbal supplements, and other methods of treatment used along with Western medicine.

Compulsion: Behavior or ritual a person feels driven to engage in to decrease distress or anxiety related to obsessions and prevent a dreaded future situation or event from occurring. Common behaviors include hand washing, counting, checking, and praying; seen in obsessive-compulsive disorder. See also **Obsessions**.

Concentration: Focusing on one subject or problem.

Concrete: Focused thinking on facts and details, a literal interpretation of messages, and an inability to generate or think abstractly/hypothetically; normal in young children; frequently seen in clients diagnosed with schizophrenia.

Confabulation: Unconsciously making up plausible (possibly believable) information to cover up for gaps in memory.

Confidentiality: A principle of professional ethics that requires anyone providing health care to limit disclosure of patient personal and treatment information. In psychiatric-mental health treatment the patient must give written permission to release information to anyone, including relatives, friends, or employers.

Congruent: General agreement, conformity, or harmony.

Consistency: Sameness—maintaining a routine, being honest, following through with promises, responding in a predictable manner, reinforcing rules uniformly, and assigning the same nurse and other mental healthcare staff to the same clients.

Contraband: Objects and substances—including anything sharp—including common objects such as pencils, pens, scissors, paperclips, staples, notebooks with metal spiral binding, glass containers, weapons, and alcohol and illegal drugs that may pose a danger to clients, members of the healthcare team, and visitors.

Coping: Use of cognitive and behavioral strategies to manage stressful situations, events, or circumstances.

Coping mechanisms: An adaptation to internal or external stress that is based on conscious or unconscious choice and that assists the individual to gain control over behavior or gives psychological comfort.

Copycat suicide: The term "copycat" is used when adolescents identify with and imitate the behavior of a peer, public figure, or teen idol who has committed suicide.

Counselor: The psychiatric-mental health nurse acts as a counselor with acquired qualification for counseling. The focus of the counseling is to help the client to achieve mutually agreed upon specific goals and outcomes. The nurse as counselor provides opportunities for the patient to express thoughts, feelings, and behaviors related to issues they are attempting to cope with.

Countertransference: When a nurse or other healthcare provider displaces or projects unconscious feelings, desires, or actions from a person in their life onto the client. This can be problematic in nursing, but it is used by psychoanalytic therapists in psychoanalysis therapy.

Covert: Hidden, latent.

Civil rights: Guaranteed rights under federal and state laws for all citizens including those with mental illness.

Critical thinking: Integrating and analyzing objective and subjective data; applying evidence and research findings along with the nursing process; also involves evaluating the quality and effectiveness of nursing practice to obtain the highest client outcomes.

Cultural awareness: Acquiring knowledge of other cultures and engaging in self-awareness and examination related to this new knowledge.

Cultural competence: Adjusting interventions and practices when possible to accommodate clients' cultural beliefs, values, and needs.

Curative factors: Therapeutic groups provide beneficial factors for group members. Yalom, a psychotherapist, identified 11 factors he described as "curative."

Cyberbullying: "Any kind of aggression perpetrated through technology—any type of harassment or bullying (teasing, telling lies, making fun of someone, making rude or mean comments, spreading rumors, or making threatening or aggressive comments) that occurs through email, a chat room, instant messaging, a website (including blogs), or text messaging." (CDC, 2010).

Cycle of violence: Predictable pattern of abuse described by Walker (1979) to occur in separate, identifiable stages with specific behavior occurring in each stage; also referred to as the cycle of "battering" in Townsend (2009, pp. 730–731).

Cytochrome P450: A protein involved in the metabolism of medications in the liver.

Day treatment: A professional program that offers coordinated interdisciplinary assessment, treatment, and rehabilitation services. Clients go to the day treatment program for approximately 6 hours a day. This type of program helps decrease the need for rehospitalization and helps prevent relapse; may also be referred to as a partial hospitalization program.

De-escalation: Verbal interventions commonly referred to as "talking down" and used to reduce or defuse a potentially or actually volatile or violent situation. These interventions include remaining calm, using empathy, limit setting, and firmness.

Defense mechanisms: An unconscious intrapsychic process serving to provide relief from emotional conflicts or anxiety.

Delusions: A fixed, false belief that is firmly maintained, is not shared by others, and is contradicted by society or any facts to the contrary. The belief is based on inferences about external reality that are the result of distorted or exaggerated thoughts. There are many different types of delusions.

Depersonalization: Feeling of strangeness or unreality related to a person's own body, body parts, their own thoughts, the self, or their environment. They feel as if they are outside their bodies and observing themselves, as if they are robots yet aware they are not; seen in schizophrenia, schizotypal personality disorder, or depersonalization disorder.

Depot injection: The intramuscular (IM) injection of medication—usually in an oil suspension or other medium—resulting in storage of medication in body fats/tissues with gradual release of the medication into circulation over several days.

Derailment: Sudden or gradual change in train of thought without blocking; disorganized, disconnected thought processes. This term may be used synonymously with loose associations.

Derealization: A feeling of detachment or separation from one's personal environment. Also, a distortion of spatial relationships between objects in the environment may occur causing the person to feel that their environment is unfamiliar or different in some way. A false perception that their environment has changed making objects appear larger or smaller to them. Some people may say they feel as if they are in a movie and things around them seem unreal. Seen in schizophrenia, dissociative disorders, or panic attacks.

Deviant behavior: Any behavior that is significantly different from what is considered typical or appropriate for a social group.

Disaster: Events that overwhelm community resources and threaten the safety and ability to function of individuals living in the community are considered to be disasters. These events may be caused by nature or be manmade, but all result in destruction and devastation of property and life, as well as psychological trauma.

Disequilibrium: Loss of physical or emotional balance (lability); a state of tension between cognitive processes.

Distractibility: Difficulty maintaining attention or being easily diverted from what is currently happening.

Dissociation: An unconscious defense mechanism in which the person temporarily experiences an altered state of consciousness and may engage in behaviors without conscious awareness. Dissociative symptoms involve changes in consciousness, motor function, and even identity to protect the self from painful emotions or psychological conflicts, including anxiety, physical or psychological trauma, or abuse. Dissociative amnesia involves memory loss for an acute precipitating event; seen in dissociative disorders and conversion disorders.

DSM-IV-TR: *Diagnostic and Statistical Manual of Mental Disorders*, (4th ed.), text revision. This manual, published by the American Psychiatric Association, is used for diagnosis, education and research related to psychiatric-mental health disorders.

Duty to warn: Also referred to as the Tarosoff ruling. Mental healthcare professionals have a duty to warn of threats to harm others. The case involved a University of California male student who confided to his therapist that he was going to kill another female student. He did not give her actual name, but she was easily identified. The therapist notified campus police who detained and questioned him, but released him because he "appeared rational." He killed the female student shortly after she returned from a trip to South America. The parents successfully sued. "The duty to protect endangered third parties is now a national standard of practice, although some jurisdictions still hold that any disclosure of confidential information is a violation of the patient's rights" (Keltner, Schwecke, & Bostrom, 2007, p. 54).

Dystonia: Involuntary muscle spasms or uncoordinated spastic muscle movements involving the face, tongue, extraocular muscles (oculogyric crisis), trachea/larynx (laryngospasm), esophagus, neck (torticollis), thorax/respiratory muscles (respiratory problems), trunk (opisthotonus or arching of the back), or pelvis (swaying or difficulty walking).

Echolalia: Repetitive, persistent repeating of words or phrases; seen in schizophrenia, particularly the catatonic subtype.

Echopraxia: Automatic imitation of another person's gestures or movements.

ECT (electroconvulsive therapy): A controlled seizure is induced by passing low-dose electric currents through one or more areas of the brain with the effect of potentially balancing neurotransmitters in the brain. The client is prepared before the procedure in the same manner as any medical–surgical procedure, including the administration of anesthesia and muscle relaxants.

Ego defense mechanisms: Unconscious mental processes theorized by Freud as one explanation for human behavior used to relieve intense emotional states such as anxiety attributed to increased conflict or tension between the superego and the id component of personality. See Appendix A for specific types.

Electroconvulsive therapy. See **ECT**.

Emotional numbing: Emotional numbing generally refers to those feelings that reflect difficulties in experiencing positive emotions. The specific symptoms that make up emotional numbing symptoms are a loss of interest in positive, activities, feeling distant from others, and experiencing difficulties having positive feelings, such as happiness or love.

Empathy: The ability to feel in ourselves or recognize the feelings experienced by someone else as if they are our own; attempting to put oneself in the place of another person; also the ability to objectively understand someone else's point of view or communicate an intention to understand another person.

Empathetic linkage: Includes empathy, but also the interpersonal transmission of feelings or emotions such as anxiety and panic.

Enuresis: Repetitive, involuntary urination in appropriate places occurring after the expected voluntary physical maturation time, chronological mental and physical age in childhood. It is frequently associated with stressful situations, delayed bladder development, or poor toilet training and is not due to a general medication condition or substances such as diuretic medication. It may occur during the day (diurinal) or at night (nocturnal) or during both times.

Environment: A group of external conditions that influence a person. These external conditions can be physical, biologic, cultural, and social.

Equilibrium: Physical, emotional (even) or cognitive stability.

Ethics: A branch of philosophy that examines how behavioral principles guide human interactions.

Ethical dilemma: A conflict between at least two decisions or potential actions that have both favorable or positive consequences and unfavorable or negative consequences.

Ethnopharmacology/Ethnopsychopharmacology: The area of pharmacology working with variations in ethnic, racial, and cultural factors regarding genetics, pharmacodynamics, and pharmacokinetics.

Euphoria: A false sense of elation, happiness or well-being; pathological elevation of mood that does not reflect the reality of the person's situation.

Expansive/elevated mood: See **Euphoria**.

External locus of control: Belief that causes or forces external or outside of the individual's control influence chances of success or failure. A client may have the view that their disease has been imposed on them by an external force or fate, and that they are not responsible for the cause or cure. A nurse may expect the client to give up control of their care to the nurse, which interferes with the client's independence.

Extrapyramidal symptoms (EPS): Side/adverse effects of antipsychotic medications including akathesia, dystonia, tardive dyskinesia, pseudoparkinsonism, and akinesia.

Fear: Emotional and physiologic responses to a recognized source of danger.

False imprisonment: Unlawfully restraining a person's individual liberty or confining a person. The confined or restrained person experiences a "reasonable" fear that force will be used to intimidate or detain them without legal justification. The implication may be implied by words, threats, or gestures.

Family violence: "Intentional intimidation, abuse or neglect of children, adults or elders by a family member, intimate partner or caretaker, in order to gain power and control over the victim" (American Academy of Family Physicians) (Varacolis & Halter, 2010, p. 585).

Feedback: Stating your perception of another person's words or actions.

Fidelity: Being loyal and committed to the client; being faithful to contracts and commitments.

Flight of ideas (FOIs): A nearly continuous flow of accelerated speech with abrupt changes from one topic to another, usually based on understandable associations, distracting stimuli, or playing on words; more reality based than "loose associations" (e.g., "How are you doing, kid, no kidding around, I'm going home . . .

home is where the heart is, the heart of the matter is I want out and that ain't hay
. . . hey Doc . . . get me out of this place.").

Flashback: Reexperiencing the psychologically distressing events of the past in terms
of memory, feelings, or perceptual experiences.

FOIs. See **Flight of ideas.**

Genuineness: Being open, honest, oneself, or authentic in interactions.

Grandiose: Delusion consisting of exaggerated perception of importance, inflated
sense of self, possessing special powers, or having special religious significance
that is not in line with reality; seen in delusional disorders and manic phases of
bipolar disorders.

Group: Three or more people meeting together who may establish an interdependent relationship and/or share some goals and norms.

Group content: Conversation or what is said during group.

Group dynamics: The interactions and interrelations among members, between
members, and between members and the group leader.

Group norm: A pattern of behavior by group members that develops over time such
as starting on time, not interrupting a member while speaking, and staying awake.
The norm provides structure for the group.

Group process: Interaction—verbal and nonverbal—that takes place among group
members, including body language, affect, who talks to whom, or who avoids whom.

Group themes: Feelings, thoughts, or ideas expressed in one meeting or across several meetings that produce a common thread.

Group therapy: Psychotherapy examining interactions among a group of clients versus individual therapy. Goals include understanding and changing how clients interact with others for the purpose of increasing insight, improving function, and
transferring new behavior to relationships with family, friends, or coworkers.

Gynecomastia: Abnormal development of breast tissue in males secondary to an imbalance in the hormone prolactin. Many antipsychotic medications inhibit the release of the neurotransmitter dopamine. Dopamine inhibits the release of
prolactin from the anterior pituitary gland. When dopamine is inhibited, there is
an excess release of prolactin leading to engorgement of breast tissue and in some
cases the expression of breast milk (galactorrhea).

Hallucinations: Response to internally generated stimuli. Various types of hallucinations include auditory (hearing), visual (seeing), tactile (feeling usually on the
skin), gustatory (taste), and olfactory (smell/odor).

Hate crimes: Crimes committed because of the perpetrator's hatred toward a racial
or other specified group (e.g., gender, religious or other belief system), or, more
broadly, if the victim is selected because of membership in a specified group.

Healing agent: A force assisting the client to move toward positive change.

Helplessness: An emotional state of powerlessness, vulnerability, or incapability resulting from the realization that a person cannot do much to prevent a negative situation from occurring or that the situation will not get better on its own. This includes low expectations about the future.

Hope: An expectation that you will have positive experiences or that a potentially negative situation will have a favorable result.

Hopelessness: Feeling as if there will be no improvement in a situation or feeling as if you will not be able to experience positive emotions.

Hyperactivity: Excessive restlessness or spontaneous gross motor activity; overactivity, distractibility.

Hyperkalemia: Abnormally elevated potassium serum or blood levels that may cause fatal cardiac arrhythmias.

Hypervigilance: Heightened state of alertness; continually scanning the room/environment for danger.

Hypnosis: A relaxed state induced by a trained therapist where suggestions are made, questions asked or requests made to remember information. The client subjectively experiences various changes in sensations, emotions, perceptions, cognition, or control over motor movements.

Hypoactive: Decreased motor movements and cognitive activity; slowing of thought and speech; may also be referred to as hypokinesis.

Hypomania: See **Bipolar II**.

Hyponatremia: Abnormally low sodium serum or blood levels that can lead to muscle twitching, seizures, or coma.

Ideas of reference: Incorrect interpretation of casual incidents and external events as having direct reference to oneself; misinterpreting the behavior of others (e.g., thinking that the newspaper headline has special significance for them; radio or TV personalities are speaking directly to them, sometimes in "code").

Illusions: Misinterpretation of external stimuli. A person sees a coat rack and perceives it instead as a person.

Incest: Sexual behavior and exploitation of a child younger than 18 years old by a biologic relative.

Incongruence: Lack of consistency, agreement, conformity, or harmony.

Insight: Conscious awareness or recognition and understanding of one's own condition.

Intelligence: Capacity for learning and rational thought; also the ability to recall and apply learning.

Intensive outpatient program: Similar to a day treatment or partial hospitalization program, but clients may attend fewer days per week and need to be more mentally stable and independent.

Intergenerational transmission: A term referring to people growing up in homes exposed to violence and abuse learning to accept and expect continued violence as adults and in the families they produce in the future, thus passing violence and abuse along to future generations.

Internal locus of control: Belief that causes or forces internal or inside of the individual's control influence chances of success or failure. A client may view themselves as powerful rather than as a victim and as a participant in the healing process. A client recognizes that their own thoughts, feelings, and behaviors have an influence on their health. A nurse respects the client's feelings and wishes and empowers the client by providing information, support, and teaching skills for the benefit of the client. The relationship honors the client's need to control their own life as much as possible.

Interpersonal: Feelings, actions or events occurring between two or more individuals.

Interpersonal therapy. See **IPT**.

Intimate partner violence: Physical, sexual, or psychological harm by a current or former partner or spouse. This type of violence can occur among heterosexual or same-sex couples and does not require sexual intimacy.

IPT (interpersonal therapy): This type of therapy focuses on the client's interpersonal relationships and the problems that occur that interfere with the maturity and security of the client. Ways to deal with these problematic relationships are explored and implemented.

Judgment: Mental act of evaluating or comparing choices within a set of values to determine what action to take.

Justice: Fair and equal treatment.

Labile: Subject to frequent and/or unpredictable, dramatic changes in mood (mood swings), affect, or behavior.

Latency: Time between a stimulus and a response; delayed verbal response.

Learned helplessness: Failure to act including lack of motivation to act after being exposed to negative events or stimuli in the environment over which the person has no control. This can lead to failure to use options they can control when other options are available.

Least restrictive alternative doctrine: A legal concept mandating that least drastic measures be taken to achieve treatment outcomes or results. For example, if a person can be safely treated in an outpatient setting, inpatient hospitalization would be considered too restrictive and unnecessarily disruptive to the person's life.

Leukocytopenia/leukopenia: Abnormal decrease in the amount of circulating WBCs (neutrophils, basophils, eosinophils).

Leukocytosis/leucocytosis: Abnormal increase in the number of circulating WBCs (neutrophils, basophils, eosinophils).

Linear: Step-by-step progression of topics or ideas.

Magical thinking: Believing that one can personally influence someone else's behavior or change events by one's own thoughts, wishes, or rituals. This type of thinking is normal in young children up to age 4 or 5 years old, but is otherwise considered abnormal.

Maladaptive behavior: Behavior that is detrimental, ineffective, and negatively affects a person's ability to adjust to a new situation, environment or level of development; includes coping skills. Thought patterns (cognitive theory vs behavioral theory or cognitive–behavioral theory) can also be maladaptive.

Mania: Excitement, overactivity, excessive preoccupation with an idea or activity, impaired judgment, and psychomotor agitation.

Maturational or developmental crisis: Predictable, critical periods/stages or turning points of "internal" origin including physical, cognitive, sexual, or instinctual change during normal growth and development that inherently have increased vulnerability and increased heightened potential for development and coping. These periods result in either psychosocial growth or regression. A crisis of this type involves value conflicts, dependency, control, capacity for emotional intimacy, and sexual identity. Examples of maturational crises include leaving home in late adolescence, entering college or starting employment, marriage, birth of first child, "empty nest" stage, retirement, or death of a loved one.

Milieu: The general environment and specifically the social environment and atmosphere that affects the development of personality and individual adjustment.

Milieu manager: Nurse in a leadership role acts as a therapeutic milieu manager. As a milieu manager, the nurse can monitor the safe physical environment and interactions between patients and healthcare team members during one-to-one interactions or group meetings. A major role for the psychiatric-mental health nurse is to maintain a safe environment for the safety of everyone and allow patients to learn new behaviors, improve coping skills, and enhance socialization for those who isolate.

Memory: Process of or ability to retain experiences, perceptions, and information.

Mental status: Global assessment of a person's behavioral, cognitive, and affective states as revealed by mental examination.

Metabolic syndrome: A collection of signs and symptoms including elevated glucose levels ($\geq$ 110), elevated cholesterol levels (triglycerides $\geq$ 150; HDL < 40 in men & < 50 in women), increased insulin levels (insulin resistance), obesity (BMI $\geq$ 25; waist circumference > 40 inches in men & > 35 inches in women) and hypertension ($\geq$ 135/85). The presence of at least three of these signs or symptoms may lead to increased risk for diabetes mellitus type 2 or cardiovascular disease; previously referred to as "Syndrome X."

Mixed episode: Having some symptoms of mania and some symptoms of depression concurrently.

Mood: Sustained internal sensations of an emotion (subjective) or state of mind exhibited through emotions and feelings.

Monotone: No change in voice pitch or tone.

Motivational enhancement therapy: This therapy is a form of CBT, is a nonconfrontational approach, and is used more often in treating clients with addictions, but may be useful working with other problems as well. The therapist expresses empathy versus taking the more neutral approach used in traditional psychotherapy.

Mutism: Absence of speech.

Negativism: Resistance or opposition verbally or nonverbally to suggestions or advice. Resistance to efforts of being moved or doing the opposite of what has been asked; seen in the catatonic subtype of schizophrenia.

Neglect: Failure to provide or act on a person's behalf resulting in medical, mental, developmental, or social problems or illness.

Neologism: A newly invented word or condensed combination of several words coined by a person to express a highly complex idea; seen in schizophrenia.

Neuroleptic: See **Antipsychotics**.

Neuroleptic malignant syndrome (NMS): A potentially fatal adverse reaction to neuroleptic (antipsychotic) medication.

Neurons: Basic nerve cells in the nervous system.

Neurotransmitters: Chemicals in the CNS that act as messengers between neurons in the synaptic junction or gap. Many different chemicals may acts as neurotransmitters including amines, peptides, and hormones.

NMS. See **Neuroleptic malignant syndrome**.

Nonmaleficence: Doing no wrong or nothing that would cause harm to the client. In bioethics this principle includes intervening in ways that may potentially cause side-effects of treatment or distress, but in the long-term will benefit the patient; maintaining a level of expertise or skill through nursing education.

Nontherapeutic: The opposite of therapeutic; anything that does not promote healing or is not beneficial.

Nursing process: Problem-solving, step-by-step, scientific approach including diagnosis, analysis, planning, implementation, and evaluation. This process is used to identify and meet client needs.

Obsessions: Recurrent, persistent, involuntary, unwanted thoughts, ideas, or impulses that cannot be removed by logical reasoning; may be accompanied by compulsions; seen in obsessive-compulsive disorder.

Orientation: State of awareness of one's self and environment according to person, time, and place.

Orientation stage: The initial stage of Peplau's therapeutic nurse–client relationship. Another name for this stage is the "introductory" stage. In some psychiatric-mental health nursing textbooks, this stage is preceded by a "preinteraction" stage; however, many authors include this step as part of the orientation stage.

Orthostatic hypotension: A sudden decrease in systolic (20 mm Hg or more), diastolic (10 mm Hg or more), or both measures of blood pressure when a person changes position (lying down, sitting, or standing). The person may also have a sudden decrease in pulse (20 beats per minute or more). Symptoms include dizziness and fainting that can lead to falling.

Overt: Open, clear, manifest.

Panic attack: A condition in which there is a discrete period of intense fear or discomfort exhibiting somatic or cognitive symptoms in the absence of real danger.

Paranoid: Suspiciousness that is not based in reality.

Parasympathetic nervous system: Part of the autonomic nervous system (ANS) that has the effect of slowing down body functions; produces a relaxation effect. See also **Autonomic nervous system**.

Parasuicidal behavior: A term used to describe behaviors including cutting of the skin or ingestion of substances that do not have a fatal outcome. Also defined as acts of deliberate self-harm that do not result in completed suicide and may or may not be intended to result in death. See also **Suicidal gesture**.

Partial hospitalization: See **Day treatment**.

Passive suicide: Behavior that is ambiguous and can be self-destructive, but not actively so. Behavior that is thought to show suicidal intent (e.g., not engaging in basic self-care or self-preservation, refusing to eat)

Perception: An awareness of objects and the environment through the five senses and meaning assigned.

Peripheral nervous system: A system of motor and sensory nerves outside of the brain and spinal cord.

Perseveration: Repetition of same word or phrase response to different stimuli or questions; seen in cognitive disorders and schizophrenia.

Pharmacodynamics: The study of the specific interactions between medications and molecules in the body including interaction with cell receptors.

Pharmacogenomics: Use of genetic knowledge provided by the International HapMap Project to customize matching of medication with individual patients with the goals of maximizing effectiveness and minimizing side-effects.

Pharmacokinetics: The study of processes involved in making medications available to the body and their removal including absorption, distribution, metabolism, and excretion.

Phobia: Persistent unrealistic fear of an object, activity or situation that results in an individual's compelling desire to avoid it.

Posttraumatic stress disorder (PTSD): A disorder in which an individual who is currently exposed to an extremely dangerous situation, as well as a life-threatening situation in the past develops a certain set of chronic symptoms. The symptoms of PTSD usually show up 3 months after the trauma or in a later stage in life. This disorder is characterized by reexperiencing an event and overreacting to stimuli that recall the event.

Postural hypotension: See **Orthostatic hypotension**.

Poverty of speech: The inability to speak or very limited speech because of decreased mental processing, confusion, aphasia, or alogia. Speech may also be adequate in amount, but conveys little information due to vagueness or use of stereotyped phrases.

Preinteraction phase: See **Orientation phase**.

Pressured speech: Increased amount of spontaneous speech, accelerated speech; loud, forceful; push of speech; seen in the manic phase of bipolar disorders, schizophrenia, or cognitive disorders.

Priaprism: Sustained, painful penile erection in males.

Pseudodementia: A condition of the elderly that includes symptoms of impaired cognitive function as well as depression; may be mistaken for actual dementia.

Pseudoparkinsonism: Signs and symptoms similar to those seen in Parkinson's disease in a person not diagnosed with Parkinson's disease. Includes slow motor movements, tremors, muscle rigidity, cogwheel rigidity, stooped posture, shuffling gait, facial masking or flattened affect, and pill rolling finger movements.

Psychiatric code: A psychiatric behavioral emergency requiring immediate response from a team of staff members and professionals who have specialized education and training in techniques of defusion/de-escalation or nonviolent crisis prevention techniques; show of force; and rapid, organized movements designed to medicate, immobilize, or seclude a patient; may be referred to as a "take down." See also **Show of force**.

Psychiatric mental health nursing field: Psychiatric-mental health nurses work in a wide array of inpatient and outpatient settings, such as full or partial hospitalization; community-based or home care programs; and local, state, and federal mental health agencies. Other settings include school/college of nursing, private practice, military, primary care office, prison/jail, home health agency, and behavioral care company/health maintenance organization (HMO).

Psychiatric-mental health nursing practice: Psychiatric-mental health nursing practice is a specialized area of nursing practice employing a wide range of explanatory theories of human behavior as a science for the purposeful use of self as its art (American Nurses' Association Scope and Standard of Practice, 2006). Psychiatric-mental health nursing is committed to promoting mental health through the assessment, diagnosis, and treatment of human responses due to mental health problems or psychiatric disorders.

Psychoactive: See **Psychotropic**.

Psychoanalysis: This type of therapy focuses on assisting clients to gain insight into and change self-destructive behavior. The childhood of clients, unconscious conflicts, and inadequate ego defense mechanisms are all explored as to how these affect current situations in clients' lives. This exploration is used to increase insight, which is crucial to changing behavior.

Psychodrama: A specialized technique of psychotherapy used to assist clients to achieve new insight and change unhealthy patterns of behaving by acting out roles in situations involving current problems for which they are being treated. Other "actors" are used to play roles of significant individuals in their lives. The therapist acts as a "director" and guides the process as well as discussing its interpretation when the drama is finished.

Psychodynamic nursing: A theoretical framework developed by Hildegard Peplau that includes self-awareness and understanding for the nurse to understand their own behavior in order to help clients identify their own difficulties; the application of the principles of interpersonal human relations to problems that occur at all levels of human experience.

Psychoeducation: Providing information on a range of topics that benefit the client and anyone else involved in the client's care; an educational approach used to shape behavior and enhance knowledge. Goals include increasing understanding and empowerment.

Psychological first aid: Techniques used to help survivors of disasters cope with intense emotional reactions that are a result of intense fear, apprehension, or uncertainty.

Psychomotor: Physical and mental processes. May be faster than normal (psychomotor agitation) or slower than normal (psychomotor retardation); seen in major depression.

Psychological triage: The process of evaluating and sorting victims by immediacy of treatment needed and directing them to immediate or delayed treatment. The goal of triage is to do the greatest good for the greatest number of victims.

Psychopathology crisis: Psychopathology (e.g., personality disorders or traits, psychotic disorders including schizophrenia) plays a role in precipitating the emotional crisis or significantly complicates or impairs successful, adaptive resolution of the crisis.

Psychopharmacology: The study of medications that affect different areas of the central nervous system including mental, emotional, and behavioral processes.

Psychotherapy: Diagnosis and treatment by an educated licensed professional psychologist, psychiatrist, social worker or advanced practice nurse (APRN) using specific communication and interpersonal techniques.

Psychotropic: Medications or other substances that significantly affect psychological processes such as thinking, perception, and emotion, causing alteration in a person's state of consciousness.

Rambling speech: Continuing to talk without a purpose or goal.

Rape: Forced sexual activity without consent; sexual assault.

Rapid cycling: Mood disturbance that changes over a short period of time; most commonly between mania and depression. In bipolar disorders rapid cycling is characterized by having four or more episodes over a 12-month period. The episodes are separated by symptom-free periods of at least 2 months.

Rapport: A relaxed, warm relationship of mutual acceptance, understanding, respect, and harmony between people.

Reality therapy: The goal of this type of therapy is to help the client break through denial and stop using irresponsible behavior to deal with the world around them and their problems.

Reality testing: Actions that test and objectively evaluate the environment including the ability to differentiate between the external and internal world; to accurately judge between what is the self and what is not. Problems with reality testing occur in psychotic states.

REBT: Behavioral psychotherapy used to identify irrational beliefs in order to challenge and change them. The therapist confronts, and teaches the patient to confront, illogical thoughts and beliefs, at times using a more confrontational approach than with CBT.

Resistance behaviors: Withstanding, defying, or acting in opposition to someone or something; may also be referred to as "testing" behaviors.

Resolution stage: The last stage of Peplau's therapeutic nurse–client relationship. This stage may also be combined with the termination stage or listed in place of the termination stage in some psychiatric-mental health nursing textbooks.

Restraints: Any method used to immobilize or reduce the ability of a patient to move their arms, legs, body, or head freely (see Joint Commission definition in Chapter 12).

Rhabdomyolysis: Acute tubular necrosis/renal failure secondary to large amount of muscle damage. May be fatal in up to 30% of cases.

Ritualistic behaviors: A form of compulsion to repeatedly carry out a stereotyped act based on rules that do not have a rational basis; having to perform a task in a specific way.

Role player: The psychiatric-mental health nurse plays a role for the client by creating simulation exercises of past, present, or future situations or incidents so the client will be able to practice new behavior in a nonthreatening environment. The patient can express thoughts, feelings, and act out a specific or real situation during role play. The benefit of this exercise is that the patient is able to build up self-confidence, learn to communicate better and in a more assertive way with others, and cope better in the given situation in the future.

Rumination: Constant preoccupation with or repetitive thoughts about a single theme. Seen in obsessive-compulsive disorder.

Seclusion: Involuntary confinement of a patient alone in a room or area (see Joint Commission definition in Chapter 12).

Secondary gain: The external gain derived from any illness such as personal attention, services, monetary gains, disability benefits, or release from an unpleasant responsibility.

Self-awareness: Learning about oneself by the examination of one's own feelings, biases, attitudes, emotions, thoughts, and actions; also includes emotional intelligence.

Self-care: Activities people perform for themselves to maintain life, health, and feelings of well-being.

Self-disclosure: Providing personal information or intimate details about oneself or one's life.

Self-mutilation: Acts of self-harm involving disfigurement but not death. Cutting is the most common type of self-mutilation, but other common methods include burning, skin piercing, or rubbing the skin to the point of forming an abrasion.

Self-system: Defined by Peplau as a product of socialization and a method of reducing anxiety. The "self" continues through personal development and changes, but seeks stability. Peplau based some of her definition on and was influenced by the work of Sullivan. The self is also defined as a personal definition that is different from that of other people.

Serotonin discontinuation syndrome: Symptoms of withdrawal from medications (SSRIs or SNRIs) affecting serum levels of the neurotransmitter serotonin.

Serotonin syndrome: A potentially fatal collection of symptoms that can occur as a result of excessive serum levels of the neurotransmitter serotonin. This syndrome can occur from the combination of more than one medication affecting serotonin levels or the combination of medications and herbal supplements.

Severe anxiety: This is the third level of anxiety in which an individual experiences difficulty in concentrating and focusing, and may have distorted thinking processes. The perceptual field is greatly reduced and the individual is unable to follow suggestions.

Sexting: Taking nude pictures of people with cell phones and then sending them.

Sexual harassment: Unwanted, unwelcome sexual behaviors or verbalizations that interfere with everyday life; considered to be sexual discrimination by the Equal Employment Opportunity Commission (EEOC).

Shaken baby syndrome: Whiplash-induced intracranial and intraocular bleeding caused by vigorous shaking of babies held by the extremities or shoulders.

Show of force/crisis team: Gathering and using the presence of several trained staff members and professionals in the immediate physical area who are ready if needed to act to subdue a person who is self-destructive or violent towards others. De-escalation or nonviolent crisis prevention techniques are used in conjunction with a show of force. Sometimes the show of force is enough to help a patient temporarily gain enough control of their own behavior and further safety measures are not needed.

Sibling abuse: Violence occurring between siblings.

Situational or dispositional crisis: Smaller scale than an adventitious crisis and occurring from an "external rather than internal" event, a situational crisis may be unanticipated or anticipated, but the resulting effect is greater than expected. Examples include divorce, loss of employment or a reduction in finances, getting an abortion, a student being placed on academic probation, etc.

Social microcosm: A small community, society, or world relating to the interactions and behavior of people as members of a group. Group members eventually behave toward each other as they do towards their family members or friends.

Social relationship: A relationship that exists for the benefit of everyone involved with the goals of increasing friendship, providing enjoyment, meeting dependency needs, and asking and receiving personal advice; subjective in nature.

Social support: Providing comfort or assistance to improve a person's coping ability.

Social support system or network: Social support provided by family, friends, neighbors, colleagues/coworkers, churches, or community organizations. The support given may be emotional or material.

Socializing agent: This role is played by the nurse while working on a one-to-one basis with a client. The focus is to identify what difficulties the client has in communicating thoughts and feelings to others. The client gets the benefits of this role by adapting an appropriate expression of behavior and affect.

Somatic: Pertaining to the body.

Stalking: "Predatory violence" may be nondelusional (a relationship existed at some point) or delusional (no relationship ever existed); involves unsolicited/unwanted contact in various forms including cyber/Internet stalking in spite of stated request to be left alone.

Standards of performance: An authoritative statement of expected practice performance by the psychiatric-mental health nurse to maintain proficiency and competency for practice as prescribed within the scope and standards of performance of psychiatric and mental health nursing by the American Nurses Association.

Standards of practice: An authoritative statement by professional organizations that describes the responsibility for which nurses are accountable for the care they provide to clients.

Stereotyped behavior: Inflexible behavior that follows a particular pattern and does not change even when conditions change; includes stereotyped, repetitive movements such as rocking, head banging, finger flicking, or tics.

Subgrouping: Forming small groups within the larger group that become preoccupied with their own interests rather than that of the group's goals. This activity can disrupt the group process and progress.

Suicidal gesture: An attempt to commit suicide, or similar self-destructive behavior, when there is a low risk of death. See also **Parasuicidal behavior**.

Suicidal ideation: Thoughts of or preoccupation with death.

Suicidal threats: Verbal statements of intent to kill oneself. Threats of suicide often precede an actual suicide attempt.

Suicide attempt: A person's deliberate act to end their own life, which is interrupted before actual death occurs.

Suicide, completed: Act of killing oneself.

Suicide survivor: A spouse, family member, friend, or anyone experiencing the loss of a loved one due to suicide.

Supportive therapy: The therapist is emotionally supportive and expresses empathy versus taking the more neutral approach used in traditional psychotherapy.

Sympathetic nervous system: Part of the autonomic nervous system (ANS) that has the effect of speeding up body functions; stress effect. See also **Autonomic nervous system**.

Synaptic junction/gap (synapse): A special junction through which neurochemical or message transmission occurs between neurons; the site of action for many psychotropic medications.

Tangential: Thoughts or speech veering from main idea and never getting back to it.

Tardive dyskinesia: Abnormal or purposeless muscle movements of the extremities, trunk, face, jaw, or oral–buccal muscles causing rocking or twisting motions, pelvic thrusting or gyrations, tremors, tongue darting or writhing, spastic facial movements, frowning, blinking, blowing, teeth grinding, lip smacking, or chewing movements as if the patient has food or gum in their mouth. This type of extrapyramidal symptom may be irreversible.

Teacher: The nurse acts as teacher to provide patient education and health teaching depending upon client's needs.

Temperament: The basis of personality. Includes characteristic intensity, emotional responsiveness, activity level, energy, ability to adapt, willingness to explore, and general mood. Biologically determined and identified early in life.

Termination stage: The third or last stage of Peplau's therapeutic nurse–client relationship depending upon the author. This stage may also be combined with the resolution stage in some psychiatric-mental health nursing textbooks.

Terrorism: Premeditated acts of violence that are politically motivated and perpetrated against civilians or private citizens.

Therapeutic: Anything that exerts a curative, healing, or beneficial effect.

Therapeutic alliance: An association between two or more people. An alliance is therapeutic in the sense that it is formed between the nurse and client for the client's benefit and is part of the therapeutic nurse–client relationship. The goal of the therapeutic alliance is the client's personal growth and healthy adaptation.

Therapeutic communication: An ongoing process of interaction using specific techniques through which meaning emerges.

Therapeutic encounter: Term used to describe any period of time the nurse and client meet, no matter how brief. The time is important and meaningful to the client.

Therapeutic factors: Therapeutic groups provide beneficial factors for group members that would not be achieved in individual psychotherapy. See also **Curative factors**.

Therapeutic listening skills: Focusing of the nurse's attention on the client and actively listening with the goal of obtaining therapeutically useful information to help the client.

Therapeutic use of self: Conscious use of a nurse's own unique personality as a therapeutic tool to assist the client to develop a positive relationship and provide structure to nursing interventions. It also involves the nurse being aware of their own values, attitudes, and beliefs regarding life and death, and acceptance of the uniqueness and differences in the client.

Thought blocking: Sudden, unconscious stop in train of thought before finishing the expression of a thought or feeling. After a brief pause the person is unable to recall what they were talking about; seen in schizophrenia and severe anxiety.

Thought broadcasting: Belief that others can "hear" their thoughts (as if over a public address or broadcasting system) or read their mind.

Thought content: What a person is thinking about; topic of conversation.

Thought insertion: Belief that others are "putting" thoughts or implanting thoughts "into" their head. Individual attributes thoughts to outside sources.

Thought removal: Belief that others are stealing or removing their thoughts.

Thought processes: Cognitive processes involved in mental activities beyond perception including remembering, reasoning, problem solving, imagining, and making judgments.

Thrombocytopenia: Abnormal decrease in the number of platelets; the most common cause of bleeding.

Thrombocytosis: Abnormal increase in the number of platelets.

Tics: Sudden, involuntary, recurrent, stereotypical muscle movements or vocal sounds. Common types include eye blinking, facial grimacing, shoulder shrugging, clearing the throat or grunting.

Transference: When a client displaces or projects unconscious feelings, desires, or actions from a person in their life onto the nurse or other healthcare provider. This can be problematic in nursing, but it is used by psychoanalytic therapists in psychoanalysis therapy.

Trust: Confidence in the worth, value, or truth of someone or something else. An important component of all types of relationships.

Unconditional positive regard: Believing in the worth and dignity of another individual; also respecting and remaining nonjudgmental of another individual.

Unintelligible/incoherent speech: Speech that is unable to be understood; disjointed or disorganized; lack of clear, orderly speech.

Unipolar: Any depressive mood disorder demonstrated by one or more episodes of major depression or a prolonged time period of depression without a history or symptoms of a bipolar disorder, hypomania, or mixed mood episodes.

Values clarification: A process through which a person can discover their own values by exploring, assessing, questioning, and choosing what their values are and how these values will influence their attitudes, emotions, and actions.

Veracity: A duty to tell the truth that protects a client's right to know about their diagnosis, treatment, and prognosis (*exception*—when doing so causes more harm than good).

Warmth: Nonverbal manner in which interest or concern is expressed.

Word salad: A mixture of words and phrases that lack comprehensive meaning or logical coherence; commonly seen in schizophrenia.

Working stage: The second stage of Peplau's therapeutic nurse–client relationship. Some authors refer to this stage as the "exploitation" stage.

Workplace violence: Includes stalking, sexual harassment, rape, emotional/verbal abuse, assault and battery, or murder.

REFERENCES

American Nurses Association. (2006). *The American Nurses Association scope and standards of psychiatric mental health nursing practice*. Washington, DC: Author.

Centers for Disease Control and Prevention (CDC). (2010). *Issue brief for educators and caregivers US*. Retrieved from www.cdc.gov/ncipc/dvp/YVP/electronic_agression_brief_for_parents.pdf

Keltner, N. L., Schwecke, L. H., & Bostrom, C. E. (2007). *Psychiatric nursing* (5th ed.). St. Louis, MO: Mosby, Elsevier.

Varcarolis, E. M., & Halter, M. J. (2010). *Foundations of psychiatric mental health nursing: A clinical approach* (6th ed.). St. Louis, MO: Saunders, Elsevier.

Nursing Care Plan

Nursing Care Plan:

Nursing Diagnosis:

Outcomes (include time frames):

Assessment Data (O = Objective, S= Subjective)	Evidence-Based Interventions	Rationales	Patient Responses

Evaluation:

Index

Pages followed by t or f denote tables and figures respectively.